Certification and Core Review for

Neonatal
Intensive Care
Nursing

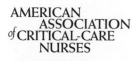

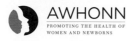

SIXTH EDITION

CERTIFICATION AND CORE REVIEW FOR
NEONATAL INTENSIVE CARE NURSING

Edited by

Robin L. Watson, RN, MN, CNS, CCRN
Clinical Infomaticist Lead
Los Angeles County Health Services
Health Services Administration
Los Angeles, California

Beth C. Diehl, DNP, NNP-BC, CCRN
Neonatal Nurse Practitioner/Transport Nurse
Johns Hopkins Hospital/Maryland Regional Neonatal Transport Program
Baltimore, Maryland

ELSEVIER

Elsevier
3251 Riverport Lane
St. Louis, Missouri 63043

Senior Content Strategist: Yvonne Alexopoulos
Content Development Specialist: Meredith Madeira
Publishing Services Manager: Deepthi Unni
Project Manager: Sindhuraj Thulasingam
Design Direction: Ryan Cook

Printed in India

Last digit is the print number: 9 8 7 6 5 4 3 2 1

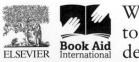

Working together
to grow libraries in
developing countries

www.elsevier.com • www.bookaid.org

Dedications

To my sisters, Sandy and Cynthy, who continue to support me, my work, and all my adventures. And to Mike Muscat, I am beyond grateful for being given the opportunity to be part of this book again. Thank you for believing in this work and my contributions to it. It has been a great ride since the book's first publication in 2001.

Robin L. Watson

To my husband, John, for his unfailing love and support; to my children and stepchildren—Andy, Theresa, Andrea, AJ, Garrett, and Tyler—for bringing joy and laughter to my life; and to all my mentors and colleagues for sharing valuable lessons about caring for fragile infants throughout my career.

Beth C. Diehl

List of Contributors

Sandra Sundquist Beauman, MSN, RNC-NIC
Manager, Clinical Trials Operations
Department of Pediatrics, Division of Neonatology
University of New Mexico Health Sciences Center
Albuquerque, New Mexico

Stephanie M. Blake, DNP, RN, NNP, NCC
Neonatal Nurse Practitioner
Pediatrics/Neonatology
Duke University Medical Center
Durham, North Carolina
Neonatal Nurse Practitioner
Pediatrics/Neonatology
Cone Health
Burlington, North Carolina
Neonatal Nurse Practitioner
Neonatology
UNC/Novant
Chapel Hill, North Carolina

Dee (Deanne) Buschbach, RN, MSN, NNP, RETIRED PNP
Consulting Associate
NNP Program, Masters Degree
Duke University School of Nursing
Durham, North Carolina

Annette Carley, DNP, MS, RN, NNP-BC PPCNP-BC
Clinical Professor
Family Health Care Nursing
UCSF School of Nursing
San Francisco, California

Theresa Carnes, BSN, RN
Perinatal Clinical Instructor
Harbor-UCLA Medical Center
Torrance, California

Kristi Coe, PhD, NNP, CNS, PNP, RN
Consulting Associate
MSN Program
Duke School of Nursing
Durham, North Carolina
Neonatal Nurse Practitioner
Neonatal Intensive Care Unit
ConeHealth
Greensboro, North Carolina

Lebanon David, DNP, NNP-BC, NPT-BC, VA-BC, NNIC
Neonatal Nurse Practitioner
Neonatal Intensive Care Unit
UT Southwestern Medical Center
Dallas, Texas
Neonatal Nurse Practitioner
Neonatal Intensive Care Unit
Parkland Health and Hospital System
Dallas, Texas
Graduate Nursing Clinical Education Specialist
Nursing Education
University of Texas Medical Branch
Galveston, Texas

Beth C. Diehl, DNP, NNP-BC, CCRN
Neonatal Nurse Practitioner/Transport Nurse
Johns Hopkins Hospital/Maryland Regional
    Neonatal Transport Program
Baltimore, Maryland

Debbie Fraser, MN, NNP, CNeoN(C), FCAN
Associate Professor
Faculty of Health Disciplines
Athabasca University
Athabasca, Alberta
Canada
Editor-in-Chief
Neonatal Network
Springer Publishing
New York, NY
Chief Nurse Planner
Academy of Neonatal Nursing
Petaluma, CA

Lindsey N. Green, DNP, MN, APRN-CNS, CCNS, RNC-NIC
Certification Practice Specialist
Certification
American Association of Critical-Care Nurses
Aliso Viejo, California
Adjunct Clinical Faculty
Nursing Education
Saint Francis Health System
Tulsa, Oklahoma
Neonatal Consultant
Independent Contractor
United States

Tosha Harris, DNP, APRN, NNP-BC
Assistant Professor
College of Nursing
University of Tennessee Health Science Center
Memphis, Tennessee

Beverly Inge-Walti, MSN, RNC-NIC, CPNP, CNS
Clinical Nurse Specialist
Neonatal Intensive Care Unit
Children's Hospital of Orange County
Orange, California

Donna Jensen, MSN, MHA, RN, RNC-NIC, PHN, CNS
Neonatal Clinical Nurse Specialist
Neonatal Intensive Care Unit
Bakersfield Memorial Hospital
Bakersfield, California

Robin Koeppel, DNP, CPNP, RNC-NIC, C-ELBW, C-NNIC
Neonatal Clinical Nurse Specialist
Neonatal Intensive Care Unit
University of California, Irvine Medical Center
Orange, California

Emily Latiolais, DNP, APRN, NNP-BC
Neonatal Nurse Practitioner
Neonatology
Pediatrix Medical Group
Fort Worth, Texas

Angela Lindbloom, BSN, MSN, ACNS-BC, RNC-NIC, NTMTC
Clinical Nurse Specialist
Neonatal Intensive Care Unit
Children's Hospital of Michigan
Detroit, Michigan

Karmen McKendree, BSN, MSN, NNP-BC
Neonatal Nurse Practitioner
Neonatal Intensive Care Unit
Johns Hopkins Hospital
Baltimore, Maryland

Lisa Miklush, PhD, RN, CNS
Adjunct Graduate Faculty
School of Nursing and Human Physiology
Gonzaga University
Spokane, Washington
Senior Content Editor
Osmosis from Elsevier

Andrea Cooke Morris, DNP, RNC-NIC, CCRN, CNS
Part-time Faculty
School of Nursing
California State University, Dominguez Hills
Carson, California

Mindy Morris, DNP, NNP-BC, CNS, RNC-NIC, C-ELBW
Co-owner
Consultant
EngageGrowThrive, LLC
Huntington Beach, California

Desi Michele Newberry, DNP, MSN, BSN
Associate Professor
College of Nursing
Duke University
Durham, North Carolina
Neonatal Nurse Practitioner
Newborn Critical Care Center
University of North Carolina
Chapel Hill, North Carolina

Tonya Oliver, BSN, MSN, NNP-BC
Neonatal Nurse Practitioner
Neonatology
Atrium Health Wake Forest Baptist
Winston Salem, North Carolina
Neonatal Nurse Practitioner
Catawba Valley Medical Center
Hickory, North Carolina

Sandra Priest, DNP, APRN, NNP-BC
NNP Program Coordinator
School of Nursing, NNP Program
University Texas Medical Branch
Galveston, Texas

Juliet K. Sasinski, MSN, RN, CNS, RNC-NIC, C-ELBW
Clinical Nurse Specialist
Neonatal Intensive Care Unit
UCLA Health
Santa Monica, California

Laura D. Selway, MSN, RN, PCNS-BC, RNC-NIC
Pediatric CNS
Neonatal Intensive Care Unit
Johns Hopkins Hospital
Baltimore, Maryland

Lorraine Arriola Shields, DNP, APRN, CNS, NNP-BC
Director of DNP Program
Associate Professor
College of Nursing
California Baptist University
Riverside, California

Timothy Matthew Snow, RN, MSN, NNP
Neonatal Nurse Practitioner
Neonatal Intensive Care
Atrium Health Wake Forest Baptist Health
Winston Salem, North Carolina
Neonatal Nurse Practitioner–Team Lead
Labor and Delivery
Atrium Health Wake Forest Baptist Health–Wilkes Medical Center
North Wilkesboro, North Carolina

Emmeline Bell Tate, BSN, MSN, NNP-BC
Neonatal Nurse Practitioner
Neonatal Intensive Care Unit
Johns Hopkins Hospital
Baltimore, Maryland

Linda Wynsma, MSN, CNS, RNC-NIC, C-ELBW
Clinical Nurse Specialist
Neonatal Intensive Care Unit
Kaiser Permanente, Downey Medical Center
Downey, California

Jenelle Mecija Zambrano, DNP, CNS, RN, CCNS
Director, Nursing Clinical Professional Development
Population Health Management
Los Angeles County Health Services
Los Angeles, California

List of Reviewers

Karen Dittman, MSN, NNP-BC
Neonatal Nurse Practitioner
Neonatal Intensive Care Unit
Johns Hopkins Hospital
Baltimore, Maryland

Beverly Inge-Walti, MSN, RNC-NIC, CPNP, CNS
Clinical Nurse Specialist
Neonatal Intensive Care Unit
Children's Hospital of Orange County
Orange, California

Lisa Lima, MSN, PNP, CNS, RNC-NIC
Advanced Practice Registered Nurse
Children's Services
Valley Presbyterian Hospital
Van Nuys, California

Angela Lindbloom, BSN, MSN, ACNS-BC, RNC-NIC, NTMTC
Registered Nurse
Neonatal Intensive Care Unit
Henry Ford Health System
Detroit, Michigan

Karen Stadd, DNP, CRNP, MSN
Neonatal Nurse Practitioner
Neonatal Intensive Care Unit
Johns Hopkins Hospital
Baltimore, Maryland

Leslie Sulpar, MSN, RNC-NIC
NICU Nurse Educator
Johns Hopkins Hospital
Baltimore, Maryland

Preface

Welcome to the sixth edition of the *Certification and Core Review for Neonatal Intensive Care Nursing*! This latest edition continues to endorse that care provided to critically ill newborns requires nurses who have specialized knowledge, skills, and experiences; certification in neonatal nursing provides validation of these specialized competencies. Accordingly, the number of questions in this edition has been increased to 950 items, divided among the chapters, to recognize the current level of cognitive complexity that exists in the neonatal intensive care arena.

Both the CCRN Certification Examination–Neonatal, offered by the American Association of Critical-Care Nurses (AACN) Certification Corporation, and the Neonatal Intensive Care Nursing certification examination, offered by the National Certification Corporation (NCC), are tools for assessing the acquisition of core knowledge essential to neonatal nursing practice.

As in the past, this edition includes an accompanying Evolve Exam Review: an online, interactive version of the text. The participant can customize the Exam Review to simulate the CCRN–Neonatal or the RNC–NIC exam and choose between a study mode and a timed examination simulation. Using the access code found inside the front cover, visit http://evolve.elsevier.com/AACN/certification/ to take advantage of this resource that is free with the purchase of the *Certification and Core Review for Neonatal Intensive Care Nursing*, 6th edition.

This book is designed to be a study guide for nurses preparing to take a national certification examination in neonatal critical care nursing as well as serving as a tool for nurses developing critical thinking skills. We hope that experienced neonatal nurses will find the *Certification and Core Review* a refresher of their professional knowledge and that clinical nurse specialists and nurse educators who are responsible for assessing the competency of neonatal nurses will refer to this resource as they design their own competency tools. The *Certification and Core Review* is an adjunct to the *Core Curriculum for Neonatal Intensive Care Nursing* and provides a mechanism for the review and study of core content for neonatal intensive care nursing practice.

Content addressed in the *Certification and Core Review* is based on the AACN Certification Corporation's Neonatal CCRN Test Plan and Neonatal CCRN Testable Nursing Actions, as well as NCC's Examination Content–Neonatal Intensive Care Nursing. These resources guided the identification of subject matter and the distribution of items for each content area. The first section of the *Certification and Core Review for Neonatal Intensive Care Nursing*, General Assessment and Management, addresses clinical issues related to assessment of the fetus and physical and gestational age assessment of the newborn, resuscitation principles, adaptation of the fetus to extrauterine life, and general management practices fundamental to the care of critically ill newborns. The second section, Pathophysiology, is divided into two subsections. The first subsection, System-Specific Disorders, addresses patient care problems primarily affecting single body systems. The second subsection, Multisystem Considerations, focuses on disorders that affect multiple organ systems. The third section, Psychosocial and Behavioral Adjustments, is dedicated to cornerstones of clinical practice beyond the realm of general assessment, management, and pathophysiology. These involve managing grief, discharge planning, and providing culturally sensitive, family-focused care. Finally, the fourth section, Professional Practice, speaks to the neonatal nurse's role in patient safety and quality improvement along with legal, ethical, and research issues emphasizing the neonatal critical care nurse's role in all areas.

All study items are multiple-choice with four options, giving readers practice selecting a correct answer amidst three distractors. The answer to each item and explanations for the correct and incorrect answers are contained within each individual chapter. Rationales for the correct and incorrect answers provide nurses with the knowledge required to prioritize, plan, and evaluate care. References supporting the correct answers and rationales are also provided. Questions are organized by topic area, so those wishing to review a particular subject can easily find the content they are seeking.

Study items address the various cognitive levels—knowledge, application, and analysis—providing readers the opportunity to recall, apply, and evaluate their knowledge of neonatal intensive care nursing. All phases of the nursing process are represented by the study items. Every effort was made to ensure that each question represents universal knowledge and reflects the core content of neonatal intensive and critical care nursing practice. None of these questions has been or will be used on any certification examination. Because certification examinations are revised frequently, all nurses who are preparing for an examination are encouraged to contact the appropriate sponsoring agency to obtain the most up-to-date materials related to the areas of knowledge being tested on specific examinations. Information about CCRN certification can be found at https://www.aacn.org/certification. For the National Certification Corporation, please visit: https://www.nccwebsite.org/certification-exams/register.

Beth C. Diehl
Robin L. Watson

AACN offers an online, subscription-based certification practice exam called "CCRN/CCRN-K Neonatal Certification Practice Exam and Questions Basic Subscription" that was developed in partnership with the company Test Run and could be seen as a competitor with this Elsevier book. More about the product is available here: https://www.aacn.org/store/books/ccrnn-t2/ccrnccrnk[1]neonatal-certification-practice-exam-and-questions-basic-subscription.

Foreword

Five previous editions of the *Core Curriculum for Neonatal Intensive Care Nursing* and the *Certification and Core Review for Neonatal Intensive Care Nursing* confirm the successful collaboration of three preeminent nursing organizations: the American Association of Critical-Care Nurses; the Association of Women's Health, Obstetric and Neonatal Nurses; and the National Association of Neonatal Nurses. Their visionary leadership identified the need for essential resources that standardize the requisite knowledge for clinical practice in the rapidly evolving field of neonatal intensive care. This text is created based on the AACN Certification Corporation test plan and the National Certification Corporation exam. (Please note that new test plans for AACN Certification Corporation exams are published periodically on the AACN website. To ensure that readers are accessing the latest test plan information, please visit www.aacn.org/certification.)

Once again, editors Robin L. Watson and Beth C. Diehl have assembled the energy, talent, and expertise of practicing nurses from these three associations to write and review study questions for neonatal nursing core content.

We applaud this singular example of how critical care nurses relentlessly and successfully foster true collaboration. With support from knowledgeable staff in each association, the editors and contributors have demonstrated the cooperation, collegiality, and quality that excellent care of critically ill infants and their families requires.

Theresa M. Davis, PhD, RN, NE-BC, CHTP, FAAN
President, American Association of Critical-Care Nurses

Jonathan Webb, MPH, MBA
Chief Executive Officer, Association of Women's Health, Obstetric and Neonatal Nurses

Rachael Zastrow, NNP-BC APNP CPNP-PC
President, National Association of Neonatal Nurses

Acknowledgments

We are honored and privileged, once again, to bring forward the sixth edition of the *Certification and Core Review for Neonatal Intensive Care Nursing*. As coeditors, we are shepherds of the material written by our terrific contributors. This book would not be possible without them. We acknowledge and thank each of them for dedicating their time and sharing their expertise with the neonatal nursing community. They are the backbone of this work. We are especially humbled that despite the burdens of emerging from the COVID-19 pandemic, contributors found the resilience and perseverance to commit to this work. Since the book's premier in 2001, contributors Linda Wynsma and Robin Koeppel have been extraordinary partners, always willing to participate and share their wealth of clinical and item-writing experience. We celebrate their tenure with this project. We are also excited to welcome 17 new contributors and hope their work on this book has been a rewarding experience. Reviewers provided insightful comments regarding content and question-and-answer construction, and we are thankful for their contributions.

Item writing—that is, writing questions and answers—requires rigor and is different from writing a narrative text. An entire field of psychology, psychometrics, is dedicated to the theory and technique of testing. Each answer option must be plausible, and only one answer option can be correct. And although negative stems like "all of the following except" are easy to write, they are confusing to test takers. Similarly, answer options that include "all of the above" are easy to write but allow learners who can identify more than one option to answer correctly, even if unsure about other options. So kudos to the contributors for transforming their knowledge into well-designed questions and answers. In addition, contributors took painstaking effort to explain why each answer option was either correct or incorrect and provided a reference to support the rationales. We applaud the contributors for their commitment to the item-writing process, ensuring questions and answers are not only clinically relevant but also constructed in a way that supports a meaningful test of knowledge.

This sixth edition would not have happened without the support of Mike Muscat, Publishing Manager at the American Association of Critical-Care Nurses—thank you, Mike, for continuing to believe in the value of this project. Yvonne Alexopoulos, Senior Content Strategist at Elsevier, provided strategy and high-level guidance throughout the process—thank you, Yvonne. We extend our appreciation to Meredith Madeira, Content Development Specialist at Elsevier. Thank you, Meredith, for managing the project and keeping us on track.

Finally, we want to acknowledge all neonatal nurses for their compassion and care for some of our most vulnerable patients. You are an inspiration for our future. For those preparing for a certification examination, we wish you well and thank you for your commitment to certified practice.

Robin L. Watson
Beth C. Diehl

Contents

GENERAL ASSESSMENT AND MANAGEMENT

Chapter 1

Assessment of Fetal Well-Being

1. A patient who is G3P2 at 33 weeks' gestation arrives at the triage unit complaining of regular uterine contractions. Her pregnancy history includes a preterm delivery at 34 weeks. Before examining her, the nurse performs electronic fetal monitoring and obtains a complete history. The patient reports no bleeding and no rupture of membranes. She has had no vaginal examinations or sexual activity for more than 24 hours. The biochemical marker useful in this situation for predicting preterm birth is:
   A. cervical ferritin.
   B. fetal fibronectin.
   C. corticotropin-releasing hormone.
   D. placental alpha-microglobulin-1.

2. A patient comes to the triage unit at 32 weeks' gestation concerned because she has been "leaking fluid" from her vagina for the past hour. She says she has felt no contractions and reports normal fetal activity. A bedside immunoassay called AmniSure is performed to determine if her membranes have ruptured. This test identifies a glycoprotein abundant in amniotic fluid. This glycoprotein is called:
   A. prolactin.
   B. alpha-fetoprotein.
   C. fetal fibronectin.
   D. placenta alpha-microglobulin-1.

3. The biophysical profile (BPP) is currently the primary method for evaluating fetal well-being through the assessment of various activities that are controlled by the central nervous system and are sensitive to oxygenation. The five variables included in the BPP are:
   A. fetal tone, fetal breathing, fetal movement, nonstress test, and amniotic fluid volume.
   B. fetal movement, fetal tone, nonstress test, amniotic fluid index, and fetal position.
   C. fetal tone, fetal position, amniotic fluid volume, fetal heart rate, and fetal activity.
   D. fetal heart rate, fetal movement, nonstress test, amniotic fluid volume, and fetal tone.

4. An appropriate gestational age for glucose screening in women who are at low risk for developing gestational diabetes in pregnancy is:
   A. 20–21 weeks' gestation.
   B. 22–23 weeks' gestation.
   C. 24–28 weeks' gestation.
   D. 32–34 weeks' gestation.

5. What is the physiologic cause of late decelerations?
   A. Fetal distress
   B. Sympathetic response to fetal activity
   C. Rapid fetal descent through the pelvis
   D. Transient hypoxemia during a uterine contraction

6. A patient who is at 42 5/7 weeks' gestation has been pushing for 90 minutes and is near delivery. Her membranes spontaneously ruptured 3 hours ago, and meconium was observed. The electronic fetal monitor demonstrates minimal fetal heart rate baseline variability. The most likely potential cause is:
   A. severe hypoxia.
   B. fetal metabolic acidemia.
   C. recent maternal methamphetamine use.
   D. response to fetal scalp stimulation.

7. When performing a BPP, which of these fetal variables should the nurse recognize as placing the fetus at high risk and in need of either delivery or repeat BPPs no fewer than two times per week?
   A. Reactive nonstress test
   B. Three body movements within 30 minutes
   C. Thirty seconds of fetal breathing within 30 minutes
   D. An amniotic fluid pocket measuring 1.5 cm in two planes perpendicular to each other

ANSWERS AND RATIONALES

1. **(B)** Fibronectins are a family of proteins found in the extracellular matrix. Fetal fibronectins (fFns) are found in fetal membranes and decidua throughout pregnancy. As the gestational sac implants and attaches to the interior of the uterus in the first half of pregnancy, fFns are normally found in cervicovaginal fluid. After 22 weeks, the presence of fFns normally is no longer detected in vaginal secretions until approximately 2 weeks before the onset of delivery, term or preterm. It is suggested that fFns be released into the cervix and the vagina when mechanical- or inflammatory-mediated damage occurs to the membranes. The presence of fFN in vaginal or cervical secretions before 35 weeks is a moderately good predictor of preterm delivery. The absence of fFN is a strong predictor that preterm delivery is unlikely within the next 7–14 days. Cervical ferritin is not a biomarker, but an inflammatory marker whose presence provides support for the theory that infection is a mediator of preterm birth. Maternal plasma concentrations of corticotropin-releasing hormone (CRH) are elevated in both term and preterm pregnancies. CRH appears to be a component of the common pathway of labor, regardless of gestation. Placental alpha-microglobulin-1 (PAMG-1) is a protein found in amniotic fluid that is a biomarker for rupture of membranes.

Reference: Singh S, Dey M, Singh S, Sasidharan S. Biochemical markers as predictor of preterm labor and their clinical relevance – the current status. *Gynecol Obstet Reprod Med.* 2022;28(3):282-289. doi:10.21613/GORM.2020.1108. Accessed 27.07.22.

2. **(D)** AmniSure detects trace amounts of PAMG-1 protein, a protein expressed by the cells of the decidua and found in the amniotic fluid. PAMG-1 is present in the blood, amniotic fluid, and cervicovaginal discharge of pregnant women. Its presence is found in vaginal secretions after the rupture of membranes, with a 99% sensitivity. The test is administered using a sterile polyester swab to obtain vaginal secretions without the need of a speculum. Prolactin is responsible for priming the breast tissue in preparation for lactation. Alpha-fetoprotein is assessed to identify neural tube defects (high) and Down syndrome (low). fFn is an extracellular glycoprotein that is thought to act as an adhesive between the fetal membranes and uterine wall and is a biomarker for predicting preterm birth.

Reference: AmniSure ROM Test (Rupture of [fetal] Membranes test). Available at: https://www.qiagen.com/us/products/diagnostics-and-clinical-research/sexual-reproductive-health/maternal-fetal-testing/amnisure-rom-test-10-min-us. Accessed September 30, 2023.

Garg A, Jaiswal A. Evaluation and management of premature rupture of members: A review article. *Cureus.* 2023;15(3):e36615. doi: 10.7759/cureus.36615.

3. **(A)** The biophysical profile (BPP) is an evaluation of fetal well-being through the use of various reflex activities that are controlled by the central nervous system (CNS) and are sensitive to hypoxia, as well as the fetal environment that can affect fetal well-being. The biophysical activities that are the first to develop are the last to disappear when asphyxia occurs. The BPP consists of assessments of five fetal variables: fetal tone, fetal movement, fetal breathing, fetal reactivity (nonstress test), and amniotic fluid volume.

References: Miller A, Miller D, Cypher R. *Mosby's Pocket Guide to Fetal Monitoring: A Multidisciplinary Approach.* 9th ed. St. Louis, MO: Elsevier; 2022:230-232.

Shviraga B, Hensley JG. Uncomplicated antepartum, intrapartum, and postpartum care. In: Verklan MT, Walden M, Forest S, eds. *Core Curriculum for Neonatal Intensive Care Nursing.* 6th ed. St. Louis, MO: Elsevier; 2021:11.

4. **(C)** Patients who are at low risk for developing gestational diabetes (<25 years, normal weight before pregnancy, not a member of a high-risk ethnic or racial group, no diabetes in a first-degree relative, no history of abnormal glucose tolerance, and no history of poor obstetric outcome) are tested between 24 and 28 weeks' gestation. Patients with risk factors (>35 years, body mass index >30, history of gestational diabetes, delivery of a large-for-gestational-age infant, polycystic ovarian syndrome, and strong family history of diabetes) should receive a plasma glucose screening at their first prenatal visit followed by one at 24–28 weeks.

Reference: American Academy of Pediatrics, The American College of Obstetricians and Gynecologists. *Guidelines for Perinatal Care.* 8th ed. Elk Grove Village, IL: American Academy of Pediatrics; 2017:116.

5. **(D)** A late deceleration is a reflex fetal response to transient hypoxemia during uterine contractions. Fetal distress is an imprecise term, and the National Institute of Child Health and Human Development Task Force has recommended that this term be abandoned. Accelerations reflect a sympathetic nervous system response and results in an increase in the fetal heart rate (FHR). Rapid descent through the pelvis may cause a parasympathetic response that results in prolonged deceleration or fetal bradycardia, but not a late deceleration.

Reference: Miller A, Miller D, Cypher R. *Mosby's Pocket Guide to Fetal Monitoring: A Multidisciplinary Approach.* 9th ed. St. Louis, MO: Elsevier; 2022:125-127.

6. **(B)** Recurrent or sustained interruption of oxygen transfer from the environment to the fetus can lead to progressive deterioration of fetal oxygenation, metabolic acidemia, and blunting of parasympathetic outflow than can reduce the moment-to-moment regulation of the FHR. In the FHR tracing, these changes can be seen as minimal to absent variability. The etiologic cause of absent variability is a severe degree of hypoxia. Methamphetamine use and scalp stimulation can elicit marked variability.

Reference: Miller A, Miller D, Cypher R. *Mosby's Pocket Guide to Fetal Monitoring: A Multidisciplinary Approach.* 9th ed. St. Louis, MO: Elsevier; 2022:118-120.

7. **(D)** Oligohydramnios, a decreased amount of amniotic fluid, is defined as a single deepest pocket of <2 cm, or an amniotic fluid index of <5 cm. Abnormalities in amniotic fluid volume often require further evaluation and can significantly impact perinatal outcome. A reactive nonstress test, 30 seconds of fetal breathing, and three body movements within 30 minutes are components of a reassuring BPP.

Reference: Miller A, Miller D, Cypher R. *Mosby's Pocket Guide to Fetal Monitoring: A Multidisciplinary Approach.* 9th ed. St. Louis, MO: Elsevier; 2022:230-234.

Chapter 2

Adaptation to Extrauterine Life

1. What shunt is responsible for the movement of blood between the right and left atrium, and in which direction does the blood primarily flow during the fetal period?
   A. Ductus arteriosus with a left-to-right shunt
   B. Foramen ovale with a left-to-right shunt
   C. Ductus arteriosus with a right-to-left shunt
   D. Foramen ovale with a right-to-left shunt

2. What vessel(s) are responsible for transporting oxygenated blood from the placenta to the fetus?
   A. Umbilical arteries
   B. Umbilical vein
   C. Aorta
   D. Inferior vena cava

3. Which of the following pressure changes would reflect a term neonate displaying symptoms of persistent pulmonary hypertension?
   A. Increase in pulmonary vascular resistance, increase in systemic vascular resistance
   B. Decrease in pulmonary vascular resistance, decrease in systemic vascular resistance
   C. Increase in pulmonary vascular resistance, decrease in systemic vascular resistance
   D. Decrease in pulmonary vascular resistance, increase in systemic vascular resistance

4. During resuscitation of a term neonate in the Labor and Delivery department, a saturation probe is placed to assess the need for supplemental oxygen. Which of the following describes the appropriate site for placement and an acceptable saturation during the first 10 minutes of life?
   A. Right hand—3-minute saturation at 74%
   B. Left hand—4-minute saturation at 72%
   C. Left foot—5-minute saturation at 75%
   D. Right hand—10-minute saturation at 80%

5. Which statement best describes the role of endogenous catecholamine released during the birth process for adaptation to occur?
   A. Premature neonates secrete lower levels of catecholamines due to their immature adrenals contributing to hypotension.
   B. Catecholamine release is responsible for glucose homeostasis, thermoregulation, increasing the blood pressure, and stimulating surfactant production.
   C. Antenatal corticosteroids administration to the mother contributes to higher catecholamine levels in the premature neonate compared with those infants whose mothers did not receive corticosteroids.
   D. Term neonates secrete higher levels of catecholamines than preterm infants; therefore they are able to regulate glucose and utilize the brown fat for thermoregulation to occur.

6. Which statement about cord blood gases is correct?
   A. There is no difference between venous and arterial cord blood gas values.
   B. Cord venous blood is the best indicator of the fetal metabolic condition before delivery.
   C. Cord arterial pH is normally higher than the cord venous pH.
   D. Cord arterial blood is the best indicator of the fetal metabolic condition before delivery.

7. Which hormone activates nonshivering thermogenesis in neonates?
   A. Epinephrine
   B. Norepinephrine
   C. Vasopressin
   D. Insulin

8. Which of the following statements correctly describes the role of surfactant?
   A. Surfactant decreases lung compliance.
   B. Surfactant is responsible for clearing the lungs of fluid.
   C. Surfactant decreases surface tension to maintain a functional residual capacity.
   D. Surfactant increases the surface tension to prevent alveolar collapse.

9. A term neonate delivered vaginally had APGAR scores of 9 at 1 minute and 9 at 5 minutes, respectively. The maternal history is significant for hepatitis B surface antigen positive. The plan of care for this neonate should include which one of the following options?
   A. Administer hepatitis B immune globulin and hepatitis B vaccine within 12 hours after birth.
   B. Administer hepatitis B vaccine and hepatitis B immune globulin within 24 hours after birth.
   C. Administer hepatitis B immune globulin at time of discharge.
   D. Administer hepatitis B vaccine at time of discharge.

10. A 36-week-gestation neonate was delivered precipitously to a 35-year-old mother. The maternal history reveals previous rapid deliveries. This pregnancy was uneventful with the exception of late preterm delivery. APGAR scores were 8 at 1 minute and 9 at 5 minutes, respectively. The infant was placed skin to skin at the time of birth and has remained on the mother's chest attempting to breastfeed. Initial vital signs: axillary temperature 36.4°C (97.6°F), heart rate 156, respiratory rate 50–60 breaths per minute with occasional increases to the 70s. Breath sounds are slightly coarse with an occasional expiratory grunt. Color is pink with mild peripheral cyanosis. Based on these initial assessment findings, follow-up care should include which of the following interventions?

A. Transfer the neonate to the special care nursery for closer observation and monitoring.

B. Consult with the pediatric provider to assess the respiratory status and peripheral cyanosis and to provide orders.

C. Keep the neonate with the mother. Continue to have the mother attempt to breastfeed. Monitor vital signs and assess glucose status.

D. Move the neonate to the warmer in the mother's room. Delay breastfeeding based on occasional grunting and intermittent respiratory rate in the 70s.

11. A term neonate is 24 hours old and rooming in with the mother. The neonate was delivered by cesarean section due to maternal arrest of labor. APGAR scores are 7 at 1 minute and 8 at 5 minutes, respectively. Membranes ruptured 12 hours before delivery and were meconium stained. Prenatal group B *Streptococcus* screen at 36 weeks was negative. Maternal temperature before delivery was 37.9°C (100.2°F). Initial neonatal assessment reveals slight pallor, decreased peripheral pulses in lower extremities, difficulty with breast latching, slight lethargy, and respiratory rate 80 breaths per minute sustained with no other work of breathing. Based on the assessment, the nurse should carry out which of the following interventions?

A. Keep the neonate with the mother, check glucose level, monitor temperature and respiratory rate, and observe for additional signs of sepsis.

B. Keep the neonate with the mother, obtain a lactation consult, and place the baby skin to skin, knowing these findings are consistent with normal transition.

C. Notify the pediatric provider and transfer the neonate to the special care nursery for observation under a radiant warmer, with suspicion of coarctation of the aorta.

D. Notify the pediatric provider and transfer the neonate to the special care nursery for observation under a radiant warmer, with the possible diagnosis of persistent pulmonary hypertension due to meconium aspiration.

12. A term neonate was just delivered with a diagnosis of gastroschisis. Delivery room management would include which one of the following?

A. Place the neonate under a radiant warmer in supine position, cover the intestines with sterile gauze, place a peripheral intravenous catheter, and administer antibiotics.

B. Place the neonate under a radiant warmer in supine position, and cover the intestines with sterile soaked normal saline gauze.

C. Place the neonate under a radiant warmer, in a sterile bowel bag tied at the axilla, and in a supported side-lying position.

D. Place the neonate under a radiant warmer in a side-lying position, place a nasogastric tube, cover the intestines with gauze, and place the infant into a sterile bowel bag tied at the axilla.

13. The neonatal nurse is called over to the Labor and Delivery department to assess a neonate in respiratory distress after an uneventful vaginal delivery. Upon arrival, the labor and delivery nurse is providing bag and mask ventilation to an apneic, dusky neonate. The abdomen has a scaphoid appearance. Breath sounds are not audible on the left side of the chest. Heart sounds are more prominent on the right side of the chest. Based on this information, the neonate most likely has which of the following conditions?

A. Congenital diaphragmatic hernia
B. Pneumothorax
C. Persistent pulmonary hypertension
D. Tracheoesophageal fistula

14. Which of the following descriptions best defines a cephalohematoma?

A. Pitting edema that extends across the suture lines
B. Collection of blood between the periosteum and the skull and does not cross the suture line
C. Premature closure of the cranial suture with a palpable suture line
D. Hemorrhage into the space between the galea aponeurotica and the periosteum and may cross the suture lines

ANSWERS AND RATIONALES

1. **(D)** The ductus arteriosus shunts blood from right to left between the pulmonary artery and the aorta during the fetal period due to the high pulmonary vascular resistance. During the fetal period, the foramen ovale allows the shunting of blood from the right atrium to the left atrium due to the high pulmonary vascular resistance and lower systemic vascular resistance.

Reference: Verklan M. Adaptation to extrauterine life. In: Verklan M, Walden M, Forest S, eds. *Core Curriculum for Neonatal Intensive Care Nursing*. 6th ed. St. Louis, MO: Elsevier; 2021:54-68.

2. **(B)** The umbilical arteries transport deoxygenated blood from the aorta to the placenta for the exchange of oxygen and carbon dioxide and removal of waste products. Oxygenated blood from the placenta is delivered to the fetus from the umbilical vein and carried to the inferior vena cava via the ductus venosus.

Reference: Verklan M. Adaptation to extrauterine life. In: Verklan M, Walden M, Forest S, eds. *Core Curriculum for Neonatal Intensive Care Nursing*. 6th ed. St. Louis, MO: Elsevier; 2021:54-68.

3. **(C)** During normal transition from fetal to extrauterine life, the pulmonary vascular resistance decreases largely in part to air entry into the lung and increase in pulmonary blood flow. Systematic vascular resistance increases with the removal of the placenta. Persistent pulmonary hypertension continues to have the increase in pulmonary vascular resistance with constriction of the pulmonary vessels. This increase in pulmonary resistance can lead to the shunting of blood through fetal channels (i.e., ductus arteriosus and foramen ovale). The shunting of blood from right to left through the fetal shunts further contributes to hypoxemia.

Reference: Verklan M. Adaptation to extrauterine life. In: Verklan M, Walden M, Forest S, eds. *Core Curriculum for Neonatal Intensive Care Nursing*. 6th ed. St. Louis, MO: Elsevier; 2021:54-68.

4. **(A)** The right arm is considered preductal, and oxygen saturation should be monitored on the right upper extremity during delivery room resuscitation because neonates may have an increase in pulmonary vascular resistance with right to left shunting. With right-to-left shunting, saturations in the lower extremities may be lower than the upper extremities depending on the insertion of the ductus arteriosus to the aorta in relation to the subclavian arteries. According to the American Academy of

Pediatrics and the neonatal resuscitation algorithm, the following chart lists the target preductal saturation after birth:

1 minute	60%–65%
2 minutes	65%–70%
3 minutes	70%–75%
4 minutes	75%–80%
5 minutes	80%–85%
10 minutes	85%–95%

Reference: Weiner GM, Zaichkin J. *Textbook of Neonatal Resuscitation.* 8th ed. Itasca, IL: American Academy of Pediatrics, American Heart Association; 2021:46.

5. **(B)** The preterm neonate secretes higher levels of catecholamines compared to the term neonate. The increase in production of endogenous catecholamines in the preterm neonate is in response to less responsive organ systems. The release of catecholamines is responsible for increasing the blood pressure at birth, the metabolism of brown fat and fatty acids to mobilize the glycogen stores for glucose homeostasis, thermoregulation, and stimulating the production of surfactant. Although the production of endogenous catecholamines in the preterm neonate is increased, these neonates often have difficulty maintaining their temperature and require glucose supplementation. The administration of antenatal steroids actually causes a decrease in production of catecholamines.

Reference: Blackburn ST. Endocrine disorders. In: Verklan M, Walden M, Forest S, eds. *Core Curriculum for Neonatal Intensive Care Nursing.* 6th ed. St. Louis, MO: Elsevier; 2021:543-567.

6. **(D)** The umbilical arterial cord blood gas values tend to be slightly more acidotic than the venous values in terms of pH and base deficits. The umbilical vein transports oxygenated blood from the placenta to the fetus. The umbilical artery transports deoxygenated blood back to the placenta for oxygenation to occur. When evaluating cord blood gases, the arterial cord blood reveals the metabolic status of the fetus before delivery and strongly correlates with perinatal asphyxia.

Reference: Barry J, Deacon J, Hernandez C, Jones D. Acid-base homeostasis and oxygenation. In: Gardner SL, Carter BS, Enzman-Hines M, Niermeyer S, eds. *Merenstein & Gardner's Handbook of Neonatal Intensive Care: An Interprofessional Approach.* 9th ed. St. Louis, MO: Elsevier; 2021:186-200.

7. **(B)** Epinephrine is produced within the adrenal glands and works with norepinephrine to produce the "fight or flight" response by increasing the supply of oxygen to the brain and muscles. It does not play a role in thermoregulation. The process of nonshivering thermogenesis is activated by the hypothalamus. Norepinephrine is a stress hormone that is activated in response to cold stress. The release of norepinephrine sends a signal to the nerve endings in the brown fat initiating metabolism. Brown fat is located in the axillary area, mediastinum, kidneys, adrenals, and nape of the neck. The primary enzyme in the brown fat that regulates nonshivering thermogenesis is thermogenin. The release of fatty acids is triggered by the norepinephrine. The energy that is produced from this metabolic process heats the blood as it circulates past the areas where the brown fat is stored. Vasopressin is created by the hypothalamus and prompts the pituitary gland to release a hormone that helps maintain blood pressure and water and electrolyte balance. It does not play a role in thermoregulation. Insulin regulates glucose. Neonates who are cold stressed are also at risk for developing hypoglycemia and should be monitored closely.

Reference: Gardner SL, Cormack BH. Heat balance. In: Gardner SL, Carter BS, Enzman-Hines M, Niermeyer S, eds. *Merenstein and Gardner's Handbook of Neonatal Intensive Care: An Interprofessional Approach.* 9th ed. St. Louis, MO: Elsevier; 2021:137-164.

8. **(C)** Surfactant is produced by type II alveolar pneumocytes and coats the inner lining of the alveoli. Surfactant decreases surface tension and allows alveoli to remain open at the end of expiration, which prevents alveolar collapse, thereby maintaining functional residual capacity. Surfactant increases lung compliance. The increase in catecholamines at birth is responsible for decreasing the production of lung fluid and improving its reabsorption through the lymphatic system. Surfactant does not clear lung fluid.

References: Gardner S, Hines M, Nyp M. Respiratory diseases. In: Gardner SL, Carter BS, Enzman-Hines M, Niermeyer S, eds. *Merenstein and Gardner's Handbook of Neonatal Intensive Care: An Interprofessional Approach.* 9th ed. St. Louis, MO: Elsevier; 2021:729-835.

Verklan M. Adaptation to extrauterine life. In: Verklan M, Walden M, Forest S, eds. *Core Curriculum for Neonatal Intensive Care Nursing.* 6th ed. St. Louis, MO: Elsevier; 2021:54-68.

9. **(A)** Both hepatitis B immune globulin and hepatitis B vaccine are to be administered within 12 hours of birth to a neonate delivered to a mother that is hepatitis B surface antigen positive. The vaccine and immunoglobulin should be administered in separate injections and sites. Term neonates whose mother is hepatitis surface antigen negative should be immunized with hepatitis vaccine at the time of discharge.

Reference: Rudd KM. Infectious diseases in the neonate. In: Verklan M, Walden M, Forest S, eds. *Core Curriculum for Neonatal Intensive Care Nursing.* 6th ed. St. Louis, MO: Elsevier; 2021:588-616.

10. **(C)** These assessment findings are expected variations during the transitional period (4–6 hours) after birth. Because the lungs are attempting to clear fluid, neonates can have moist-sounding breath sounds, intermittently elevated respiratory rates, and occasional grunting. Transfer to the special care nursery/neonatal intensive care unit should be considered if the neonate has a sudden deterioration in respiratory status, difficulty maintaining temperature outside of skin-to-skin care, or changes in neurologic status. The pediatric provider should be contacted if the respiratory status changes with sustained grunting, increased work of breathing, and/or central color change. Peripheral acrocyanosis is normal finding during the transition period after birth due to vasomotor instability. The risk of aspiration increases when neonates are consistently tachypneic, with other signs of respiratory distress (grunting, flaring, and/or retracting). Oral feeding should be delayed if those factors are present and persist. Glucose monitoring is indicated for late preterm infants because they have inadequate glycogen stores and increased glucose utilization to maintain temperature after birth.

References: Lee HK, Oh E. Care of the well newborn. In: Cloherty J, Eichenwald EC, Hansen AR, Martin C, Stark AR, eds. *Cloherty and Stark's Manual of Neonatal Care.* 8th ed. Philadelphia, PA: Wolters Kluwer; 2017:106-111.

Verklan MT. Adaptation to extrauterine life. In: Verklan M, Walden M, Forest S, eds. *Core Curriculum for Neonatal Intensive Care Nursing.* 6th ed. St. Louis, MO: Elsevier; 2021:54-68.

Verklan MT. Care of the late preterm infant. In: Verklan M, Walden M, Forest S, eds. *Core Curriculum for Neonatal Intensive Care Nursing.* 6th ed. St. Louis, MO: Elsevier; 2021:388-393.

11. **(C)** Coarctation of the aorta has the classic finding of decreased perfusion and pulses in the lower extremities. These neonates can develop "comfortable" tachypnea, temperature instability, and fatigue with PO feeding. Congenital heart disease should be suspected when neonates present with an increase in respiratory rate in the absence of any other respiratory signs of distress and/or cyanosis. The pediatric provider should be notified immediately and the neonate transferred to the nursery for further evaluation. Severity of impaired perfusion can increase as the ductus arteriosus begins to physiologically close 1–2 days after birth. Septic neonates can present with signs and symptoms of infection within 12–24 hours of birth. Clinical findings of sepsis

can include hypoglycemia, poor feeding, lethargy, temperature instability, respiratory distress, weak pulses in all extremities, and cyanosis. Normal transition occurs in the first 4–6 hours after birth, so this neonate has completed transition to extrauterine life. The poor perfusion in the lower extremities and tachypnea suggest a pathologic process for which the neonate should be assessed. Severe meconium aspiration that leads to persistent pulmonary hypertension usually presents itself in the delivery room and is usually not associated with decreased perfusion in the lower extremities. Respiratory distress presents with tachypnea and an increase work of breathing.

References: Sadowski SL, Verklan MT. Cardiovascular disorders. In: Verklan M, Walden M, Forest S, eds. *Core Curriculum for Neonatal Intensive Care Nursing*. 6th ed. St. Louis, MO: Elsevier; 2021:460-503.

Verklan MT. Adaptation to extrauterine life. In: Verklan M, Walden M, Forest S, eds. *Core Curriculum for Neonatal Intensive Care Nursing*. 6th ed. St. Louis, MO: Elsevier; 2021:58-76.

12. **(C)** At the time of delivery, protection of the intestines is important as well as minimizing insensible water loss from the exposed surfaces. The neonate should be placed in a sterile bowel bag to allow for visualization of the intestines. In the absence of a sterile bowel bag, another option to protecting the intestines includes covering the intestines with warm sterile saline–soaked gauze that covers the exposed intestines and then applying a plastic covering over the gauze to prevent evaporation and heat loss. If gauze is used, it must maintain moisture to prevent adherence and damage to the viscera. The disadvantage of saline-soaked gauze is that it does not allow for visualization of the perfusion of the bowel. Care must be taken to maintain perfusion to the intestines. A side-lying position with support is acceptable. Placement of a peripheral intravenous line and nasogastric tube are not necessary in the delivery room and can be delayed until the neonate is transferred to the nursery.

Reference: Bradshaw WT. Gastrointestinal disorders. In: Verklan M, Walden M, Forest S, eds. *Core Curriculum for Neonatal Intensive Care Nursing*. 6th ed. St. Louis, MO: Elsevier; 2021:504-542.

13. **(A)** A scaphoid abdomen is the classic appearance of a neonate with a congenital diaphragmatic hernia. The majority of diaphragmatic hernias occur on the left side, resulting in breath and heart sounds auscultated on the right side of the chest. The degree of respiratory distress varies depending on the size of the herniation and underlying pulmonary hypoplasia. Respiratory distress can increase when the neonate is bag-and-mask ventilated because air can enter the stomach, pass to the intestine (located in the pleural cavity), and interfere with lung expansion. Bag-and-mask ventilation should be stopped and the neonate intubated if assisted ventilation is required. Placing an orogastric tube to decompress the stomach can help with ventilation. Respiratory distress is also evident with a pneumothorax. Breath sounds are diminished or absent on the affected side, however, the abdomen will appear normal on assessment. The presence of a scaphoid abdomen is a hallmark assessment pointing to a different diagnosis. Although respiratory distress can occur in an infant with a tracheoesophageal (TE) fistula, the presence of excessive oral secretions and inability to advance on orogastric tube are usually the primary presenting symptoms. Persistent pulmonary hypertension can present with profound respiratory distress but will generally have audible breath sounds on both sides unless complicated with a pneumothorax. Infants with a diaphragmatic hernia often have some degree of persistent pulmonary hypertension, due to pulmonary hypoplasia.

References: Bradshaw WT. Gastrointestinal disorders. In: Verklan M, Walden M, Forest S, eds. *Core Curriculum for Neonatal Intensive Care Nursing*. 6th ed. St. Louis, MO: Elsevier; 2021:504-542.

Verklan MT. Adaptation to extrauterine life. In: Verklan M, Walden M, Forest S, eds. *Core Curriculum for Neonatal Intensive Care Nursing*. 6th ed. St. Louis, MO: Elsevier; 2021:58-76.

Gentle S, Travers C, Carlo WA. Respiratory system. In: Kenner C, Altimier BB, Boykova MV, eds. *Comprehensive Neonatal Nursing*. 6th ed. New York: Springer Publishing Inc.; 2020:127-146.

Gallagher ME, Pacetti AS, Lovvorn HN, Carter BS. Neonatal surgery. In: Gardner SL, Carter BS, Enzman-Hines M, Niermeyer S, eds. *Merenstein and Gardner's Handbook of Neonatal Intensive Care: An Interprofessional Approach*. 9th ed. St. Louis, MO: Elsevier; 2021:996-1038.

14. **(B)** A cephalohematoma is a collection of blood between the periosteum and the skull that does not cross the suture line. It may enlarge during the 24 hours after birth and may take several weeks to months to spontaneously resolve. These neonates are at a higher risk for developing hyperbilirubinemia as the collection of blood is reabsorbed into circulation. A caput succedaneum is caused from pressure on the fetal skull by the cervix during labor. A common characteristic of a caput succedaneum is pitting edema that extends across the suture lines, and is described as a "boggy" edema. Edema generally resolves within a few days. Craniosynostosis is the premature closure of the cranial sutures and is not evident at birth. A hemorrhage into the space between the galea aponeurotica and the periosteum is a subgaleal hemorrhage. It is characterized by a rapid accumulation of blood in the subgaleal space, with an increasing head circumference, neurologic changes, and symptoms of hypovolemia and shock.

Reference: Cavaliere TA. Assessment of the newborn and infant. In: Kenner C, Altimier BB, Boykova MV, eds. *Comprehensive Neonatal Nursing*. 6th ed. New York: Springer; 2020:65-104.

Chapter 3

Neonatal Resuscitation

1. A neonate, delivered through thick meconium, initially has poor muscle tone and inadequate breathing. Which of the following actions is the most appropriate initial step:
   A. Place the neonate on the mother's chest and dry the neonate.
   B. Intubate and suction the trachea of the neonate.
   C. Place the neonate on the radiant warmer and perform the initial steps of resuscitation.
   D. Place the neonate on the radiant warmer and begin positive pressure ventilation (PPV).

2. A neonate is cyanotic, grunting, and has a barrel chest and scaphoid abdomen. The nurse auscultates bowel sounds on the left side of the chest accompanied by diminished breath sounds. Based on this assessment, this neonate is most likely to have which of the following conditions?
   A. Left pneumothorax
   B. Tracheoesophageal fistula
   C. Meconium aspiration syndrome
   D. Congenital diaphragmatic hernia

3. The most effective method to manage respiratory distress in an infant with suspected diaphragmatic hernia in the delivery room is via:
   A. high-flow nasal cannula.
   B. bag-and-mask ventilation/PPV.
   C. continuous positive airway pressure (CPAP).
   D. intubation and endotracheal tube ventilation.

4. Following the resuscitation of a term, 3-kg neonate delivered after a motor vehicle accident, the neonate is noted to be pale with an oxygen saturation of 95%. The heart rate is 170 beats per minute and the blood pressure is 34/22 mm Hg with a mean of 28 mm Hg. The neonate's tone is diminished. The bedside blood glucose level is 83 mg/dL and the initial venous cord gas is 7.12 with a base deficit of –8. Which of the following is the most appropriate initial action?
   A. Administer 30 mL normal saline bolus.
   B. Administer 6 mL dextrose 10% in water (D10W).
   C. Administer 30 mL O-negative blood.
   D. Initiate an infusion of 6 mEq 4.2% sodium bicarbonate.

5. When preparing for the delivery of a neonate with prenatally diagnosed hydrops and a pleural effusion, the resuscitation team should be prepared to take which initial action?
   A. Perform a pericardiocentesis.
   B. Administer a normal saline bolus.
   C. Perform a thoracentesis.
   D. Place an umbilical arterial catheter.

6. A term neonate is born via normal spontaneous vaginal delivery. The neonate is noted to be cyanotic when quiet but becomes pink when crying. The most likely diagnosis for this infant is:
   A. choanal atresia.
   B. Pierre Robin syndrome.
   C. congenital cardiac disease.
   D. respiratory distress syndrome.

7. Despite continuous positive pressure ventilation (PPV) via an endotracheal tube in the Delivery room, a neonate is persistently cyanotic with an oxygen saturation of 75%. The heart rate remains less than 100 beats per minute. Breath sounds can be heard over both the lung fields and the stomach. The stomach is distended. The end tidal CO_2 detector has not changed color. Which is the most likely location of the endotracheal tube?
   A. At the carina
   B. In the esophagus
   C. In the right mainstem bronchus
   D. Midway between the vocal cords and carina

8. The initial use of epinephrine in neonatal resuscitation for bradycardia less than 60 beats per minute is recommended in which of the following scenarios?
   A. After completing the initial steps and 30 seconds of optimizing ventilations
   B. After completing the initial steps, 30 seconds of optimizing ventilations and 60 seconds of chest compressions
   C. If the neonate is not responding to volume resuscitation
   D. Immediately upon delivery if the heart rate cannot be auscultated

9. After an emergent cesarean section for an umbilical cord prolapse, a term neonate requires intubation and chest compressions for 3 minutes. Apgar scores at 1, 5, and 10 minutes are 0, 3, and 4, respectively. At 12 minutes of age, the neonate remains hypotonic with no spontaneous respirations. This neonate is most at risk for:
   A. hyperglycemia.
   B. increased urinary output.
   C. right ventricular hypertrophy.
   D. hypoxic ischemic encephalopathy.

10. A 32-week preterm neonate born at a community facility has a heart rate of 130 beats per minute. The neonate is breathing spontaneously with moderate retractions. The oxygen saturation on room air is 75% at 4 minutes of life. Which of the following is the most appropriate next step for the nurse?
    A. Continue to monitor respiratory status.
    B. Provide CPAP at 5 cm H_2O, 30% fraction of inspired oxygen.
    C. Intubate and administer surfactant.
    D. Provide PPV via T-piece resuscitator.

11. A term, appropriate-for-gestational-age neonate is born via a vacuum-assisted vaginal delivery after a prolonged second stage of labor. During the first few hours after delivery, the neonate needs to be observed closely for which of the following conditions?
    A. Fractured clavicle
    B. Facial nerve palsy
    C. Caput succedaneum
    D. Subgaleal bleeding

12. A neonate, born through thick meconium, is taken to the warmer and initial steps are performed. PPV via bag and mask is given, but the chest rise is minimal, and gasping is noted. Repositioning the mask and head, suctioning and opening the airway, and increasing the pressure (MR SOPA) do not achieve effective ventilation. Auscultation of the breath sounds reveal rhonchi bilaterally. The appropriate next step would be to:
    A. perform direct laryngoscopy and endotracheal suctioning.
    B. reposition the mask and head again and continue to give PPV.
    C. perform chest physiotherapy to dislodge the meconium in the bronchioles.
    D. perform transillumination to rule out a pneumothorax.

13. A woman with a history of stillbirth delivery due to erythroblastosis fetalis is seen by a perinatologist. The most helpful prenatal test that will guide the resuscitation team at delivery is:
    A. amniocentesis.
    B. Kleihauer–Betke.
    C. glycosylated hemoglobin.
    D. high-resolution ultrasonography.

14. Which of the following differentiates secondary apnea from primary apnea?
    A. A decrease in heart rate
    B. Cessation of breathing
    C. Need for vigorous stimulation
    D. Need for assisted ventilation

ANSWERS AND RATIONALES

1. (C) Due to the presence of meconium and the clinical condition at birth, the neonate should be taken to the warmer and have initial steps performed to clear any secretions/meconium from the mouth and nose. Following the initial steps, if the neonate continues to have inadequate breathing or a heart rate of less than 100 beats per minute, positive pressure ventilation (PPV) should be begun. Intubation is indicated if the neonate requires continued resuscitation following initial steps and PPV. Intubation for tracheal suctioning is no longer recommended prior to PPV.

References: Aziz K, Lee HC, Escobedo MB, et al. Part 5: Neonatal Resuscitation – 2020 American Heart Association guidelines for cardiopulmonary resuscitation and emergency cardiovascular care. *Circulation.* 2020;142(suppl 2):S524-S550. doi:10.1161/CIR0000000000000902.

Weiner GM, Zaichkin J, Kattwinkel J, et al., eds. *Textbook of Neonatal Resuscitation.* 8th ed. Itasca, IL: American Academy of Pediatrics; 2021:52-55.

2. (D) The most common presenting signs of a congenital diaphragmatic hernia are barrel chest, scaphoid abdomen, diminished breath sounds, and bowel sounds heard in the chest cavity. The most common presenting signs of a left pneumothorax include diminished or absent breath sounds on the left side. Bowel sounds in the chest are not characteristic of a pneumothorax. Symptoms of a TE fistula are respiratory distress and excessive salivation. Although meconium aspiration syndrome can present with respiratory distress and a barrel chest, bowel sounds will not be heard in the chest cavity.

Reference: Bradshaw WT. Gastrointestinal disorders. In: Verklan MT, Walden M, Forest S, eds. *Core Curriculum of Neonatal Intensive Care Nursing.* 6th ed. St. Louis, MO: Elsevier; 2021:531-533.

3. (D) Intubation is the treatment of choice for stabilization of the patient with congenital diaphragmatic hernia. High-flow nasal cannula, bag-and-mask ventilation, and continuous positive airway pressure (CPAP) would potentially result in gastrointestinal distension and further compromise respiratory status by limiting lung expansion.

References: Bradshaw WT. Gastrointestinal disorders. In: Verklan MT, Walden M, Forest S, eds. *Core Curriculum of Neonatal Intensive Care Nursing.* 6th ed. St. Louis, MO: Elsevier; 2021:531-533.

Weiner GM, Zaichkin J, Kattwinkel J, et al., eds. *Textbook of Neonatal Resuscitation.* 8th ed. Itasca, IL: American Academy of Pediatrics; 2021:255.

4. (A) Pallor despite adequate oxygenation, tachycardia, hypotension, hypotonia, and metabolic acidosis are all signs of hypovolemic shock. Normal saline is the preferred fluid to correct hypovolemia and facilitate tissue perfusion. Giving a bolus of glucose-containing fluids to a neonate who is not hypoglycemic may precipitate hyperglycemia and aggravate metabolic acidosis. Giving O-negative blood would be an option in this case of known hemorrhage but may delay necessary volume expansion. While giving sodium bicarbonate was at one time considered to be a standard treatment for metabolic acidosis, that is no longer the case. Providing one or more normal saline boluses will generally resolve acidosis related to hypovolemia.

Reference: Bagwell GA. Resuscitation and stabilization of the newborn and infant. In: Kenner C, Altimier LB, Boykova M, eds. *Comprehensive Neonatal Nursing Care.* 6th ed. New York: Springer; 2020:59-60.

5. (C) With a pleural effusion related to hydrops, pleural fluid may be present to such a degree that it prevents adequate chest expansion. An emergency thoracentesis may be necessary. A pericardiocentesis may be necessary should a pericardial effusion be present; it would generally require ultrasound guidance. Although normal saline would assist with volume expansion and tissue perfusion, respiratory support is the top priority. An umbilical arterial catheter for monitoring blood pressures and arterial blood gases can be placed after initial stabilization.

Reference: Bradshaw WT. Gastrointestinal disorders. In: Verklan MT, Walden M, Forest S, eds. *Core Curriculum of Neonatal Intensive Care Nursing.* 6th ed. St. Louis, MO: Elsevier; 2021:531-533.

6. (A) Choanal atresia commonly presents with cyanosis upon delivery due to the blockage that resolves with crying. Pierre Robin syndrome presents with cyanosis, stridor, and apnea. The jaw is characteristically small and recessed, which results in obstruction of the airway by the tongue. Neonates with congenital cardiac disease would generally become more cyanotic with crying and stress. Respiratory distress syndrome (RDS) is most frequently seen in premature neonates. In addition to cyanosis, infants with RDS normally have other signs of respiratory distress such as retractions, grunting, and flaring.

References: Weiner GM, Zaichkin J, Kattwinkel J, et al., eds. *Textbook of Neonatal Resuscitation.* 8th ed. Itasca, IL: American Academy of Pediatrics; 2021:253.

Pappas BE, Robey DL. Neonatal delivery room resuscitation. In: Verklan MT, Walden M, Forest S, eds. *Core Curriculum of Neonatal Intensive Care Nursing.* 6th ed. St. Louis, MO: Elsevier; 2021:83.

7. (B) Signs of inadvertent esophageal intubation include auscultation of breath sounds over the stomach, abdominal distension, and a poor response to resuscitation. When intubated midway between the trachea and carina (the correct position) or at the carina, breath sounds will be of equal intensity on both sides and the neonate will respond to resuscitation with increased heart rate and oxygenation. In addition, the end tidal CO_2 detector would likely change color. Signs of inadvertent right mainstem intubation include a failure to respond to resuscitation and absent or diminished breath sounds over the left side of the chest. Breath sounds can be heard over the right side of the chest.

Reference: Weiner GM, Zaichkin J, Kattwinkel J, et al., eds. *Textbook of Neonatal Resuscitation.* 8th ed. Itasca, IL: American Academy of Pediatrics; 2021:135-138.

8. (B) The most effective means of correcting bradycardia in the neonate is optimizing ventilation. If bag and mask are not effective, it is recommended to insert an advanced airway. However, if the heart rate remains less than 60 beats per minute after optimizing ventilation for 30 seconds and providing 60 seconds of chest compressions, current literature supports the use of epinephrine. Volume expansion is utilized when blood loss is known or suspected (as evidenced by signs of shock such as not paleness, delayed capillary refill, and/or weak pulses). Volume is also indicated if the neonate has a persistently low heart rate after optimizing ventilations, performing chest compressions, and administering epinephrine. If the baby does not respond to volume expansion, the team needs to step back and reevaluate the quality of ventilation and compressions. Inability to auscultate the heart rate immediately following delivery may be due to fetal compromise or poor technique. Even with fetal compromise, performing the initial steps of resuscitation are indicated.

References: Aziz K, Lee HC, Escobedo MB, et al. Part 5: Neonatal Resuscitation – 2020 American Heart Association guidelines for cardiopulmonary resuscitation and emergency cardiovascular care. *Circulation.* 2020;142(suppl 2):S524-S550. doi:10.1161/CIR0000000000000902.

Weiner GM, Zaichkin J, Kattwinkel J, et al., eds. *Textbook of Neonatal Resuscitation.* 8th ed. Itasca, IL: American Academy of Pediatrics; 2021:189-191.

9. (D) Infants with hypoxic ischemic encephalopathy have many intrapartum risk factors. This scenario reflects a cord accident, low Apgar scores, and a prolonged resuscitation. Clinical presentation of severe encephalopathy includes continued marked hypotonia and prolonged need for mechanical ventilation. Although initially blood glucose rises with stress, glucose stores are depleted rapidly during a prolonged resuscitation, resulting in hypoglycemia. If the kidneys experience hypoxia during a prolonged resuscitation, early signs of ischemia or decreased renal perfusion would be low urinary output. Right ventricular hypertrophy is often seen in many congenital cardiac defects, including pulmonary stenosis and tetralogy of Fallot.

Reference: Ditzenberger G. Neurologic disorders. In: Verklan MT, Walden M, Forest S, eds. *Core Curriculum of Neonatal Intensive Care Nursing*. 6th ed. St. Louis, MO: Elsevier; 2021:649-652.

10. **(B)** Because this preterm neonate has moderate retractions and a relatively low oxygen saturation at 4 minutes of life, respiratory support is indicated. Providing CPAP at a FiO$_2$ of 21–30% is a noninvasive form of respiratory support that is particularly helpful for premature neonate who are breathing spontaneously and has an adequate heart rate but increased work of breathing and a low oxygen saturation. PPV is appropriate if the neonate is not breathing sufficiently, demonstrating apnea, or has a heart rate of less than 100 beats per minute. Intubating the premature neonate and providing early surfactant may be helpful if other forms of respiratory support are not effective. Surfactant administration in the delivery room remains controversial; particularly if the team is not skilled with administration.

References: Aziz K, Lee HC, Escobedo MB, et al. Part 5: Neonatal Resuscitation – 2020 American Heart Association guidelines for cardiopulmonary resuscitation and emergency cardiovascular care. *Circulation*. 2020;142(suppl 2):S524-S550. doi:10.1161/CIR0000000000000902.

Pappas BE, Robey DL. Neonatal delivery room resuscitation. In: Verklan MT, Walden M, Forest S, eds. *Core Curriculum of Neonatal Intensive Care Nursing*. 6th ed. St. Louis, MO: Elsevier; 2021;79.

11. **(D)** The most life-threatening complications of vacuum deliveries are intracranial bleeds or subgaleal hemorrhages. The incidence of subgaleal hemorrhages with vacuum is only 0.59%, but mortality is 17–25%. Signs of a subgaleal bleed include apnea or tachypnea, hypotension, and signs of hypovolemic shock. Because the shearing of the emissary vein happens during delivery, these signs can rapidly develop within minutes to hours after birth. A fractured clavicle would occur most frequently with a large-for-gestational-age neonate with shoulder dystocia at the time of delivery. Facial nerve palsy would occur most frequently after the use of forceps. Although a caput succedaneum is a known complication related to the use of vacuum, it is a benign condition and usually resolves within a few days of birth.

Reference: Ditzenberger G. Neurologic disorders. In: Verklan MT, Walden M, Forest S, eds. *Core Curriculum of Neonatal Intensive Care Nursing*. 6th ed. St. Louis, MO: Elsevier; 2021:641-642.

12. **(A)** Direct laryngoscopy and endotracheal suctioning are not routinely required for all neonates born through thick meconium. However, if there are signs of inadequate ventilation while providing PPV, intubation is indicated as the fifth step of MR SOPA (M-Mask adjustment, R-Reposition airway, S-Suction Mouth and Nose, O-Open mouth, P-Pressure Increase, A-Alternative Airway). If there is meconium blocking the upper airway, continuing to perform MR SOPA will not facilitate a positive response to PPV. While chest physiotherapy may be useful for an intubated neonate with meconium aspiration syndrome to facilitate movement of debris from the smaller to larger bronchi, it has the potential for decreasing oxygenation in the acutely ill neonate, and its use in the delivery room is not evidence-based. A pneumothorax is a possibility if a neonate does not respond to resuscitation or has an acute decompensation. However, breath sounds are generally diminished on the side where the pneumothorax has occurred.

References: Aziz K, Lee HC, Escobedo MB, et al. Part 5: Neonatal Resuscitation – 2020 American Heart Association guidelines for cardiopulmonary resuscitation and emergency cardiovascular care. *Circulation*. 2020;142(suppl 2):S524-S550. doi:10.1161/CIR0000000000000902.

Weiner GM, Zaichkin J, Kattwinkel J, et al., eds. *Textbook of Neonatal Resuscitation*. 8th ed. Itasca, IL: American Academy of Pediatrics; 2021:246-248.

Gardner SL, Enzman-Hines M, Nyp M. Respiratory diseases. In: Gardner SL, Carter BS, Enzman-Hines M, Niermeyer S, eds. *Merenstein & Gardner's Handbook of Neonatal Intensive Care: An Interprofessional Approach*. 9th ed. St. Louis, MO: Elsevier; 2021:745-748.

13. **(D)** Amniocentesis can determine the karyotype of the fetus, bilirubin level, and reduce uterine fluid volume but will not predict the neonate's condition at time of delivery. The Kleihauer-Betke test identifies fetal cells in the maternal blood and can be useful in determining whether the mother needs Rh IgG but will not predict the neonate's condition at the time of delivery. The glycosylated hemoglobin test, known as A1C, determines the mother's blood glucose over a 3-month period and is not related to erythroblastosis fetalis. High-resolution ultrasonography is useful for determining ascites, pericardial and pleural effusion, and other conditions in the fetus before delivery. The test gives the resuscitation team the ability to anticipate what degree of resuscitation may be needed.

References: Bagwell G. Hematologic disorders. In: Kenner C, Lott J, eds. *Comprehensive Neonatal Nursing Care*. 5th ed. New York: Springer; 2014: 347-349.

Bradshaw WT. Gastrointestinal disorders. In: Verklan MT, Walden M, Forest S, eds. *Core Curriculum of Neonatal Intensive Care Nursing*. 6th ed. St. Louis, MO: Elsevier; 2021:531-533.

14. **(D)** The heart rate decreases and breathing cessation occurs in both primary and secondary apnea; both types of apneas require stimulation. In secondary apnea, the neonate will not respond to stimulation alone and requires assisted ventilation to shorten the time to the onset of spontaneous breathing. Without effective PPV, biochemical deterioration quickly follows the last gasp of breath.

Reference: Niermeyer S, Clark SB. Care at birth. In: Gardner SL, Carter BS, Enzman-Hines M, Niermeyer S, eds. *Merenstein & Gardner's Handbook of Neonatal Intensive Care: An Interprofessional Approach*. 9th ed. St. Louis, MO: Elsevier; 2021:68-70.

Chapter 4

Physical Assessment

1. Exposure to magnesium sulfate before delivery increases the likelihood that the newborn will develop which of the following postdelivery?
   A. Exaggerated deep tendon reflexes
   B. Hypotension and hypoglycemia
   C. Hypotonia and respiratory depression
   D. Thrombocytopenia and anemia

2. A newborn infant born at 35 weeks' gestation plots at the third percentile for weight, length, and head circumference. The most likely explanation for this finding is:
   A. chronic fetal distress.
   B. intrauterine infection.
   C. maternal hypertension.
   D. Rh isoimmunization.

3. A 3.2-kg, 37-week-gestation infant is admitted to the neonatal intensive care unit (NICU) related to respiratory distress. The infant was delivered by cesarean section for maternal hypertension; Apgar score was 6 at 1 minute and 8 at 5 minutes. On admission the infant's respiratory rate is 90 breaths per minute with moderate retractions and occasional grunting. A chest radiograph showed increased vascular markings with expansion to the 10th rib. This infant most likely has:
   A. meconium aspiration.
   B. respiratory distress syndrome.
   C. group B strep pneumonia.
   D. transient tachypnea of the newborn.

4. A term infant who is small for gestational age is noted to have several anomalies, including low-set ears, low posterior hairline with a webbed neck, broad chest with widely spaced nipples, and edema of the hands and feet. These findings are most likely related to:
   A. trisomy 18.
   B. Down syndrome (trisomy 21).
   C. Turner syndrome.
   D. Klinefelter syndrome.

5. A term infant presents at birth with tachypnea and increased work of breathing. The infant's oxygen saturation is 78–80% despite being given 100% oxygen. Congenital heart disease is suspected. Which of the following defects is most likely to cause these symptoms?
   A. Aortic stenosis
   B. Coarctation of the aorta
   C. Patent ductus arteriosus
   D. Transposition of the great vessels

6. The nurse practitioner is examining the eyes of a late preterm infant prior to discharge and notes the absence of the red reflex in the infant's left eye. The most likely explanation for this finding is:

   A. congenital cataracts.
   B. coloboma.
   C. retinopathy of prematurity.
   D. strabismus.

7. An infant is admitted to the NICU for management of neonatal opioid withdrawal syndrome secondary to maternal methadone use. Symptoms of methadone withdrawal typically present within which time frame?
   A. Less than 24 hours
   B. 24–28 hours
   C. 48–72 hours
   D. 5–7 days

8. In assessing a 5-day-old infant with a history of maternal methadone use, the nurse would expect to find:
   A. constipation.
   B. hypothermia.
   C. skin excoriation.
   D. excessive sleepiness.

9. A term infant is noted to have low-set ears, a short neck with excessive skin, Brushfield spots, a large tongue, and simian creases. This infant is at increased risk of:
   A. coarctation of the aorta.
   B. duodenal atresia.
   C. polycystic kidneys.
   D. tracheoesophageal fistula.

10. An otherwise healthy term infant is found to have eight cafe au lait spots scattered over his trunk and extremities. This infant should be investigated for the presence of what condition?
    A. Klippel-Trénaunay-Weber syndrome
    B. Neurofibromatosis
    C. Sturge-Weber syndrome
    D. Tuberous sclerosis

11. After a vaginal delivery a newborn infant is noted to have an enlarged fluctuant nontender scrotal sac. The left scrotum is larger than the right. There is no tenderness, but the scrotum appears bruised. The most likely explanation for this finding is:
    A. ascites.
    B. hydrocele.
    C. inguinal hernia.
    D. testicular torsion.

12. A 5-day-old, 35-week infant presents with a temperature of 37.8°C and moderate jaundice. He has been exclusively breastfed and is otherwise well. The infant's mother was group B strep negative, and membranes were ruptured for 4 hours before a spontaneous vaginal delivery. What is the most likely explanation for these findings?

A. Dehydration
B. Herpes encephalitis
C. Intracranial hemorrhage
D. Sepsis

13. During routine assessment of a 2-day-old term newborn, a holosystolic murmur is heard over the apex. The murmur is described as "harsh and machinelike" in quality and does not radiate. The infant is otherwise asymptomatic and has no family history of congenital heart disease or other medical problems. What is the most likely cause of this murmur?
A. Coarctation of the aorta
B. Patent ductus arteriosus
C. Tricuspid atresia
D. Ventricular septal defect

14. A mother reports that her week-old daughter "has her own breast milk." On examination, the infant has enlarged breast tissue and a milky secretion, but the chest otherwise appears normal. Education for the mother is based on the knowledge that:
A. this is normal and will self-resolve.
B. this is indicative of mastitis and should be treated with antibiotics.
C. blood work should be drawn to assess hormone levels.
D. this is a sign of a chromosomal abnormality.

15. Bilious vomiting requires immediate evaluation for:
A. duodenal atresia.
B. Hirschsprung disease.
C. meconium ileus.
D. midgut volvulus.

16. Bounding femoral pulses are most likely indicative of:
A. coarctation of the aorta.
B. interrupted aortic arch.
C. patent ductus arteriosus.
D. ventricular septal defect.

17. A small-for-gestational-age infant is born with several anomalies, including micrognathia, a cleft lip, overlapping digits, rocker bottom feet, and cutis aplasia. The most likely explanation for this constellation of anomalies is:
A. Pierre Robin sequence.
B. trisomy 13.
C. trisomy 21.
D. Turner syndrome.

18. The presence of central cyanosis is assessed in which part of the body?
A. Face
B. Fingertips
C. Tongue
D. Trunk

19. A 41-week infant is delivered by cesarean section for failure to progress. The baby is large for gestational age with head, length, and weight at the 95th percentile. On examination, the newborn is centrally pink, in no respiratory distress, and has good tone. There is no caput or molding of the head. However, on palpation, several soft spots that recoil with pressure are noted over the back of the head. The most likely explanation for this finding is:

A. craniotabes.
B. DiGeorge syndrome.
C. premature fusion of the sutures.
D. depressed skull fracture.

20. During an examination of a newborn, the nurse palpates a firm abdominal mass midline just below the umbilicus and above the symphysis pubis. The most likely cause of this mass is:
A. enlarged bladder.
B. umbilical hernia.
C. rectus diastasis.
D. meconium plug.

21. The Ortolani test is used in assessing for what condition?
A. Brachial plexus injury
B. Clavicular fracture
C. Talipes equinovarus
D. Developmental dysplasia of the hip

22. A small-for-gestational-age infant is born with hypoplasia of the arm with cicatricial scarring and microphthalmia. The most likely cause of these findings is congenital infection caused by:
A. cytomegalovirus.
B. rubella.
C. toxoplasmosis.
D. varicella.

23. A 10-day-old infant born at 34 weeks by spontaneous vaginal delivery after 12 hours of ruptured membranes develops a vesicular rash over the occiput. In addition to culturing the lesion, the nurse should anticipate that this infant will require which of the following urgent tests?
A. Computerized tomography
B. Electroencephalography
C. Lumbar puncture
D. Magnetic resonance imaging

24. Which of the following is part of a routine assessment for a well newborn?
A. Blood pressure measurement
B. Fundoscopy
C. Percussion
D. Red reflex examination

25. Umbilical hernias are more common in which of the following population groups?
A. African American
B. Asian
C. Caucasian
D. Native American

26. The mother of an infant born at 39 weeks' gestation asks about her infant's ability to focus on a picture of a human face. The nurse's response is based on the knowledge that a term newborn can be expected to briefly fixate on objects at a distance of how many inches?
A. 10–12
B. 12–14
C. 14–16
D. 16–18

27. When performing a Ballard Assessment, the nurse would expect to see moderate flexion of all four limbs and a popliteal angle of 100 degrees at which gestational age range?
    A. 29–31 weeks
    B. 32–33 weeks
    C. 34–36 weeks
    D. 38–40 weeks

28. An infant born at 34 weeks gestational age has a small, recessed mandible, cleft palate, and a tongue that is displaced to the rear of the mouth at birth. These findings are suggestive of:
    A. fetal alcohol syndrome.
    B. fetal Dilantin exposure.
    C. Pierre Robin sequence.
    D. trisomy 13.

29. An infant is born by vaginal delivery complicated by moderate shoulder dystocia. The infant is noted to have an asymmetric Moro reflex, and his arm is adducted and internally rotated. The wrist is flexed. What is the most likely cause?
    A. Bell palsy
    B. Erb palsy
    C. Phrenic nerve paralysis
    D. Fractured humerus

30. A 1-month-old infant born at 27 weeks' gestation has developed two soft, raised, bright-red tumors, one on the chest and one on the arm. These lesions have grown in size over the past 10 days from when they were first noted. The mother asks the nurse if these lesions will continue to grow. The nurse's response is based on the knowledge that this type of lesion will:
    A. continue to grow as the child grows.
    B. grow for 6 months and then involute.
    C. remain at the current size through childhood.
    D. require treatment to halt the growth.

31. A 2-day-old, full-term male infant has a history of low Apgar scores, poor urine output, and hypertonicity. The infant was noted to have two episodes of apnea accompanied by lip smacking and eye deviations. These episodes are most likely:
    A. benign familial seizures.
    B. sleep myoclonus.
    C. subtle seizures.
    D. tonic–clonic seizures.

32. An infant was born at 31 weeks' gestation and treated with continuous positive airway pressure for 10 days. At 2 weeks the infant was noted to have difficulty feeding and high-pitched inspiratory stridor. What is the most likely cause?
    A. Laryngomalacia
    B. Vocal cord paralysis
    C. Laryngeal atresia
    D. Subglottic stenosis

33. A newborn presents with failure to thrive, liver failure, a coppery-brown skin rash, and a purulent nasal discharge. The mother and infant should be tested for:
    A. syphilis.
    B. cytomegalovirus.
    C. herpes.
    D. hepatitis B.

34. A 2-day-old infant is noted to have significant jaundice. His blood work shows decreased hemoglobin, hyperbilirubinemia, and a positive direct antigen test. These findings are most likely a result of:
    A. biliary atresia.
    B. immune-mediated hemolysis.
    C. hereditary spherocytosis.
    D. thalassemia.

35. The nurse caring for a 2-day-old African American infant notices a scattered rash on the infant's face and trunk. The rash consists of a mix of vesicles, pustules, and brown macules. The infant is afebrile and feeding well. The rash most likely represents:
    A. milia.
    B. erythema toxicum.
    C. neonatal candidiasis.
    D. transient neonatal pustular melanosis.

36. Congenital heart disease is more likely to be present in infants with which of the following malformations?
    A. Gastroschisis
    B. Omphalocele
    C. Pyloric stenosis
    D. Hirschsprung disease

37. A term newborn presents with a large port-wine stain over the forehead and eyelid. This infant is at risk for:
    A. clotting deficits.
    B. hearing loss.
    C. thrombocytopenia.
    D. underlying hemangiomas.

38. A newborn infant presents with cyanosis. On examination, the nurse hears a murmur at the left upper sternal border, but hears nothing else unusual. What cardiac defect is most likely responsible for these findings?
    A. Tetralogy of Fallot
    B. Atrial septal defect
    C. Transposition of the great arteries (vessels)
    D. Ventricular septal defect

39. A 4-day-old infant born by spontaneous vaginal delivery at 29 weeks' gestation develops a markedly erythematous area around the umbilicus with a cluster of blisters, some of which are desquamating, leaving areas of raw skin. The most likely cause of this skin condition is an infection due to:
    A. *Candida*.
    B. *Klebsiella*.
    C. Herpes simplex.
    D. *Staphylococcus aureus*.

40. A 1-day-old infant is noted to have a petechial rash over his scalp, face, and trunk. The nurse caring for this infant should anticipate an order to check the infant's:
    A. clotting time.
    B. hemoglobin.
    C. platelets.
    D. white blood cell count.

41. When assessing a newborn infant, the nurse notes that the infant has sclerae that appear blue. This infant should have additional evaluation for which of the following conditions?
    A. DiGeorge syndrome
    B. Muscular dystrophy
    C. Osteogenesis imperfecta
    D. Systemic lupus erythematosus

42. During labor, a fetus at 37 weeks' gestation is noted to have sustained bradycardia with a heart rate of 72–84 beats per minute. After an emergency cesarean section, the infant is pink with good respiratory efforts and good tone. The heart rate remains 82–88 beats per minute. Which of the following maternal conditions explains this heart rate pattern?
    A. Diabetes
    B. Preeclampsia
    C. Chorioamnionitis
    D. Systemic lupus erythematosus

43. After a pregnancy complicated by polyhydramnios, the newborn should be assessed for which of the following conditions?
    A. Pyloric stenosis
    B. Prune belly syndrome
    C. Posterior urethral valves
    D. Tracheoesophageal fistula

44. A 2-day-old term infant sleeps poorly and has a moderate emesis with multiple feedings, is jittery, and has loose stools with perianal excoriation. These findings are likely related to in utero exposure to:
    A. alcohol.
    B. cocaine.
    C. oxycodone.
    D. selective serotonin reuptake inhibitors.

45. A 3-day-old infant born after induction at 41 weeks' gestation has a birthweight of 4.2 kg. The infant has coarse facial features, a large anterior fontanel with a normal head circumference, an umbilical hernia, and a history of poor perfusion and feeding. This infant should be further assessed for:
    A. congenital adrenal hyperplasia.
    B. congenital hypothyroidism.
    C. Down syndrome.
    D. Prader-Willi syndrome.

46. A murmur caused by pulmonic stenosis would best be heard over which of the following anatomical landmarks?
    A. Second intercostal space, left sternal border
    B. Second intercostal space, right sternal angle
    C. Fourth intercostal space, left sternal angle
    D. Fifth intercostal space, midclavicular line

47. After a vaginal delivery complicated by a prolonged second stage, a term infant is noted to have bruising over the occiput with a small firm mass on the right side of the sagittal suture. The mass does not cross the suture line. This is likely a:
    A. skull fracture.
    B. cephalohematoma.

C. subdural hematoma.
D. subgaleal hemorrhage.

48. A 2-week-old premature neonate has vesiculopapular lesions with an erythematous base in her groin. Small white pustules can be seen on the lower abdomen. The most likely cause of this rash is:
    A. *Candida albicans*.
    B. diaper dermatitis.
    C. Herpes simplex.
    D. *S. aureus*.

49. At 6 days of age a 34-week-gestation neonate is noted to have edema of the eyes with reddened conjunctiva and yellow discharge. This most likely cause of these findings is:
    A. blocked lacrimal duct.
    B. *Chlamydia trachomatis* infection.
    C. corneal abrasion.
    D. herpes simplex infection.

50. In addition to hypoglycemia, an infant of a diabetic mother should be assessed for the development of:
    A. hypernatremia.
    B. hypocalcemia.
    C. hyponatremia.
    D. thrombocytopenia.

51. During a routine assessment after a spontaneous vaginal birth at term gestation, the neonate is pink when crying but demonstrates central cyanosis when quiet. Breath sounds are equal, and there is no tachypnea. The most likely cause of these findings is:
    A. bilateral choanal atresia.
    B. congenital heart disease.
    C. tracheoesophageal fistula.
    D. persistent pulmonary hypertension of the newborn.

52. The mother of a healthy full-term newborn asks about the hymenal tag that was noted while changing her daughter's diaper. The nurse's response is based on the knowledge that:
    A. newborn screening should be done to rule out congenital adrenal hyperplasia.
    B. chromosome analysis should be done to rule out further anomalies.
    C. removal of the tag will be done after a few months.
    D. tags are benign and resolve spontaneously.

53. After therapeutic cooling for hypoxic ischemic encephalopathy, the nurse notes a 1-cm area of induration on the infant's upper back and a second small, firm nodule over the sacrum. Which of the following electrolyte values should be monitored in this infant?
    A. Calcium
    B. Magnesium
    C. Potassium
    D. Sodium

ANSWERS AND RATIONALES

1. **(C)** Magnesium sulfate crosses the placenta and may cause hypermagnesemia. Signs of elevated serum magnesium include respiratory depression, hypotonia, poor suck, weakness, and lethargy. Magnesium depresses rather than exaggerates deep tendon reflexes. Magnesium does affect blood pressure levels. Magnesium does not alter blood glucose levels, interfere with platelet or red cell production, or cause red blood cell hemolysis.

Reference: Hurst HM. Antepartum-intrapartum complications. In: Verklan MT, Walden M, Forest S, eds. *Core Curriculum for Neonatal Intensive Care Nursing.* 6th ed. St. Louis, MO: Elsevier; 2021:20-34.

2. **(B)** Symmetric intrauterine growth restriction (IUGR) begins early in gestation and is most often caused by intrauterine infection or genetic abnormalities. Chronic fetal distress is implicated as a cause of asymmetric growth restriction, resulting in a larger head circumference in comparison to length and weight. Maternal hypertension causes asymmetric IUGR. Rh isoimmunization is not known to cause growth restriction.

Reference: Trotter C. Gestational age assessment. In: Tappero EP, Honeyfield ME, eds. *Physical Assessment of the Newborn.* 6th ed. New York: Springer Publishing; 2019:23-43.

3. **(D)** Transient tachypnea is more common in late preterm infants and term infants born by cesarean section. Infants with transient tachypnea of the newborn have chest radiographic findings that include overexpansion, haziness, increased vascular markings, and fluid in the fissure. Meconium aspiration is more common in post-term infants. Radiographic findings in meconium aspiration include hyperinflation and patchy infiltrates. Infants with respiratory distress syndrome present at birth or within hours with clinical signs of respiratory distress that include tachypnea, grunting, retractions, and cyanosis accompanied by increasing oxygen requirements. The chest radiograph is characterized by atelectasis, air bronchograms, and diffuse granular infiltrates that often progress to severe bilateral opacity. Group B *Streptococcus* is the most common cause of congenital pneumonia and, although possible, is less likely in infants born by cesarean section with intact membranes and in the absence of risk factors such as maternal fever.

Reference: Fraser D. Respiratory distress. In: Verklan MT, Walden M, Forest S, eds. *Core Curriculum for Neonatal Intensive Care Nursing.* 6th ed. St. Louis, MO: Elsevier; 2021:394-416.

4. **(C)** Infants with Turner syndrome, which occurs in phenotypic females, are usually small for gestational age with a broad chest, widely spaced nipples, edema of the extremities, and a short-webbed neck. Features of trisomy 18 include a prominent occiput, low-set malformed ears, small eyes and jaw, clenched hands with overlapping fingers, and rocker-bottom feet. Down syndrome, or trisomy 21, can feature Brushfield spots, small ears, simian creases, excess skin at the nape of the neck, up slanting palpebral fissures, hypotonia, large protruding tongue, and cardiac anomalies. Klinefelter syndrome occurs in males and results in long limbs, elbow dysplasia, and clinodactyly involving the fifth finger. Hypospadias, hypogonadism, and cryptorchidism are usually present.

Reference: Lubbers L. Congenital anomalies. In: Verklan MT, Walden M, Forest S, eds. *Core Curriculum for Neonatal Intensive Care Nursing.* 6th ed. St. Louis, MO: Elsevier; 2021:654-677.

5. **(D)** Transposition of the great vessels occurs when the aorta arises from the right ventricle and the pulmonary artery arises from the left ventricle. Marked cyanosis is a presenting feature of transposition because the aorta carries deoxygenated blood from the right ventricle to the systemic circulation. Aortic stenosis reduces blood flow to the body. In isolation, aortic stenosis is usually asymptomatic at birth. Signs of poor systemic blood flow such as pallor, mottling, and poor perfusion may develop when the ductus arteriosus closes. Coarctation or constriction of the aorta may occur anywhere in the aorta but most often occurs around the junction of the aorta and the ductus arteriosus. Symptoms vary according to the location of the constriction, but cyanosis is usually not seen in infants with an isolated coarctation. Patent ductus arteriosus is an acyanotic heart defect resulting from a failure of the ductus arteriosus to close after birth.

Reference: Swanson R, Erickson L. Cardiovascular diseases and surgical interventions. In: Gardner SL, Carter BS, Hines ME, Niermeyer S, eds. *Merenstein & Gardner's Handbook of Neonatal Intensive Care: An Interprofessional Approach.* 9th ed. St. Louis, MO: Elsevier; 2021:836-885.

6. **(A)** The absence of a red reflex indicates that some disease process is blocking passage of light through the lens to the retina. This finding is seen in congenital cataracts, retinoblastoma, and glaucoma. Infants with strabismus have misalignment of the red reflex due to deviation of the eye, however, the red reflex is still visible. Coloboma is a congenital absence of ocular tissue, often seen in the lens or iris. Retinopathy of prematurity (ROP) is seen in premature infants and is very rare after 32 weeks of gestation. The red reflex is usually visible in infants with ROP unless retinal detachment is present.

Reference: Johnson P. Head, eyes, ears, nose, mouth and neck assessment. In: Tappero EP, Honeyfield ME, eds. *Physical Assessment of the Newborn.* 6th ed. New York: Springer; 2019:71.

7. **(C)** Methadone withdrawal usually presents between 48 and 72 hours after birth, later than other opioids. The half-life of methadone is longer than other opioids. Methadone maintenance is usually given daily; less than 24 hours is too soon for symptoms of withdrawal to appear. Between 24 and 28 hours after delivery methadone is still present in the infant's bloodstream; therefore signs of withdrawal will not be seen. Five to seven days exceeds the time by which withdrawal symptoms most commonly appear.

Reference: Wallen L, Gleason C. Prenatal drug exposure. In: Gleason C, Juul S, eds. *Avery's Diseases of the Newborn.* 10th ed. Philadelphia, PA: Elsevier; 2018:126-144.

8. **(C)** Symptoms of neonatal opioid withdrawal syndrome (NOWS) include excoriation, diarrhea, tachypnea, and hyperthermia. Infants experiencing NOWS tend to have higher than normal body temperatures, often because of excessive motor activity. NOWS infants experience jitteriness, tremors, and excessive motor activity. Poor sleep is common; excessive sleepiness would not be expected.

Reference: Wallen L, Gleason C. Prenatal drug exposure. In: Gleason C, Juul S, eds. *Avery's Diseases of the Newborn.* 10th ed. Philadelphia, PA: Elsevier; 2018:126-144.

9. **(B)** The feature suggests Down syndrome. Duodenal atresia occurs in 2–5% of infants with Down syndrome. Heart defects common to infants with Down syndrome include endocardial cushion defects, ventricular septal defects, patent ductus arteriosus, atrial septal defects, and tetralogy of Fallot. Coarctation of the aorta is not commonly found in infants with Down syndrome. Infants with Down syndrome are not at increased risk of renal anomalies. Esophageal atresia is more common in infants with Down syndrome; however, TE fistula is not highly associated with Down syndrome.

Reference: Haldeman-Englert C, Saitta S, Zackai E. Chromosomal disorders. In: Gleason C, Juul S, eds. *Avery's Diseases of the Newborn.* 10th ed. Philadelphia, PA: Elsevier; 2018:211-223.

10. **(B)** The presence of six or more large café au lait macules is associated with neurofibromatosis type 1. A port wine stain on the leg can be a marker for Klippel-Trénaunay-Weber syndrome. Sturge-Weber syndrome is suspected when the infant has a port wine stain over the trigeminal area of the face. An ash leaf–shaped birthmark raises the suspicion of tuberous sclerosis.

Reference: Witt C. Neonatal dermatology. In Verklan MT, Walden M, Forest S, eds. *Core Curriculum for Neonatal Intensive Care Nursing.* 6th ed. St. Louis, Elsevier; 2021:678-690.

11. **(B)** Hydroceles are common in newborn infants and usually present as a unilateral nontender mass that can be transilluminated. Peritoneal fluid can drain into the scrotum via the inguinal canal; however, ascites in an otherwise healthy newborn is uncommon. An inguinal hernia is uncommon at birth and is more likely to feel firm rather than fluctuant. Testicular torsion can present at birth with scrotal enlargement, typically firm and painful.

Reference: Walker V. Newborn evaluation. In: Gleason C, Juul S, eds. *Avery's Diseases of the Newborn.* 10th ed. Philadelphia, PA: Elsevier; 2018:289-331.

12. **(A)** Poor oral intake is common in late preterm infants and can lead to dehydration. Five days is a typical time frame for low milk intake to result in dehydration. Fever is a common presentation of dehydration. Herpes encephalitis usually presents between 14 and 21 days of life with neonatal seizures. Intracranial hemorrhage is unusual in infants >32 weeks of life and most commonly presents with changes in tone, activity, or fullness of the fontanel. The risk of sepsis is increased in late preterm infants and should be considered in the differential diagnosis. A negative swab for group B *Streptococcus* along with a short duration of rupture of membranes decreases the likelihood of sepsis in this neonate.

Reference: Taylor J, Wright J, Woodrum D. Newborn nursery care. In: Gleason C, Juul S, eds. *Avery's Diseases of the Newborn.* 10th ed. Philadelphia, PA: Elsevier; 2018:312-331.

13. **(D)** Ventricular septal defects are the most common congenital heart defects in newborns and usually present with a harsh holosystolic murmur that does not radiate. Coarctation of the aorta is usually asymptomatic until the ductus arteriosus closes. At that time the infant may display signs of decreased systemic circulation. In healthy term infants the ductus arteriosus normally closes in the first 24–48 hours of life. The murmur associated with a patent ductus arteriosus (PDA) is systolic and is best heard over the upper left sternal border and sometimes radiates to the axilla. Infants with tricuspid atresia always have some degree of cyanosis and may have a murmur if other shunts or lesions are present.

Reference: Swanson R, Erickson L. Cardiovascular diseases and surgical interventions. In: Gardner SL, Carter BS, Hines ME, Niermeyer S, eds. *Merenstein & Gardner's Handbook of Neonatal Intensive Care: An Interprofessional Approach.* St. Louis, MO: Elsevier; 2021:644-688.

14. **(A)** The influence of maternal estrogen can cause engorgement with so-called "witch's milk"; this secretion is short lived, and the enlargement will disappear after a few months. Mastitis would have enlargement and secretions but would also be accompanied by redness and hardness. Persistent breast enlargement beyond the newborn period may require further investigation; however, there is nothing in the history of this infant to suggest that blood work for hormone levels or chromosomal study is warranted.

Reference: Fraser D. Chest and lung assessment. In: Tappero EP, Honeyfield ME, eds. *Physical Assessment of the Newborn.* 6th ed. New York: Springer Publishing; 2019:79-92.

15. **(D)** Bilious emesis can be indicative of midgut volvulus. The presence of a volvulus compromises circulation to the gut, which can result in ischemia and necrosis of the intestine without surgical intervention. The duodenum is located superior to the bile duct; therefore, obstruction results in emesis of gastric secretions that are mucus or yellow in color rather than bilious. Hirschsprung disease or the absence of ganglion in the large bowel results in constipation and distention of the large bowel. It is not a surgical emergency. Meconium ileus may result in bile-stained emesis but is not a surgical emergency.

Reference: Goodwin M. Abdominal assessment. In: Tappero EP, Honeyfield ME, eds. *Physical Assessment of the Newborn.* 6th ed. New York: Springer Publishing; 2019:111-120.

16. **(C)** A PDA causes right to left shunting, resulting in additional blood flow to the aorta. This causes peripheral pulses to feel full and bounding. Coarctation of the aorta and interrupted aortic arch are associated with weak femoral pulses. A ventricular septal defect is more likely to be asymptomatic aside from an audible murmur.

Reference: Goodwin M. Abdominal assessment. In: Tappero EP, Honeyfield ME, eds. *Physical Assessment of the Newborn.* 6th ed. New York: Springer Publishing; 2019:111-120.

17. **(B)** Clinical findings in trisomy 13 include cutis aplasia, overlapping digits, low-set ears, cleft palate, microcephaly, microphthalmia, polydactyly, rocker-bottom feet, and numerous organ abnormalities, including cardiac defects, holoprosencephaly, and genitourinary abnormalities. Pierre Robin sequence is characterized by micrognathia resulting in upper airway compromise. Low-set ears are found in infants with Down syndrome; however, the other anomalies listed are not common to Down syndrome. Turner syndrome findings include a broad chest with widely spaced nipples, lymphedema of the hands and feet, a short-webbed neck, and low-set ears. Cutis aplasia, polydactyly, and rocker-bottom feet are not features of Turner syndrome.

Reference: Haldeman-Englert C, Saitta S, Zackai E. Chromosome disorders. In: Gleason C, Juul S, eds. *Avery's Diseases of the Newborn.* 10th ed. Philadelphia, PA: Elsevier; 2018:211-232.

18. **(C)** The tongue and mucus membranes best reflect blood oxygen levels. This is especially true in non-Caucasian infants where skin pigmentation can mask the presence of cyanosis. Periorbital and perioral cyanosis is common in the first 24 hours of life and does not correlate well with arterial blood oxygen levels. Acrocyanosis of the hands and feet is considered normal in the first 24–48 hours of life and does not correlate well with central oxygen levels. Mottling of the trunk is a common response to cold stress in newborns and does not reflect central oxygenation.

Reference: Walker V. Newborn evaluation. In: Gleason C, Juul S, eds. *Avery's Diseases of the Newborn.* 10th ed. Philadelphia, PA: Elsevier; 2018:289-331.

19. **(A)** Craniotabes are soft spots on the skull that collapse and recoil with pressure. They are usually found in the parietal and occipital region and are thought to result from bone reabsorption due to pressure of the skull against the maternal pelvis. Infants with 22q deletion or DiGeorge syndrome usually have microcephaly and a long face with a prominent nose and small mouth and chin. Fusion of the sutures causes a misshapen skull. With fusion the skull may appear more triangular in shape, widened, oblique, or narrow depending on which suture is fused. Depressed skull fractures are uncommon and are usually secondary to excessive force such as forceps or extreme molding. A single area of depression could represent a depressed skull fracture. Multiple areas of depression would not be a feature of a depressed skull fracture.

Reference: Tappero E. Physical assessment. In: Verklan MT, Walden M, Forest S, eds. *Core Curriculum for Neonatal Intensive Care Nursing.* 6th ed. St. Louis, MO: Elsevier; 2021:99-130.

20. **(A)** An enlarged bladder is the most common cause of a subumbilical abdominal mass. An umbilical hernia is usually periumbilical and would be visible on the surface of the abdomen. Rectus diastasis refers to a separation of the muscle due to weakness of the fascia. It appears as a visible bulge or ridge running down the abdomen, usually midline. A meconium plug may be palpable as an abdominal mass but would most likely be felt along the descending colon in the left lower quadrant.

Reference: Walker V. Newborn evaluation. In: Gleason C, Juul S, eds. *Avery's Diseases of the Newborn.* 10th ed. Philadelphia, PA: Elsevier; 2018:289-331.

21. **(D)** An asymmetric Moro reflex is suggestive of a brachial plexus injury, as is the classic waiter's tip hand and arm position. A fractured clavicle is suspected when the infant displays an asymmetric moro in the presence of a history of shoulder dystocia. Palpation may result in a finding of crepitus or a mass over the

clavicle. An x-ray is done to make the diagnosis of a clavicular fracture. Clubfoot, or talipes equinovarus, is diagnosed when the foot is turned in. This deformity may be fixed or positional. Gentle range of motion is used to determine the severity of the deformity. The Ortolani test is used in conjunction with the Barlow test to assess for developmental dysplasia of the hip.

Reference: Walker V. Newborn evaluation. In: Gleason C, Juul S, eds. *Avery's Diseases of the Newborn*. 10th ed. Philadelphia, PA: Elsevier; 2018:289-331.

22. **(D)** Cicatricial scarring is a classic finding in congenital varicella. Limb hypoplasia and microphthalmia are also described with this infection. Congenital cytomegalovirus infection is characterized by hepatosplenomegaly and a characteristic "blueberry muffin" rash. Signs of congenital rubella infections include microphthalmia but also other findings such as cataracts, glaucoma, chorioretinitis, and congenital heart disease. Toxoplasmosis infection in symptomatic newborns is characterized by chorioretinitis and intracerebral calcifications.

Reference: Pammi M, Brand C, Weisman LE. Infection in the neonate. In: Gardner SL, Carter BS, Hines ME, Niermeyer S, eds. *Merenstein & Gardner's Handbook of Neonatal Intensive Care: An Interprofessional Approach*. St. Louis, MO: Elsevier; 2021:692-728.

23. **(C)** A computed tomography scan may be warranted if CNS disease is suspected but would not be done routinely in the absence of neurologic symptoms. An electroencephalogram should be performed if seizures are suspected. Lumbar puncture is performed in all suspected cases of neonatal herpes simplex virus disease, whereas the other tests are reserved for central nervous system (CNS) involvement. A magnetic resonance imaging may be done if CNS disease is suspected but is not urgently done for infants with skin and eye disease.

Reference: Schleiss MR, Marsh KJ. Viral infections of the fetus and newborn. In: Gleason C, Juul S, eds. *Avery's Diseases of the Newborn*. 10th ed. Philadelphia, PA: Elsevier; 2018:472.

24. **(D)** Blood pressure is not routinely checked in healthy newborns. Fundoscopy is not currently part of the standard of care. Percussion is of limited utility. Red reflex examination should be done for all newborns.

Reference: Walker V. Newborn evaluation. In: Gleason C, Juul S, eds. *Avery's Diseases of the Newborn*. 10th ed. Philadelphia, PA: Elsevier; 2018:289-331.

25. **(A)** Umbilical hernia is found in 30% of term African American infants. Umbilical hernias are rare in Asian, Caucasian, and Native American infants.

Reference: Goodwin M. Abdominal assessment. In: Tappero EP, Honeyfield ME, eds. *Physical Assessment of the Newborn*. 6th ed. New York: Springer Publishing; 2019:111-120.

26. **(A)** Newborns can focus on objects at a distance of 10–12 in. but have decreased visual acuity at greater distances. An object 12–14 in. from the newborn's face will not be seen as clearly as one 10–12 in. away. Fourteen inches and beyond is too distant for an infant to clearly visualize.

Reference: Vittner D, McGrath JM. Behavioral assessment. In: Tappero EP, Honeyfield ME, eds. *Physical Assessment of the Newborn*. 6th ed. New York: Springer Publishing; 2019:193-218.

27. **(C)** Infants between 29 and 31 weeks have limited flexion and a popliteal angle of 140 degrees. Thirty-two- to thirty-three-week infants have a popliteal angle of 120 degrees and slight flexion of all four limbs. Popliteal angle of 100 degrees occurs in infants of 34–36 weeks of gestation, and four-limb flexion is typical of 36 weeks. Term infants have a popliteal angle of 90 degrees and full flexion of all four limbs.

Reference: Trotter C. Gestational age assessment. In: Tappero EP, Honeyfield ME, eds. *Physical Assessment of the Newborn*. 6th ed. New York: Springer Publishing; 2019:23-43.

28. **(C)** Fetal alcohol syndrome results in a number of mid-face defects but is not associated with cleft palate. Defects associated with Dilantin exposure include sacral agenesis, vertebral, cardiac, and renal anomalies. Infants with Pierre Robin sequence have significant mandibular hypoplasia which results in a posteriorly located tongue and cleft palate. Features of trisomy 13 include cleft palate but not micrognathia or tongue displacement.

Reference: Bennett M, Meier SR. Assessment of the dysmorphic infant. In: Tappero EP, Honeyfield ME, eds. *Physical Assessment of the Newborn*. 6th ed. New York: Springer Publishing; 2019:219-239.

29. **(B)** Shoulder dystocia places the infant at increased risk of Erb palsy, an injury to the brachial plexus. With Erb palsy the Moro reflex is asymmetric, and the arm and wrist are positioned in what is referred to as *waiter's tip*. Bell palsy results from damage to the facial nerve caused by pressing against the maternal pelvis. Phrenic nerve paralysis may be unilateral or bilateral. Unilateral damage, usually on the right side, is more common. Symptoms include respiratory distress due to diaphragm impact. Fracture of the humerus would result in an asymmetric Moro but would not cause the wrist to be flexed and the arm pronated.

Reference: Tappero EP. Musculoskeletal assessment. In: Tappero EP, Honeyfield ME, eds. *Physical Assessment of the Newborn*. 6th ed. New York: Springer Publishing; 2019:139-166.

30. **(B)** The lesion being described is an infantile or strawberry hemangioma. This lesion, more common in premature infants, usually grows for 6–12 months and then spontaneously involutes. Port wine stains grow in proportion to the growth of the child. Both port wine stains and strawberry hemangiomas continue to enlarge during infancy. Some clinicians elect to treat strawberry hemangiomas with oral or topical propranolol; however, treatment is not necessarily needed for the lesion to regress.

Reference: Tappero EP, Honeyfield ME, eds. *Physical Assessment of the Newborn*. 6th ed. New York: Springer Publishing; 2019:279.

31. **(C)** Subtle seizures are the most common type of seizures in premature infants and manifest as lip smacking, eye deviations, stiffening, arching, and changes in vital signs. Benign familiar seizures present in a similar fashion to subtle seizures but without the risk factors of low Apgar scores. Neonatal myoclonus manifests as episodes of repetitive jerking or jitteriness that does not stop with passive restraint. The movements seen in tonic–clonic seizures include stiffening and repetitive jerking.

Reference: Hall AS, Reavey DA. Neurologic disorders. In: Gardner SL, Carter BS, Hines ME, Niermeyer S, eds. *Merenstein & Gardner's Handbook of Neonatal Intensive Care: An Interprofessional Approach*. St. Louis, MO: Elsevier; 2021:929-968.

32. **(A)** Laryngomalacia is the most common cause of stridor in infants and typically presents in the first month of life. Risk factors include prematurity and respiratory support. Vocal cord paralysis does not typically present with stridor. Laryngeal atresia is present from birth. Subglottic stenosis may be present at birth or may develop as a result of intubation and prolonged mechanical ventilation.

Reference: Keller R, Hirose S, Farmer DL. Surgical disorders of the chest and airways. In: Gleason C, Juul S, eds. *Avery's Diseases of the Newborn*. 10th ed. Philadelphia, PA: Elsevier; 2018:695-723.

33. **(A)** Purulent or bloody nasal discharge and a copper-colored maculopapular rash that goes on to blister and peel are classic findings of congenital syphilis. Most infants with cytomegalovirus are asymptomatic at birth. Those who do present with symptoms have a blueberry muffin rash and hepatosplenomegaly. Congenitally acquired herpes presents with skin lesions or scars, microphthalmia and microcephaly, or hydranencephaly. Skin rash and nasal discharge are not findings in hepatitis B infection.

Reference: Lane ER, Chisholm KM, Murray KF. Disorders of the liver. In: Gleason C, Juul S, eds. *Avery's Diseases of the Newborn*. 10th ed. Philadelphia, PA: Elsevier; 2018:1098-1112.

34. **(B)** A positive direct antiglobulin test (DAT) is an indication of the presence of maternal antibodies causing hemolysis. A low hemoglobin and elevated bilirubin would be expected. Biliary atresia presents with an elevated direct bilirubin and a normal hemoglobin. A positive DAT would not be expected. Hemolytic anemia is a finding in hereditary spherocytosis but the DAT would be negative. Some types of thalassemia present at birth with hemolysis, anemia, and jaundice. The DAT would be negative.

Reference: Christensen RD. Neonatal erythrocyte disorders. In: Gleason C, Juul S, eds. *Avery's Diseases of the Newborn*. 10th ed. Philadelphia, PA: Elsevier; 2018:1152-1179.

35. **(D)** Pustular melanosis is more common in infants with pigmented skin. This benign rash consists of a mixture of vesicles and pustules and pigmented macules. The vesicles and pustules resolve quickly; however, the macules may remain for several months. Milia are small white cysts appearing most often over the nose and chin of the newborn. Erythema toxicum is a pustular rash on an erythematous base. It tends to fade in one location and reappear in another. Cutaneous candida forms a beefy red rash with satellite lesions. It is found in the groin, diaper area, and occasionally in other skin folds such as the axilla.

Reference: Khorsand K, Sidbury R. Common newborn dermatoses. In: Gleason C, Juul S, eds. *Avery's Diseases of the Newborn*. 10th ed. Philadelphia, PA: Elsevier; 2018:1503-1510.

36. **(B)** Only 10–15% of infants with gastroschisis have associated anomalies, and those are usually other gastrointestinal malformations. Among infants with omphalocele, 50% have accompanying cardiac defects. The incidence of pyloric stenosis is 3 in 1000 live births, but associated anomalies are rare.

Hirschsprung disease may be associated with colonic atresia or imperforate anus, but congenital heart disease is not reported with Hirschsprung disease.

Reference: Bradshaw WT. Gastrointestinal disorders. In: Verklan MT, Walden M, Forest S, eds. *Core Curriculum for Neonatal Intensive Care Nursing*. 6th ed. St. Louis, MO: Elsevier; 2021.

37. **(D)** Port wine stains over the trigeminal area may indicate the presence of Sturge-Weber syndrome. Features of Sturge-Weber include endothelial proliferation and calcifications of small veins in the brain or eye. Unlike cavernous hemangiomas, port wine stains do not cause problems with platelet consumption or clotting. Hearing loss is not associated with facial port wine stains. The presence of a port wine stain does not increase the risk of low platelets.

Reference: Witt C. Neonatal dermatology. In: Verklan MT, Walden M, Forest S, eds. *Core Curriculum for Neonatal Intensive Care Nursing*. 6th ed. St. Louis, MO: Elsevier; 2021:678-690.

38. **(A)** Tetralogy of Fallot is the most common cyanotic heart defect. A grade II–IV murmur is heard over the left upper sternal border. Atrial septal defects are characterized by splitting of the second heart sound and do not usually result in cyanosis. Transposition of the great arteries (vessels) causes cyanosis but is not associated with murmur. A ventricular septal defect typically presents with a murmur heard at the left lower sternal border but is an acyanotic lesion.

Reference: Goff D. Cardiovascular system. In: Kenner C, Altimier LB, Boykova MV, eds. *Comprehensive Neonatal Nursing Care*. 6th ed. New York: Springer Publishing; 2020:147-178.

39. **(D)** Scalded skin syndrome is an infection caused by *Staphylococcus aureus*. Occurring most often in the diaper area or around the umbilicus, it consists of vesicles that may coalesce to form bullae. When the vesicles rupture, they leave areas of denuded skin resembling a burn. *Candida* skin infection usually occurs in the diaper area and is characterized by white or yellow pustules on an erythematous base. *Klebsiella*, a waterborne pathogen, usually causes pneumonia and is not implicated in newborn skin infections. The rash seen in skin infections caused by the herpes simplex virus is often vesicular and may occur first over the area of the body presenting at birth.

Reference: Witt C. Neonatal dermatology. In: Verklan MT, Walden M, Forest S, eds. *Core Curriculum for Neonatal Intensive Care Nursing*. 6th ed. St. Louis, MO: Elsevier; 2021:678-690.

40. **(C)** If platelets were normal, a test of clotting factors may be appropriate. When significant blood loss accompanies thrombocytopenia, anemia may result but is not a contributing factor. A diffuse petechial rash is suggestive of thrombocytopenia. A low platelet count would be an expected finding. Abnormalities in clotting factors could result in a petechial rash; however, this is much less common than thrombocytopenia. Low white blood cell counts are found in newborns with infection, but infection is not a common cause of petechiae.

Reference: Tappero E. Physical assessment. In Verklan MT, Walden M, Forest S. eds. *Core Curriculum for Neonatal Intensive Care Nursing*, 6th ed. St. Louis, Elsevier; 2021:99-130.

41. **(C)** Blue sclera is a marker for osteogenesis imperfecta, or brittle bone disease. A deficiency of collagen results in a thin sclera and increased visibility of the underlying blood vessels. Features of DiGeorge syndrome, or 22q deletion, include microcephaly and a long face with a prominent nose and small mouth and chin but not blue sclera. There are several types of muscular dystrophies. Muscle weakness is the predominant feature. Rare in the neonatal period, systemic lupus erythematosus (SLE) may occur as a result of exposure to maternal SLE antibodies. Clinical signs in the newborn include skin rash and heart block.

Reference: Bennett M, Meier SR. Assessment of the dysmorphic infant. In: Tappero EP, Honeyfield ME, eds. *Physical Assessment of the Newborn*. 6th ed. New York: Springer Publishing; 2019:219-239.

42. **(D)** During pregnancy, antilupus antibodies cross the placenta, resulting in neonatal lupus erythematosus (NLE), which is characterized by congenital heart block, a cutaneous lupus rash, and pancytopenia. These antibodies persist in the neonatal circulation for several weeks after delivery, followed by resolution of the NLE. Maternal diabetes predisposes the fetus and newborn to cardiomyopathy. Sustained bradycardia is not a feature of cardiomyopathy. Preeclampsia is sometimes treated with magnesium sulfate, which can cause respiratory depression in the newborn. Bradycardia is not associated with preeclampsia. Chorioamnionitis usually presents with an increased heart rate and decreased heart rate variability.

Reference: Vargo L. Cardiovascular assessment. In: Tappero EP, Honeyfield ME, eds. *Physical Assessment of the Newborn*. 6th ed. New York: Springer Publishing; 2019:93-110.

43. **(D)** The presence of an esophageal atresia in an infant with TE fistula prevents the fetus from swallowing amniotic fluid. Polyhydramnios occurs as a result. Pyloric stenosis presents with projectile vomiting after feeding. An olive-sized mass may be palpated in the epigastric region. Symptoms usually begin after 3 weeks of age. Prune belly syndrome includes weakness of the abdominal musculature and urinary tract abnormalities, which may cause oligohydramnios rather than polyhydramnios. The presence of posterior urethral valves results in obstruction of the flow of urine from the bladder. In cases of severe obstruction, the volume of amniotic fluid is reduced, not increased.

Reference: Bradshaw WT. Gastrointestinal disorders. In: Verklan MT, Walden M, Forest S, eds. *Core Curriculum for Neonatal Intensive Care Nursing*. 6th ed. St. Louis, MO: Elsevier; 2021:504-540.

44. **(C)** The onset of alcohol withdrawal is usually seen between birth and 12 hours of age and includes hypertonia, tremors, and a poor feeding pattern. Excessive crying and exaggerated sucking are reported. Restlessness, irritability, and tremors have been described in cocaine-exposed newborns. These effects are thought to be direct effects of the drug rather than signs of withdrawal. After an

initial period of hyper-alertness, infants often become drowsy or lethargic. Narcotic opioid exposure in pregnancy results in symptoms of withdrawal, usually beginning about 48 hours after delivery. Symptoms include increased activity, irritability, tremors, tachypnea, diarrhea, poor feeding, and vomiting. Reported effects of selective serotonin reuptake inhibitors on newborns include seizures, respiratory distress, hypoglycemia, and poor feeding.

Reference: D'Apolito K. Perinatal substance abuse. In: Verklan MT, Walden M, Forest S, eds. *Core Curriculum for Neonatal Intensive Care Nursing.* 6th ed. St. Louis, MO: Elsevier; 2021:38-53.

45. **(B)** Signs of congenital hypothyroidism are not always obvious at birth. The disorder is often diagnosed during routine newborn screening. When present, signs include a large fontanel, umbilical hernia, coarse facial features, thick skin, and delayed bone age. Poor perfusion, hypothermia, and poor feeding may also be present. Several forms of congenital adrenal hyperplasia (CAH) exist, with the most common being a deficiency of 21-OHD (Hydroxylase deficiency). Signs of CAH in females include abnormal genitalia. Males may remain undiagnosed until 7–24 days of life when symptoms such as hypoglycemia, hyponatremia, hypotension, and shock develop. Infants with Down syndrome have a variety of abnormal features, including low-set ears, redundant nuchal skin, simian creases, and Brushfield spots. Umbilical hernia and coarse facial features are not associated with Down syndrome. Prader-Willi syndrome is a rare genetic disease with features including hypogonadism, lethargy, hypotonia, and feeding difficulty.

Reference: Blackburn S. Endocrine disorders. In: Verklan MT, Walden M, Forest S, eds. *Core Curriculum for Neonatal Intensive Care Nursing.* 6th ed. St. Louis, MO: Elsevier; 2021:543-567.

46. **(A)** The pulmonic valve is best heard at the second intercostal space, left sternal angle. The aortic valve is best heard at the second intercostal space, right sternal angle. The landmarks for the tricuspid valve are the fourth intercostal space and the left sternal angle. The mitral area is found at the fifth intercostal space, midclavicular line.

Reference: Vargo L. Cardiovascular assessment. In: Tappero EP, Honeyfield ME, eds. *Physical Assessment of the Newborn.* 6th ed. New York: Springer Publishing; 2019:93-110.

47. **(B)** A cephalohematoma is a collection of blood under the periosteum. Most commonly found over the parietal or occipital bones, a cephalohematoma is bounded by suture lines. It is usually present at birth but increases in size over the first few hours after delivery. Skull fractures are rare in newborns. When present, they may be linear or depressed. Linear fractures are often asymptomatic, whereas with depressed fractures, an indentation over the affected bone may be palpated. A subdural hematoma is a collection of blood in the subdural space within the cranium. Presentation is one of altered tone, altered alertness, or seizures. A subgaleal hemorrhage results from a tear in a blood vessel in the subgaleal space. It is more common after vacuum or forceps delivery and presents with a fluctuant mass over the back of the head, with bruising extending to the ears and sometimes to the eyes. It is a medical emergency.

Reference: Johnson PJ. Head, eyes, ears, nose, mouth and neck assessment. In: Tappero EP, Honeyfield ME, eds. *Physical Assessment of the Newborn.* 6th ed. New York: Springer Publishing; 2019:61-78.

48. **(A)** Premature infants are at increased risk of developing cutaneous candida. A candida rash is most often found in the groin and consists of lesions over an erythematous base with satellite lesions extending beyond the groin. Diaper dermatitis is beefy red and most often seen in the perianal area. Satellite lesions are not common to diaper dermatitis. Skin disease caused by herpes usually starts over the part of the body presenting at birth. It is vesicular in nature but does not form an erythematous base or satellite lesions. Staphylococcal infections are more common around the umbilicus or in the diaper area. The rash consists of

vesicles that coalesce to form bullae. The infant with a staphylococcal infection is usually febrile and unwell.

Reference: Witt C. Neonatal dermatology. In: Verklan MT, Walden M, Forest S, eds. *Core Curriculum for Neonatal Intensive Care Nursing.* 6th ed. St. Louis, MO: Elsevier; 2021:678-690.

49. **(B)** Chlamydia infection may cause mild conjunctivitis but is also known to cause significant edema and purulent discharge. The onset of symptoms is usually between 5 and 7 days. A blocked lacrimal duct may cause mild edema and yellow discharge but does not cause reddened conjunctiva. Unilateral blockage is more common than bilateral. Symptoms of a corneal abrasion include conjunctivitis and clear discharge. An abrasion would be unilateral rather than bilateral. Herpes infection of the eye typically presents with keratoconjunctivitis, inflammation of the cornea, and conjunctiva. Some edema may be present; purulent discharge is not an initial finding.

Reference: Fraser D, Diehl-Jones W. Ophthalmologic and auditory disorders. In: Verklan MT, Walden M, Forest S, eds. *Core Curriculum for Neonatal Intensive Care Nursing.* 6th ed. St. Louis, MO: Elsevier; 2021:813-831.

50. **(B)** Hypernatremia usually results from dehydration. An infant of a diabetic mother (IDM) is not at risk of hypernatremia. Maternal diabetes in pregnancy results in a delay in the newborn's production of parathyroid hormone (PTH). As a result of this suppression in PTH production, hypocalcemia can occur. Hyponatremia is usually dilutional, resulting from fluid retention. Renal losses of sodium in premature infants can also cause hyponatremia. IDMs are not at increased risk of hyponatremia. Maternal diabetes can result in polycythemia in the infant, but thrombocytopenia is not associated with maternal diabetes.

Reference: Bell SG. Fluid and electrolyte management. In: Verklan MT, Walden M, Forest S, eds. *Core Curriculum for Neonatal Intensive Care Nursing.* 6th ed. St. Louis, MO: Elsevier; 2021:131-143.

51. **(A)** Because neonates are obligate nose breathers, bilateral obstruction of the nose results in cyanosis at rest. During crying the neonate breathes through the mouth, bringing oxygen into the lungs. Cyanosis secondary to congenital heart disease is more likely to be persistent or to worsen with crying when oxygen demands are higher. Features of TE fistula include excessive oral secretions and increased work of breathing secondary to aspiration of secretions. Cyanosis at rest is not a feature of TE fistula. Persistent pulmonary hypertension of the newborn (PPHN) causes persistent hypoxia and increased work of breathing. Improved oxygenation with crying is not a finding in PPHN.

Reference: Johnson PJ. Head, eyes, ears, nose, mouth and neck assessment. In: Tappero EP, Honeyfield ME, eds. *Physical Assessment of the Newborn.* 6th ed. New York: Springer Publishing; 2019:61-78.

52. **(D)** Hymenal tags are commonly seen in newborn females and usually disappear spontaneously within a few weeks of delivery. Congenital adrenal hyperplasia can cause the genitalia in female infants to appear masculine. This most often affects the clitoris and labia. If the remainder of the genitourinary examination is normal, ambiguous genitalia can be ruled out and chromosome analysis is not necessary. Surgical removal of a hymenal tag is not necessary and would not be the first line of management should the tag persist.

Reference: Cavaliere TA. Genitourinary assessment. In: Tappero EP, Honeyfield ME, eds. *Physical Assessment of the Newborn.* 6th ed. New York: Springer Publishing; 2019:121-137.

53. **(A)** These nodules are the result of subcutaneous fat necrosis, a complication of cooling. In the presence of multiple nodules, the risk of hypercalcemia is increased. Magnesium, potassium, and sodium values are not affected by the presence of subcutaneous fat necroses.

Reference: Witt C. Neonatal dermatology. In: Verklan MT, Walden M, Forest S, eds. *Core Curriculum for Neonatal Intensive Care Nursing.* 6th ed. St. Louis, MO: Elsevier; 2021:678-690.

Chapter 5

Gestational Age Assessment

1. Low birth weight is classified as birth weight less than:
   A. 500 g.
   B. 700 g.
   C. 1000 g.
   D. 2500 g.

2. Length measurement entails measuring the infant:
   A. head to toe.
   B. crown to heel.
   C. crown to rump.
   D. shoulder to shoulder.

3. Large for gestational age is birth weight:
   A. at the 50th percentile.
   B. less than the 10th percentile.
   C. greater than the 90th percentile.
   D. between the 10th and 90th percentiles.

4. Small for gestational age is birth weight:
   A. at the 50th percentile.
   B. less than the 10th percentile.
   C. greater than the 90th percentile.
   D. between the 10th and 90th percentiles.

5. Appropriate for gestational age is birth weight:
   A. at the 50th percentile.
   B. less than the 10th percentile.
   C. greater than the 90th percentile.
   D. between the 10th and 90th percentiles.

6. An infant is born at 36 weeks' gestation. This infant is considered to be:
   A. term.
   B. postterm.
   C. late preterm.
   D. extremely preterm.

7. When assessing a premature infant born at 27 weeks' gestation, the nurse expects to find:
   A. no lanugo.
   B. sparse lanugo.
   C. lanugo with balding areas.
   D. lanugo covering the entire body.

8. When assessing an infant with intrauterine growth restriction, the nurse can anticipate finding that the infant's:
   A. skin is covered in vernix.
   B. head is disproportionately large for the infant's trunk.
   C. umbilical cord is thickened with abundant Wharton jelly.
   D. anterior fontanelles are small with overlapping cranial sutures.

9. A physical assessment performed on a newborn infant notes that the skin of the infant is cracking and pale in some areas, the areolae are raised with 10-mm buds, and the pinna is formed, firm, does not have thick cartilage, and springs back promptly from being folded. Based on these physical assessment findings, this infant is:
   A. term.
   B. preterm.
   C. late preterm.
   D. postterm.

10. After the initial assessment of the newborn infant, the infant's weight, length, and head circumference are plotted out on a growth chart. The growth chart shows that the infant's weight is at the 15th percentile, length is at the 20th percentile, and head circumference is at the 30th percentile. These results indicate that the infant:
    A. is small for gestational age.
    B. is large for gestational age.
    C. is appropriate for gestational age.
    D. has intrauterine growth restriction.

11. A 4000-g male infant has just been delivered via cesarean section due to fetal distress. The infant is born through thick meconium. At the initial assessment, the infant's skin is noted to be leathery, cracked, and wrinkled. The infant's scrotum is noted to be pendulous with the testes completely descended with rugae. The nurse assessing this infant can anticipate that this infant is:
    A. preterm.
    B. late preterm.
    C. term.
    D. postterm.

12. A gestational age examination has just been performed on a newborn infant. The infant was noted to be in flexed position. The assessment shows that the square window angle is 0 degrees and the popliteal angle is 90 degrees, and the scarf sign evaluation shows increased resistance to crossing the midline. The infant's skin is noted to be cracking with no veins visible. Creases over the entire sole of the plantar surface are noted. Based on these findings, which of the following gestational ages would this infant be likely to be?
    A. 24 weeks' gestation
    B. 32 weeks' gestation
    C. 36 weeks' gestation
    D. 40 weeks' gestation

13. The correct way to assess the scarf sign in an infant is to:
    A. position the infant supine, flex the arms for 5 seconds, then fully extend the infant's arms by pulling the hands downward, and then release.
    B. position the infant supine, take the infant's hand and pull it across the infant's chest and around the neck as far posterior as possible toward the opposite shoulder, and observe the elbow position in relation to the midline of the infant's body.
    C. flex the infant's hand on the forearm between the examiner's thumb and index finger, use enough pressure to get full flexion, and visually measure the angle between the hypothenar eminence and the ventral aspect of the forearm.
    D. position the infant supine with the pelvis flat on a surface, hold the infant's thigh in knee-chest position with the left index finger and thumb, place the right index finger behind the infant's ankle and extend the leg gently, and measure the angle between the lower leg and thigh.

14. The correct way to assess the arm recoil of an infant is to:
    A. position the infant supine, flex the arms for 5 seconds, then fully extend the infant's arms by pulling the hands downward, and then release.
    B. position the infant supine, take the infant's hand and pull it across the infant's chest and around the neck as far posterior as possible toward the opposite shoulder, and observe the elbow position to the midline of the infant's body.
    C. flex the infant's hand on the forearm between the examiner's thumb and index finger, use enough pressure to get full flexion, and visually measure the angle between the hypothenar eminence and the ventral aspect of the forearm.
    D. position the infant supine with the pelvis flat on a surface, hold the infant's thigh in knee-chest position with the left index finger and thumb, place the right index finger behind the infant's ankle and extend the leg gently, and measure the angle between the lower leg and thigh.

15. After plotting a newborn's weight, length, and head circumference by gestational age on a standardized growth chart, the nurse shows the mother the growth chart. The mother asks what the percentiles on the chart mean. Which of the following is the best teaching point to explain at this moment?
    A. Babies who plot between the 10th and the 90th percentiles have grown in utero as expected.
    B. Babies who plot between the 10th and the 90th percentiles often have more problems than other babies.
    C. Babies who plot above the 90th percentile are bigger and therefore always are healthier than other babies.
    D. Babies who plot below the 10th percentile have grown larger than expected and can have problems with blood glucose level.

16. The mother of an infant born at 28 weeks' gestation tells the nurse that she is very worried because her baby's ears do not look normal. Which of the following is the best explanation to give her?
    A. As a baby matures, the pinnae of the ears will mature, and the cartilage will eventually firm up.
    B. A preterm baby's ears are not formed yet, and this is what leads to deafness in preterm infants.
    C. Preterm babies do not have any cartilage in the pinnae of their ears, causing their ears to have no shape.
    D. Growth and development stop at birth, so preterm infants have flatter ears than term babies, but their hearing is intact.

17. The nurse is performing a gestational age assessment on a premature infant. Observations will likely include which of the following?
    A. Vernix in the axilla only
    B. Very few visible veins on the abdomen
    C. Palpable breast buds with raised and stippled areolae
    D. Smooth plantar surfaces and large amounts of lanugo over the shoulders and back

18. Which of the following statements is true of growth curves?
    A. Growth curves should be gestational age and gender specific.
    B. All growth curves are the same and can be used for all infants.
    C. Growth curve measurements include birth weight, length, and abdominal girth.
    D. Growth curves are only applicable to infants born between 24 weeks' and 40 weeks' gestation.

19. Which of the following is a true statement about the neurologic portion of the gestational age examination?
    A. Posture and flexion decrease with advancing gestational age and muscle mass.
    B. The square window angle increases with advancing gestational age due to increasing muscle tone.
    C. The values of neurologic indicators are not accurate in preterm infants of less than 30 weeks' gestation.
    D. Gestational examination scoring can be altered by neurologic disorders and asphyxia injury and therefore may not be reliable.

20. A 40-week, 2000-g infant is admitted to the neonatal intensive care unit. The nurse should assess for:
    A. birth trauma.
    B. polycythemia.
    C. hyperglycemia.
    D. respiratory distress syndrome.

21. Which of the following problems is a full-term, large-for-gestational-age infant at highest risk for developing?
    A. Hypothermia
    B. Hyponatremia
    C. Hypokalemia
    D. Hypoglycemia

22. An extremely low-birth-weight infant born at less than 25 weeks' gestation can be scored using the New Ballard Score gestational age examination. Which of the following findings is expected in an infant born at less than 25 weeks' gestation?
    A. Eyes are open.
    B. Lanugo is sparse.
    C. Skin is dry and paperlike.
    D. Plantar creases are absent.

23. A gestational age examination of a 44 weeks' gestation infant is done using the New Ballard Score. Which statement best describes the examination findings the nurse anticipates finding?
    A. Skin has superficial peeling, the ears are stiff, and the labia majora do not cover the clitoris.
    B. Skin has few visible veins, the ears are well curved with ready recoil, and lanugo is thinning.

C. Plantar creases extend to two-thirds of the feet, the ears are firm with instant recoil, and breast areolae are stippled.

D. Skin is leathery, cracked, and wrinkled, plantar creases cover the entire sole of the foot, and lanugo is mostly absent.

24. What maternal factor is a risk factor for an infant being born large for gestational age?
    A. Preeclampsia
    B. Systemic lupus erythematosus
    C. Cocaine use throughout pregnancy
    D. Diabetes with poor glucose control

25. General considerations for accurate use of a gestational age assessment tool, such as the Dubowitz score or New Ballard Score, include which of the following?
    A. Perform the examination at 7 days of life for best accuracy.
    B. Perform the examination within 24–48 hours of life for best accuracy.
    C. Gestational age assessment is most accurate when performed on infants in a deep sleep state.
    D. The combined score of the physical and neurologic components has a lower correlation than either component used separately.

26. A 4.5-kg infant born at 38 weeks' gestation is most at risk for which of the following?
    A. Hypothermia
    B. Polycythemia
    C. Hyperglycemia
    D. Fractured clavicle

27. Which of the following statements demonstrates the nurse's understanding of gestational age?
    A. "An infant born at 40 weeks' gestation is classified as a postterm infant and must be monitored closely for signs of respiratory distress."
    B. "It's important to monitor the 35-week gestational age infant, especially because this infant is preterm and may be at risk for higher morbidity and mortality."
    C. "This 43-week gestational age infant is a term neonate and is at decreased risk for experiencing any morbidities or mortality."
    D. "This 38-week gestational age infant is preterm and is at increased risk for experiencing higher morbidity than those born at term."

28. The mother of a newborn born at 24 weeks' gestation is worried about her infant's eyes being fused. Which statement indicates the nurse's understanding of fused eyes?
    A. "Fused eyelids in a newborn means the newborn will be blind."
    B. "Fused eyelids at this point in time is normal, and they will open between 26 and 28 weeks' gestation."
    C. "Fused eyelids at this point in time indicates congenital anomalies and requires an extensive workup to be done."
    D. "Fused eyelids at this point in time is normal. Eyelids usually open at 36 weeks' gestation."

ANSWERS AND RATIONALES

1. **(D)** Low birth weight is classified as birth weight less than 2500 g. Very low birth weight is classified as birth weight less than 1500 g. Extremely low birth weight is classified as birth weight less than 1000 g.

Reference: Tappero E. Physical assessment. In: Verklan MT, Walden M, Forest S, eds. *Core Curriculum for Neonatal Intensive Care Nursing.* 6th ed. St. Louis, MO: Elsevier; 2021:104.

2. **(B)** Measuring the infant crown to heel is the correct way to determine length. Measuring head to toe does not ensure an accurate length because the toes can flex or extend, which causes the length measurement to potentially vary. Measuring crown-to-rump is used to establish proportionality when length falls below norms. Measuring the infant shoulder to shoulder determines the infant's width, not the infant's length.

Reference: Tappero E. Physical assessment. In: Verklan MT, Walden M, Forest S, eds. *Core Curriculum for Neonatal Intensive Care Nursing.* 6th ed. St. Louis, MO: Elsevier; 2021:105.

3. **(C)** An infant whose weight is greater than the 90th percentile is a large-for-gestational-age (LGA) infant. An infant whose weight is between the 10th and 90th percentiles is an appropriate-for-gestational-age (AGA) infant. An infant whose weight is less than the 10th percentile is a small-for-gestational-age (SGA) infant.

Reference: Tappero E. Physical assessment. In: Verklan MT, Walden M, Forest S, eds. *Core Curriculum for Neonatal Intensive Care Nursing.* 6th ed. St. Louis, MO: Elsevier; 2021:108.

4. **(B)** An infant whose weight is less than the 10th percentile is a SGA infant. An infant whose weight is between the 10th and 90th percentiles is an AGA infant. An infant whose weight is greater than the 90th percentile is a LGA infant.

Reference: Tappero E. Physical assessment. In: Verklan MT, Walden M, Forest S, eds. *Core Curriculum for Neonatal Intensive Care Nursing.* 6th ed. St. Louis, MO: Elsevier; 2021:108.

5. **(D)** An infant whose weight is between the 10th and 90th percentiles is an AGA infant. Although an infant whose weight is at the 50th percentile is an AGA infant, a wider range of weight is considered AGA. An infant whose weight is less than the 10th percentile is a SGA infant. An infant whose weight is greater than the 90th percentile is a LGA infant.

Reference: Tappero E. Physical assessment. In: Verklan MT, Walden M, Forest S, eds. *Core Curriculum for Neonatal Intensive Care Nursing.* 6th ed. St. Louis, MO: Elsevier; 2021:108.

6. **(C)** Late-preterm infants are those whose gestational age falls between 34 and 36 6/7 weeks. Term infants are infants whose gestational age falls between 37 and 42 weeks. Postterm infants are those whose gestational age greater than 42 weeks. "Extremely preterm" is not a recognized gestational category.

Reference: Tappero E. Physical assessment. In: Verklan MT, Walden M, Forest S, eds. *Core Curriculum for Neonatal Intensive Care Nursing.* 6th ed. St. Louis, MO: Elsevier; 2021:104.

7. **(D)** Lanugo covers the entire body from 20 to 28 weeks' gestation and does not start disappearing until 28 weeks' gestation.

Reference: Tappero E. Physical assessment. In: Verklan MT, Walden M, Forest S, eds. *Core Curriculum for Neonatal Intensive Care Nursing.* 6th ed. St. Louis, MO: Elsevier; 2021:104.

8. **(B)** A head disproportionately large for the trunk is the typical appearance of an infant with intrauterine growth restriction (IUGR). An infant with IUGR is born with little or no vernix on

the skin. The umbilical cord of an infant with IUGR is thin with decreased Wharton jelly. The anterior fontanelles of an infant with IUGR are typically large with cranial sutures wide or overlapping.

Reference: Tappero E. Physical assessment. In: Verklan MT, Walden M, Forest S, eds. *Core Curriculum for Neonatal Intensive Care Nursing*. 6th ed. St. Louis, MO: Elsevier; 2021:109-110.

9. **(A)** As gestation progresses beyond 38 weeks, the subcutaneous tissue decreases. The term infant's skin is cracking and pale in areas with no visible veins, but not leathery or wrinkled. At term gestation, the breast tissue nodule measures up to 10 mm. The pinna is formed, firm, and springs back promptly from being folded. In the preterm infant, the skin is usually transparent, breast tissue is imperceptible or barely imperceptible, and the pinna has little cartilage, which causes the pinna to stay folded on itself. In the late-preterm infant, the subcutaneous tissue has not decreased to the point of causing the skin to wrinkle, the breast tissue nodule measures only 1–2 mm, and the pinna may or may not stay folded on itself, depending on the gestational age. In the postterm infant, the skin is leathery or wrinkled and the cartilage in the pinna is thick.

Reference: Tappero E. Physical assessment. In: Verklan MT, Walden M, Forest S, eds. *Core Curriculum for Neonatal Intensive Care Nursing*. 6th ed. St. Louis, MO: Elsevier; 2021:102.

10. **(C)** An infant whose weight is between the 10th and 90th percentiles is an AGA infant. An infant whose weight is less than the 10th percentile is a SGA infant. An infant whose weight is greater than the 90th percentile is a LGA infant. The growth chart does not determine if an infant has IUGR. IUGR infants may or may not be SGA.

Reference: Tappero E. Physical assessment. In: Verklan MT, Walden M, Forest S, eds. *Core Curriculum for Neonatal Intensive Care Nursing*. 6th ed. St. Louis, MO: Elsevier; 2021:108.

11. **(D)** Increased cesarean section rates and meconium aspiration are associated with term and postterm infants. The postterm infant's skin is leathery, cracked, and wrinkled. In the postterm infant male, the scrotum becomes more pendulous and is completely covered with rugae. The testes have completely descended. The preterm infant's skin is gelatinous, red, and translucent with visible veins. In the premature infant male, the scrotum is not completely covered with rugae and the testes have not yet descended into the scrotum. The late-preterm infant's skin is smooth and pink with few visible veins and has superficial peeling. In the late-preterm infant male, the scrotum is not completely covered with rugae and the testes have descended high into the scrotum. The term infant's skin is cracking and pale in areas with no visible veins, but not leathery or wrinkled. In the term infant male, the scrotum is completely covered with rugae and the testes are completely descended, but not pendulous.

Reference: Tappero E. Physical assessment. In: Verklan MT, Walden M, Forest S, eds. *Core Curriculum for Neonatal Intensive Care Nursing*. 6th ed. St. Louis, MO: Elsevier; 2021:104.

12. **(D)** For the term infant, the square window angle would be 0 degree, the popliteal angle would be 90 degrees, and in scarf sign testing, the elbow could not be pulled over the infant's body. The term infant's skin is cracking and pale in areas with no visible veins, but not leathery or wrinkled as it is in the postterm infant. At 24 weeks' gestation, the infant's posture would be hypotonic, the square window would be greater than 90 degrees and popliteal angle at least 160 degrees. There would be little resistance to pulling the arm across the chest. The skin would be gelatinous red and translucent, and there would be no creases on the plantar surface. At 32 weeks, the infant's posture would have minimal flexion, the square window would be between 45 and 60 degrees,

and popliteal angle would be between 120 and 140 degrees. There would be some resistance to pulling the arm across the chest. The skin would have some cracking and visible veins. The plantar surface would have creases covering up to two-thirds of the surface. For the late-preterm infant, the square window angle would be about 45 degrees, the popliteal angle would be 110–140 degrees, and in scarf sign testing, the elbow could be pulled to the midline of the infant's body. The infant's posture would be slightly flexed, skin would be cracking with rare visible veins, and anterior transverse creases would be noted on the plantar surface.

Reference: Tappero E. Physical assessment. In: Verklan MT, Walden M, Forest S, eds. *Core Curriculum for Neonatal Intensive Care Nursing*. 6th ed. St. Louis, MO: Elsevier; 2021:102-103.

13. **(B)** Positioning the infant supine, taking the infant's hand and pulling it across the infant's chest and around the neck as far posterior as possible toward the opposite shoulder, and observing the elbow position relative to the midline of the infant's body is the correct way to test for the scarf sign. Positioning the infant supine, flexing the infant's arms for 5 seconds, then fully extending the infant's arms by pulling the hands downward and releasing is the technique for performing the arm recoil test. Flexing the infant's hand on the forearm between the examiner's thumb and index finger, using enough pressure to get full flexion, and visually measuring the angle between the hypothenar eminence and the ventral aspect of the forearm is the correct way to perform the square window test. Positioning the infant supine with the pelvis flat on a surface, holding the infant's thigh in knee–chest position with the left index finger and thumb, placing the right index finger behind the infant's ankle and extending the leg gently, and measuring the angle between the lower leg and thigh is the correct way of determining popliteal angle.

Reference: Tappero E. Physical assessment. In: Verklan MT, Walden M, Forest S, eds. *Core Curriculum for Neonatal Intensive Care Nursing*. 6th ed. St. Louis, MO: Elsevier; 2021:102.

14. **(A)** Positioning the infant supine, flexing the infant's arms for 5 seconds, then fully extending the infant's arms by pulling the hands downward and releasing is the technique for performing the arm recoil test. Positioning the infant supine, taking the infant's hand and pulling it across the infant's chest and around the neck as far posterior as possible toward the opposite shoulder, and observing the elbow position relative to the midline of the infant's body is the correct way to test for the scarf sign. Flexing the infant's hand on the forearm between the examiner's thumb and index finger, using enough pressure to get full flexion, and visually measuring the angle between the hypothenar eminence and the ventral aspect of the forearm is the correct way to perform the square window test. Positioning the infant supine with the pelvis flat on a surface, holding the infant's thigh in knee–chest position with the left index finger and thumb, placing the right index finger behind the infant's ankle and extending the leg gently, and measuring the angle between the lower leg and thigh is the correct way of determining popliteal angle.

Reference: Tappero E. Physical assessment. In: Verklan MT, Walden M, Forest S, eds. *Core Curriculum for Neonatal Intensive Care Nursing*. 6th ed. St. Louis, MO: Elsevier; 2021:102.

15. **(A)** Babies who fall between the 10th and 90th percentiles are AGA infants, which means that they have grown in utero as expected and are therefore at less risk for problems such as hypoglycemia, infection, and poor neurodevelopmental outcomes. Babies who fall above the 90th percentile are LGA infants and at risk for birth trauma and hypoglycemia. Babies who fall below the 10th percentile have not grown as expected and may need further evaluation to assess the possible cause(s) of abnormal growth. These babies can have problems with blood glucose level (e.g., hypoglycemia).

Reference: Tappero E. Physical assessment. In: Verklan MT, Walden M, Forest S, eds. *Core Curriculum for Neonatal Intensive Care Nursing*. 6th ed. St. Louis, MO: Elsevier; 2021:105-108.

16. **(A)** As a baby matures, the pinnae of the ears will mature, and the cartilage will eventually firm up. Growth and development continue after birth, so preterm babies will develop cartilage in their ears. Before 34 weeks, the pinna has little cartilage and will stay folded on itself. The internal structure of a preterm infant's ears will form normally. Hearing loss in preterm infants may be related to exposure to ototoxic antibiotics (e.g., aminoglycosides).

Reference: Tappero E. Physical assessment. In: Verklan MT, Walden M, Forest S, eds. *Core Curriculum for Neonatal Intensive Care Nursing*. 6th ed. St. Louis, MO: Elsevier; 2021:104.

17. **(D)** Preterm infants have smooth plantar surfaces, which develop creases as they mature, and large amounts of lanugo over the shoulders and back, which will eventually slough off into the amniotic fluid as they get close to term. Vernix presents during the third trimester and decreases with increasing gestational age. The skin of preterm infants is thin with little subcutaneous fat, which allows veins to be visible on the abdomen. Palpable breast buds and stippling of the areolae would be apparent in the full-term infant.

Reference: Tappero E. Physical assessment. In: Verklan MT, Walden M, Forest S, eds. *Core Curriculum for Neonatal Intensive Care Nursing*. 6th ed. St. Louis, MO: Elsevier; 2021:104.

18. **(A)** Growth curves should be gestational age and gender specific for weight, length, and head circumference. Therefore not all growth curves are the same. Abdominal girth is not one of the measurements captured on the growth curve. Newborn growth curves can be used for infants born from 24 to 43 weeks' gestation.

Reference: Tappero E. Physical assessment. In: Verklan MT, Walden M, Forest S, eds. *Core Curriculum for Neonatal Intensive Care Nursing*. 6th ed. St. Louis, MO: Elsevier; 2021:104-108.

19. **(D)** Neurologic examination findings can be altered by neurologic disorders or asphyxic injury, which can affect tone and responsiveness, and therefore may not be reliable. Posture and flexion increase with advancing gestational age, as tone and muscle mass increase; however, counterintuitively, the wrist and ankle joints increase in flexibility, which decreases the number of degrees of the square window angle when tested with gentle pressure. The values of neurologic indicators are accurate in preterm infants; the tools account for gestational age.

Reference: Tappero E. Physical assessment. In: Verklan MT, Walden M, Forest S, eds. *Core Curriculum for Neonatal Intensive Care Nursing*. 6th ed. St. Louis, MO: Elsevier; 2021:102-104.

20. **(B)** An infant born at 40 weeks' gestation weighing 2000 g is well below the 10th percentile for weight and would be classified as small for gestational age (SGA). Potential problems for which SGA infants are at risk include polycythemia, hypoglycemia, hypothermia, hypoxia, and infection. LGA infants are at risk for birth trauma. Premature infants are at risk for respiratory distress syndrome.

Reference: Tappero E. Physical assessment. In: Verklan MT, Walden M, Forest S, eds. *Core Curriculum for Neonatal Intensive Care Nursing*. 6th ed. St. Louis, MO: Elsevier; 2021:109-110.

21. **(D)** Full-term infants who are LGA are at risk for birth trauma, polycythemia, and hypoglycemia and have an increased risk of being born by cesarean section. Preterm infants and infants with IUGR are at risk for hypothermia. Sodium and potassium homeostasis are not affected by size classification.

Reference: Tappero E. Physical assessment. In: Verklan MT, Walden M, Forest S, eds. *Core Curriculum for Neonatal Intensive Care Nursing*. 6th ed. St. Louis, MO: Elsevier; 2021:110-111.

22. **(D)** Extremely premature infants do not have plantar creases. Creases first appear on the anterior portion of the foot, between 28 and 30 weeks of gestation. At the earliest gestations, the eye–ear maturity sign is based on fusion of the eyelids. The extremely premature infant can be expected to have fused eyelids. Lanugo covers the body of the fetus from 20 to 28 weeks' gestation. As the fetus matures, the skin becomes dry and paperlike. The skin of an extremely premature infant is sticky, friable, gelatinous, and transparent.

Reference: Tappero E. Physical assessment. In: Verklan MT, Walden M, Forest S, eds. *Core Curriculum for Neonatal Intensive Care Nursing*. 6th ed. St. Louis, MO: Elsevier; 2021:102-104.

23. **(D)** Infants whose gestational age is greater than 42 weeks are postterm. In postterm infants, the skin is leathery, cracked, and wrinkled, plantar creases cover the entire foot sole, and the skin is mostly bald of lanugo. The size of fat deposits in the labia majora has increased so that the clitoris is completely covered. Additionally, the ears of postterm infants are stiff with thick cartilage and the breast areolae are full with 5- to 10-mm buds.

Reference: Tappero E. Physical assessment. In: Verklan MT, Walden M, Forest S, eds. *Core Curriculum for Neonatal Intensive Care Nursing*. 6th ed. St. Louis, MO: Elsevier; 2021:102-104.

24. **(D)** Poorly controlled maternal glucose levels result in fetal hyperglycemia, hyperinsulinemia, and subsequent macrosomia. Preeclampsia can lead to poor placental perfusion and asymmetric growth restriction. Maternal systemic lupus erythematosus is an autoimmune disease associated with IUGR. Infants exposed to cocaine have a higher incidence of low birth weight, smaller head circumference, and prematurity.

Reference: Tappero E. Physical assessment. In: Verklan MT, Walden M, Forest S, eds. *Core Curriculum for Neonatal Intensive Care Nursing*. 6th ed. St. Louis, MO: Elsevier; 2021:110-111.

25. **(B)** The best accuracy is obtained when the gestational age examination is performed on infants in an awake and alert state and within 24–48 hours of life. Neonatal assessment tools should be used from birth to 5 days, before physical characteristics change. The combined score of the physical and neurologic components has a higher correlation than either component used separately.

Reference: Tappero E. Physical assessment. In: Verklan MT, Walden M, Forest S, eds. *Core Curriculum for Neonatal Intensive Care Nursing*. 6th ed. St. Louis, MO: Elsevier; 2021:102.

26. **(D)** This infant is full term and LGA. Full-term LGA infants are at risk for birth trauma, such as a fractured clavicle and brachial plexus. SGA infants, not LGA infants, are at risk for hypothermia due to limited fat stores, increased glucose utilization and ineffective free fatty acid and triglyceride oxidation. Additionally, SGA infants are at risk for polycythemia due to increased red blood cell production in utero caused by chronic hypoxia or endocrine/metabolic or chromosomal disorder. LGA are at risk for hypoglycemia, not hyperglycemia, as a result of potential abnormal glucose metabolism after birth.

Reference: Tappero E. Physical assessment. In: Verklan MT, Walden M, Forest S, eds. *Core Curriculum for Neonatal Intensive Care Nursing*. 6th ed. St. Louis, MO: Elsevier; 2021:110-111.

27. **(B)** An infant born at 35 weeks' gestation is considered a late preterm infant and is at risk for higher morbidity and mortality due to prematurity. Potential complications of the late preterm infant include hypothermia, respiratory distress syndrome, sepsis, hyperbilirubinemia, hypoglycemia, and feeding difficulties. Term infants are those born on the first day of the 38th week to the last day of the 42nd week and are at decreased risk for morbidity and mortality compared to the other gestational age classifications.

Post-term infants are classified as infants born from the first day of the 43rd week and are at increased risk for experiencing morbidities and mortalities.

Reference: Tappero E. Physical assessment. In: Verklan MT, Walden M, Forest S, eds. *Core Curriculum for Neonatal Intensive Care Nursing.* 6th ed. St. Louis, MO: Elsevier; 2021:109.

28. **(B)** Fused eyelids normally open between 26 and 28 weeks' gestation. Fused eyelids at 24 weeks' gestation are not associated with blindness or indicate congenital anomalies.

Reference: Tappero E. Physical assessment. In: Verklan MT, Walden M, Forest S, eds. *Core Curriculum for Neonatal Intensive Care Nursing.* 6th ed. St. Louis, MO: Elsevier; 2021:104.

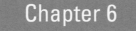

Chapter 6

Thermoregulation

1. Conduction is heat transfer by which of the following mechanisms?
   A. Air currents
   B. Direct contact
   C. Water vaporization from the skin
   D. Infrared energy transfer from a warm to a cooler object not in direct contact

2. Convection is heat transfer by which of the following mechanisms?
   A. Air currents
   B. Direct contact
   C. Water vaporization from the skin
   D. Infrared energy transfer from a warm to a cooler object that is not in direct contact

3. Evaporation is heat transfer by which of the following mechanisms?
   A. Air currents
   B. Direct contact
   C. Water vaporization from the skin
   D. Infrared energy transfer from a warm to a cooler object that is not in direct contact

4. Radiation is heat transfer by which of the following mechanisms?
   A. Air currents
   B. Direct contact
   C. Water vaporizing from the skin
   D. Infrared energy transfer from a warm to a cooler object that is not in direct contact

5. A nurse orienting to the neonatal intensive care unit (NICU) asks the preceptor why double-walled incubators are used in the NICU instead of single-walled incubators. Which of the following statements by the preceptor reflects an accurate understanding of the mechanisms of heat transfer?
   A. "Double-walled incubators direct air between the inner and outer incubator walls to reduce the amount of heat loss by radiation to the incubator walls."
   B. "Double-walled incubators direct air between the inner and outer incubator walls to reduce the amount of heat loss by conduction to the incubator walls."

   C. "Double-walled incubators direct air between the inner and outer incubator walls to reduce the amount of heat loss by convection to the incubator walls."
   D. "Double-walled incubators direct air between the inner and outer incubator walls to reduce the amount of heat loss by evaporation to the incubator walls."

6. Infants are at risk for hyperthermia due to which of the following characteristics?
   A. Limited glycogen stores
   B. Limited brown fat stores
   C. Large body surface area
   D. Limited ability to dissipate heat

7. Maintaining a neutral thermal environment for the neonate is important due to which of the following?
   A. It increases the metabolic rate.
   B. It limits the ability to maintain normothermia.
   C. It maximizes glucose consumption.
   D. It promotes minimal consumption of oxygen.

8. Which of the following places an infant at risk for hypothermia?
   A. Increase in muscle tone
   B. Increased glycogen stores
   C. Increased brown fat stores
   D. Increased body surface area

9. Which of the following places an infant at risk for hyperthermia?
   A. Infection
   B. Prematurity
   C. Gastroschisis
   D. Small-for-gestational-age

10. A premature infant has just been delivered vaginally. The nurse thoroughly dries the infant, places them on a warming mattress, applies a knit cap, and transports the infant to the nursery via an incubator. Which of these interventions reduces conductive heat loss?
    A. Thorough drying
    B. Applying a knit cap
    C. Placing on a warming mattress
    D. Transporting to the nursery via an incubator

11. A premature infant has just been delivered via cesarean section and is placed on a prewarmed radiant warmer. The nurse dries the infant thoroughly, places a warming mattress under the infant, and positions the infant away from drafts. Which of these interventions reduces convective heat loss?
    A. Thoroughly drying the infant
    B. Prewarming the radiant warmer
    C. Placing the infant away from drafts
    D. Placing the infant on a warming mattress

12. A mother has just given birth via normal spontaneous vaginal delivery. The nurse thoroughly dries the infant and places the infant directly on the mother's chest for skin-to-skin (kangaroo) care and then covers the infant with a blanket. The action of placing the infant on the mother's skin is specific to reducing which type of heat loss?
    A. Radiant
    B. Convective
    C. Conductive
    D. Evaporative

13. The infant will respond physiologically to cold stimuli by which of the following mechanisms?
    A. Increasing glycogen stores
    B. Storing brown adipose tissue
    C. Peripheral vasoconstriction
    D. Decreasing oxygen consumption

14. Upon initial assessment of a preterm infant, the nurse determines that the infant is tachycardic and irritable, shows signs of dehydration, and appears flushed. The serum sodium concentration is 152 mEq/L. These findings are consistent with which of the following conditions?
    A. Hypothermia
    B. Hyperthermia
    C. Hyponatremia
    D. Normothermia

15. A premature neonate has just been born at 24 weeks' gestation with a birth weight of 525 g. Which of the following statements demonstrates that the nurse understands how to use a polyethylene wrap?
    A. "I need to make sure that the entire baby is dried thoroughly before I apply the polyethylene wrap."
    B. "I need to make sure that I cover the baby's head and body with the polyethylene wrap before I dry the baby."
    C. "I need to make sure that I apply the polyethylene wrap once the baby gets to the nursery from the delivery room."
    D. "I need to make sure that I remove the polyethylene wrap once the baby's temperature is stable in a humidified environment for 1 hour."

16. An infant is being cared for in an incubator on servo-control mode. Which of the following increases the risk of hyperthermia?
    A. Dislodged skin temperature probe
    B. Skin temperature probe covered by an insulated probe cover
    C. Placement of the skin temperature probe away from brown adipose tissue areas
    D. Continuous monitoring of the skin temperature using a servo-controlled incubator

17. A term infant has just been admitted to the nursery and has been placed on a prewarmed radiant warmer. Which of the following statements made by the admitting nurse demonstrates correct understanding of how to operate the radiant warmer?
    A. "It's important to make sure the radiant warmer alarms are off when it's in use."
    B. "Once the radiant warmer has finished prewarming, it can be turned off."
    C. "Once I put the temperature probe on the patient, I need to switch the radiant warmer mode from manual to servo-controlled."
    D. "I need to switch the radiant warmer mode from servo-controlled to manual once I place the temperature probe on the patient."

18. Strategies to decrease heat loss in a neonate include:
    A. cooling all medical gas sources.
    B. transporting neonates in an open warmer.
    C. encouraging parental skin-to-skin contact.
    D. placing a neonate's incubator under the air vent.

19. One way to reduce convective heat loss in a neonate is to:
    A. prewarm the incubator.
    B. thoroughly dry the neonate at the time of delivery.
    C. transport a newly born infant via an incubator.
    D. warm the stethoscope before examining the neonate.

20. Humidification helps maintain neutral thermal environments for very low-birth-weight and extremely low-birth-weight infants by:
    A. reducing radiant heat loss.
    B. decreasing conductive heat gain.
    C. increasing evaporative heat loss.
    D. reducing transepidermal water loss.

21. Which of the following statements demonstrates the nurse's understanding of the role of subcutaneous fat in thermoregulation?
    A. "The more mature the neonate, the less body heat is maintained."
    B. "The more premature the neonate, the less subcutaneous fat is available."
    C. "Heat is maintained because heat is transferred from organs to the skin surface."
    D. "Neonates maintain heat because subcutaneous fat accounts for 50% of the neonate's body fat."

22. Which of the following statements by the nurse reflects an accurate understanding of weaning an infant from an incubator to an open crib?
    A. "Once an infant is over 1200 g, I can start weaning from an incubator to an open crib."
    B. "I need to monitor the infant's temperature and weight gain after weaning to an open crib."
    C. "As long as the infant maintains an axillary temperature above 33°C, they can remain in the open crib."
    D. "Before moving an infant to an open crib, I should maintain the incubator's temperature above 32°C."

23. A neonate's main mechanism for generating heat is:
    A. crying.
    B. flexing.

C. shivering.

D. nonshivering thermogenesis.

24. Placing a newly born infant on a nonwarmed mattress in the delivery room would lead to heat loss by which of the following mechanisms?
A. Radiation
B. Convection
C. Conduction
D. Evaporation

25. At the delivery of a term infant, the infant is thoroughly dried, wrapped in a nonwarmed blanket, and transferred to the nursery without a cap via an open crib. In the nursery, the infant is placed under a prewarmed radiant warmer, which is located by the unit's cold windows. The initial temperature of the infant indicates that the infant is hypothermic. The low temperature most likely resulted from:
A. conductive, convective, and radiant heat loss.
B. convective, radiant, and evaporative heat loss.
C. conductive, radiant, and evaporative heat loss.
D. conductive, convective, and evaporative heat loss.

26. Which of the following places a neonate at risk for hyperthermia?
A. Prematurity
B. Cardiac defect
C. Hypoglycemia
D. Large abdominal wall defects

27. One strategy to prevent heat loss in the neonate due to evaporation is to:
A. use a radiant warmer.
B. use a double-walled incubator.
C. dry the neonate with warm blankets.
D. cover the weighing scale with a prewarmed blanket.

28. One strategy to prevent heat loss in the neonate due to conduction is to:
A. use a radiant warmer.
B. use a double-walled incubator.
C. dry the neonate with warm blankets.
D. cover the weighing scale with a prewarmed blanket.

ANSWERS AND RATIONALES

1. **(B)** Conduction is heat transfer from direct contact when a cooler object is in direct contact with the newborn. An infant placed on a cold scale will lose heat via conduction to the scale. Convection is heat transfer via air currents. Evaporation is the loss of heat via the conversion of liquid into vapor. Radiation is the transfer of radiant energy (heat) without direct contact through absorption and emission of infrared rays.

Reference: Brand MC, Shippey HA. Thermoregulation. In: Verklan MT, Walden M, Forest S, eds. *Core Curriculum for Neonatal Intensive Care Nursing.* 6th ed. St. Louis, MO: Elsevier; 2021:86-88.

2. **(A)** Convection is heat transfer from the skin surface via air currents or drafts. Heat loss depends on the air's velocity and temperature. Conduction is heat transfer from direct contact. Evaporation is heat transfer due to water vaporizing from the skin or respiratory tract into the surrounding air. Radiation is the transfer of radiant energy (heat) without direct contact through absorption and emission of infrared rays.

Reference: Brand MC, Shippey HA. Thermoregulation. In: Verklan MT, Walden M, Forest S, eds. *Core Curriculum for Neonatal Intensive Care Nursing.* 6th ed. St. Louis, MO: Elsevier; 2021:86-88.

3. **(C)** Evaporation is heat transfer due to water vaporizing from the skin or respiratory tract into the surrounding air. Convection is heat transfer via air currents. Conduction is heat transfer via direct contact. Radiation is the transfer of radiant energy (heat) without direct contact through absorption and emission of infrared rays. An infant placed near cold windows will lose heat via radiation to the windows.

Reference: Brand MC, Shippey HA. Thermoregulation. In: Verklan MT, Walden M, Forest S, eds. *Core Curriculum for Neonatal Intensive Care Nursing.* 6th ed. St. Louis, MO: Elsevier; 2021:86-88.

4. **(D)** Radiation is the transfer of radiant energy (heat) without direct contact through absorption and emission of infrared rays. Convection is heat transfer via air currents. Conduction is heat transfer from direct contact. Evaporation is heat transfer due to water vaporizing from the skin or respiratory tract into the surrounding air.

Reference: Brand MC, Shippey HA. Thermoregulation. In: Verklan MT, Walden M, Forest S, eds. *Core Curriculum for Neonatal Intensive Care Nursing.* 6th ed. St. Louis, MO: Elsevier; 2021:86-88.

5. **(A)** Radiant heat loss occurs when heat is transferred from the infant's skin to a cooler object not in direct contact. Double-walled incubators minimize radiant heat loss because the inner wall is not exposed to the outside temperature. Heat loss through evaporation occurs when moisture on the skin or respiratory tract vaporizes into the surrounding air. An example of evaporative heat loss is when a newly born infant is not thoroughly dried after delivery. Conduction is heat loss to a cooler object in direct contact with the newborn. An example of conductive heat loss is when an infant is placed on a cold scale. Convection is heat transfer from the skin surface via air currents or drafts. An example of heat loss via convection is when an infant is placed near an air vent in an open crib.

Reference: Brand MC, Shippey HA. Thermoregulation. In: Verklan MT, Walden M, Forest S, eds. *Core Curriculum for Neonatal Intensive Care Nursing.* 6th ed. St. Louis, MO: Elsevier; 2021:86-88.

6. **(D)** Infants do not have the full capability to dissipate heat, which makes them prone to hyperthermia. A large body surface area and limited glycogen and brown fat stores increase the infant's risk of hypothermia.

Reference: Brand MC, Shippey HA. Thermoregulation. In: Verklan MT, Walden M, Forest S, eds. *Core Curriculum for Neonatal Intensive Care Nursing.* 6th ed. St. Louis, MO: Elsevier; 2021:88-90.

7. **(D)** A neutral thermal environment minimizes oxygen and glucose consumption, and decreases metabolic rate. A neutral thermal environment enables the neonate to maintain normothermia.

Reference: Brand MC, Shippey HA. Thermoregulation. In: Verklan MT, Walden M, Forest S, eds. *Core Curriculum for Neonatal Intensive Care Nursing.* 6th ed. St. Louis, MO: Elsevier; 2021:93-94.

8. **(D)** Increased body surface area, in combination with decreased brown fat stores, decreased subcutaneous fat, and decreased glycogen stores, makes the infant prone to experiencing hypothermia. Increased muscle tone, glycogen, and brown fat stores decrease the infant's risk of hypothermia.

Reference: Brand MC, Shippey HA. Thermoregulation. In: Verklan MT, Walden M, Forest S, eds. *Core Curriculum for Neonatal Intensive Care Nursing.* 6th ed. St. Louis, MO: Elsevier; 2021:88-90.

9. **(A)** Infection increases the infant's body temperature. Because the infant has limited ability to dissipate heat, the infant is at risk of hyperthermia. Prematurity, gastroschisis, and small size for gestational age increase the infant's risk of hypothermia.

Reference: Brand MC, Shippey HA. Thermoregulation. In: Verklan MT, Walden M, Forest S, eds. *Core Curriculum for Neonatal Intensive Care Nursing.* 6th ed. St. Louis, MO: Elsevier; 2021:88-90.

10. **(C)** Placing the infant on a warming mattress reduces the potential for heat loss to occur from direct contact. Thoroughly drying the infant reduces evaporative heat loss. Applying a knit cap on the infant reduces convective heat loss. Transporting the infant via an incubator versus an open crib will decrease convective loss from being exposed to air currents.

Reference: Brand MC, Shippey HA. Thermoregulation. In: Verklan MT, Walden M, Forest S, eds. *Core Curriculum for Neonatal Intensive Care Nursing.* 6th ed. St. Louis, MO: Elsevier; 2021:86-88.

11. **(C)** Placing the infant away from drafts decreases the potential for heat loss to occur due to air currents. Prewarming the radiant warmer reduces heat loss via radiation. Thoroughly drying the infant reduces evaporative heat loss. Placing the infant on a warming mattress reduces conductive heat loss.

Reference: Brand MC, Shippey HA. Thermoregulation. In: Verklan MT, Walden M, Forest S, eds. *Core Curriculum for Neonatal Intensive Care Nursing.* 6th ed. St. Louis, MO: Elsevier; 2021:86-88.

12. **(C)** The infant is receiving warmth from direct contact with the mother's skin. This decreases conductive heat loss.

Reference: Brand MC, Shippey HA. Thermoregulation. In: Verklan MT, Walden M, Forest S, eds. *Core Curriculum for Neonatal Intensive Care Nursing.* 6th ed. St. Louis, MO: Elsevier; 2021:86-88.

13. **(C)** The body responds to cold stimuli by peripherally vasoconstricting to decrease the amount of heat loss. The body also responds to cold stimuli by depleting glycogen stores, increasing the consumption of brown adipose tissue, and increasing oxygen consumption.

Reference: Brand MC, Shippey HA. Thermoregulation. In: Verklan MT, Walden M, Forest S, eds. *Core Curriculum for Neonatal Intensive Care Nursing.* 6th ed. St. Louis, MO: Elsevier; 2021:87-89.

14. **(B)** Signs of hypothermia do not include dehydration and hypernatremia. The hypothermic infant would be pale from vasoconstriction as opposed to flushed from vasodilation. Signs of normothermia do not include tachypnea, tachycardia, irritability, dehydration, a flushed look, and hypernatremia. Hyponatremia will not clinically exhibit the same symptoms of hyperthermia.

Reference: Brand MC, Shippey HA. Thermoregulation. In: Verklan MT, Walden M, Forest S, eds. *Core Curriculum for Neonatal Intensive Care Nursing.* 6th ed. St. Louis, MO: Elsevier; 2021:88-90.

15. **(D)** Once the infant's temperature is stable in a humidified environment for 1 hour, the polyethylene wrap must be removed. This reduces the potential for the infant to experience hyperthermia. Only the infant's head should be dried before placing the infant in the polyethylene wrap. The infant's head should not be covered with the polyethylene wrap. The polyethylene bag should be used once the infant is born, before drying, to reduce evaporative heat loss.

Reference: Brand MC, Shippey HA. Thermoregulation. In: Verklan MT, Walden M, Forest S, eds. *Core Curriculum for Neonatal Intensive Care Nursing.* 6th ed. St. Louis, MO: Elsevier; 2021:93-94.

16. **(A)** A dislodged skin temperature probe will sense the ambient temperature and attempt to bring the temperature to the skin temperature set on the incubator, which could lead to hyperthermia. A skin temperature probe covered by an insulated probe cover enables continuous monitoring of the infant's skin temperature, which decreases the potential for hyperthermia. The placement of the skin temperature probe away from brown adipose tissue areas enables accurate continuous monitoring of skin temperature, which decreases the potential for hyperthermia. The continuous monitoring of the skin temperature using a servo-controlled incubator decreases the potential for hyperthermia.

Reference: Brand MC, Shippey HA. Thermoregulation. In: Verklan MT, Walden M, Forest S, eds. *Core Curriculum for Neonatal Intensive Care Nursing.* 6th ed. St. Louis, MO: Elsevier; 2021:93-94.

17. **(C)** Once the infant is placed on the radiant warmer, changing the mode from manual to servo-controlled will decrease the risk that the infant will become overheated. Alarms should not be turned off, particularly when equipment is in use. The warmer needs to be on; turning it off causes the radiant warmer to lose heat obtained during the prewarming process. The radiant warmer should be set to servo-controlled mode when it is being used to warm an infant.

Reference: Brand MC, Shippey HA. Thermoregulation. In: Verklan MT, Walden M, Forest S, eds. *Core Curriculum for Neonatal Intensive Care Nursing.* 6th ed. St. Louis, MO: Elsevier; 2021:93-94.

18. **(C)** Parental skin-to-skin contact decreases heat loss through conduction of heat from parent to infant. Warming all medical gas sources is a strategy to decrease heat loss. Transporting neonates in an enclosed incubator would decrease the potential for heat loss. Placing a neonate's incubator under the air vent would contribute to heat loss via convection.

Reference: Brand MC, Shippey HA. Thermoregulation. In: Verklan MT, Walden M, Forest S, eds. *Core Curriculum for Neonatal Intensive Care Nursing.* 6th ed. St. Louis, MO: Elsevier; 2021:86-88.

19. **(C)** Transporting an infant via an incubator will avoid exposing the infant to drafts, thereby reducing convective heat loss. Prewarming the incubator will reduce heat loss by radiation. Thoroughly drying the neonate will reduce evaporative heat loss. Warming the stethoscope before examining the neonate decreases conductive heat loss.

Reference: Brand MC, Shippey HA. Thermoregulation. In: Verklan MT, Walden M, Forest S, eds. *Core Curriculum for Neonatal Intensive Care Nursing.* 6th ed. St. Louis, MO: Elsevier; 2021:86-88.

20. **(D)** Humidification reduces transepidermal water loss, which therefore reduces evaporative heat loss. Humidification decreases evaporative heat loss, increases conductive heat gain, and does not influence radiant heat transfer.

Reference: Brand MC, Shippey HA. Thermoregulation. In: Verklan MT, Walden M, Forest S, eds. *Core Curriculum for Neonatal Intensive Care Nursing.* 6th ed. St. Louis, MO: Elsevier; 2021:93-94.

21. **(B)** The availability of subcutaneous fat decreases with prematurity. Subcutaneous fat serves as insulation for the body. As a neonate matures, the neonate is better able to maintain body heat. Heat loss results from the transferring of heat from organs to skin surface. Subcutaneous fat accounts for 16% of body fat in neonates.

Reference: Brand MC, Shippey HA. Thermoregulation. In: Verklan MT, Walden M, Forest S, eds. *Core Curriculum for Neonatal Intensive Care Nursing.* 6th ed. St. Louis, MO: Elsevier; 2021:91.

22. **(B)** Monitoring the infant's temperature and weight gain after weaning to an open crib is important to ensure that the infant tolerates the transition and is able to maintain temperature and weight gain while being in an open environment. Weaning from an incubator to an open crib should occur after an infant is medically stable and weighs 1600 g or more. The incubator's temperature should be slowly weaned to 28°C–29°C as a thermal challenge

before moving the infant to an open crib. An infant should be able maintain a normal axillary temperature of 36.5°C or higher after weaning. If the infant cannot maintain a normal temperature, they should be moved back into an incubator.

Reference: Brand MC, Shippey HA. Thermoregulation. In: Verklan MT, Walden M, Forest S, eds. *Core Curriculum for Neonatal Intensive Care Nursing*. 6th ed. St. Louis, MO: Elsevier; 2021:93-94.

23. **(D)** Nonshivering thermogenesis produces heat through the metabolism of the brown adipose tissue and is the main method to generate heat. Crying is not the main method to generate heat. Flexing helps maintain heat yet is not the main method for generating heat. Shivering helps generate heat yet is not the primary method for generating heat.

Reference: Brand MC, Shippey HA. Thermoregulation. In: Verklan MT, Walden M, Forest S, eds. *Core Curriculum for Neonatal Intensive Care Nursing*. 6th ed. St. Louis, MO: Elsevier; 2021:87f, 91.

24. **(C)** Placing a newly born infant on a nonwarmed mattress in the delivery room would lead to heat loss by conduction. In conduction, heat is lost when a neonate comes in contact with a cold surface. Convection is heat transfer via air currents. Evaporation is the loss of heat via the conversion of liquid into vapor. Radiation is the transfer of radiant energy without direct contact through absorption and emission of infrared rays.

Reference: Brand MC, Shippey HA. Thermoregulation. In: Verklan MT, Walden M, Forest S, eds. *Core Curriculum for Neonatal Intensive Care Nursing*. 6th ed. St. Louis, MO: Elsevier; 2021:86-88.

25. **(A)** Use of a nonwarmed blanket promoted conductive heat loss, transfer of the infant without a cap promoted convective heat loss, and placement of the warmer by the cold windows promoted radiant heat loss. The infant was dried thoroughly, which reduced the risk of evaporative heat loss.

Reference: Brand MC, Shippey HA. Thermoregulation. In: Verklan MT, Walden M, Forest S, eds. *Core Curriculum for Neonatal Intensive Care Nursing*. 6th ed. St. Louis, MO: Elsevier; 2021:86-88.

26. **(B)** A neonate with a cardiac defect is at risk for experiencing hyperthermia due to the inability to dissipate heat. Prematurity places infants at risk for hypothermia due to decreased brown fat and glycogen stores, poor muscle tone, and high transepidermal water loss. Hypoglycemia places infants at risk for hypothermia due to decreased glucose availability needed for thermogenesis. Large abdominal wall defects place infants at risk for hypothermia, as the open defect presents a permeable surface for rapid fluid losses and increased evaporative heat loss.

Reference: Brand MC, Shippey HA. Thermoregulation. In: Verklan MT, Walden M, Forest S, eds. *Core Curriculum for Neonatal Intensive Care Nursing*. 6th ed. St. Louis, MO: Elsevier; 2021:87-88, 92-93.

27. **(C)** Transepidermal water loss occurs due to evaporation of amniotic fluid and accounts for 25% of neonatal heat loss in the delivery room. Drying a neonate with warmed blankets in the delivery room is a strategy that prevents heat loss due to evaporation. Using a radiant warmer is a strategy that prevents heat loss due to convection. Using a double-walled incubator is a strategy that prevents heat loss due to radiation. Covering the weighing scale with a prewarmed blanket is a strategy that prevents heat loss due to conduction.

Reference: Brand MC, Shippey HA. Thermoregulation. In: Verklan MT, Walden M, Forest S, eds. *Core Curriculum for Neonatal Intensive Care Nursing*. 6th ed. St. Louis, MO: Elsevier; 2021:86-88.

28. **(D)** Covering the weighing scale with a prewarmed blanket is a strategy that prevents heat loss that would occur from direct contact with the cold surface of the scale. Using a radiant warmer is a strategy that prevents heat loss due to convection. Using a double-walled incubator is a strategy that prevents heat loss due to radiation. Drying a neonate with warmed blankets in the delivery room is a strategy that prevents heat loss due to evaporation.

Reference: Brand MC, Shippey HA. Thermoregulation. In: Verklan MT, Walden M, Forest S, eds. *Core Curriculum for Neonatal Intensive Care Nursing*. 6th ed. St. Louis, MO: Elsevier; 2021:86-88.

Chapter 7

Fluids and Electrolytes

1. A 6-day-old term infant presents with a palate anomaly, systolic murmur, and hypertelorism. Laboratory values reflect the following: calcium 6.3 mg/dL, ionized calcium 3.4 mg/dL, phosphorus 5 mg/dL, and magnesium 2.6 mg/dL. The nurse should anticipate the most likely etiology is:
   A. hypomagnesemia related to Potters syndrome.
   B. chromosomal deletion on chromosome 22 at the q11.2 locus (DiGeorge syndrome).
   C. trisomy 18.
   D. Treacher-Collins syndrome.

2. A 6-hour-old term infant with perinatal asphyxia required extensive resuscitation at birth. The serum potassium is 6.6 mEq/L. The elevated potassium level is a result of the shift of potassium from the:
   A. extracellular space to the intracellular space secondary to metabolic alkalosis.
   B. extracellular space to the intracellular space secondary to metabolic acidosis.
   C. intracellular space to the extracellular space secondary to metabolic alkalosis.
   D. intracellular space to the extracellular space secondary to metabolic acidosis.

3. A former 25-week-gestation infant, now 3 months old, has been diagnosed with bronchopulmonary dysplasia/chronic lung disease. This infant has been receiving phenytoin (Dilantin) for a seizure disorder. Furosemide (Lasix) is now ordered. The nurse should anticipate which of the following side effects?
   A. Hypercalcemia
   B. Phenytoin (Dilantin) toxicity
   C. Decreased diuretic response
   D. Hyperglycemia

4. An infant's basic metabolic panel was obtained by venous puncture and the serum potassium level is 6.8 mEq/L. Which of the following is the most appropriate initial action by the nurse?
   A. Redraw serum potassium using an arterial puncture.
   B. Notify the provider for discontinuation of any potassium-containing fluids, nutritional supplements, and medications.
   C. Notify the provider to obtain an order for an electrocardiogram.
   D. Notify the parents of an impending critical situation.

5. An infant's serum sodium is 128 mEq/L. The urinary output is 6.2 mL/kg/h. The nurse should anticipate which of the following changes to the plan of care?
   A. Decrease in the total daily fluid quantity
   B. Administration of a normal saline (NS) bolus
   C. Administration of sodium bicarbonate
   D. Initiation of oral sodium supplements

6. An infant's electrocardiograph demonstrates ventricular tachycardia, peaked T waves, and a widened QRS complex. The nurse should assess the infant for which of the following electrolyte abnormalities?
   A. Hypokalemia
   B. Hyperkalemia
   C. Hypocalcemia
   D. Hypercalcemia

7. A 35-year-old gravida 2, para 1-0-0-1 woman with HELLP (hemolysis, elevated liver enzymes, and low platelets) syndrome was administered magnesium sulfate. When formulating the plan of care for the infant at birth, the nurse should anticipate which of the following symptoms?
   A. Lethargy and hypotonia
   B. Diarrhea and flaccidity
   C. Tremors and irritability
   D. Hyperreflexia progressing to seizures

8. A 30-week-gestation infant weighs 2500 g (5 lb, 8 oz) at birth; on day of life four, the infant weighs 2050 g (4 lb, 8 oz). The infant is cared for in an open crib with normal body temperatures, heart rate, and respiratory rate. Total fluid intake is 110 mL/kg/day; blood glucose is consistently 50 mg/dL. The nurse should perform which of the following actions?
   A. Obtain order for blood cultures and complete blood count (CBC).
   B. Increase amount of total fluid intake.
   C. Place the infant in an incubator.
   D. Obtain an order for serum sodium.

9. A 14-day-old former 27-week-gestation infant has serum sodium of 136 mEq/L. The total fluid goal is 120 mL/kg/day of total parenteral nutrition (TPN) and emulsified fats. Urinary output is 2.3 mL/kg/h. During rounds the medical team plans to increase the sodium slightly in the TPN. Which of the following statements reflects the physiologic reason for the intervention?
   A. Urine output is not within acceptable range.
   B. Preterm infants have immature renal concentration function.
   C. Infant is receiving too much free water in the TPN.
   D. The additional sodium will prevent dilutional hyponatremia.

10. A 12-day-old former 27-week-gestation infant is advancing on enteral feeding, receiving nasal continuous airway pressure +6 cm with oxygen 25–40% and had two apneic events overnight. Current capillary blood gas (CBG) shows pH 7.28, PaCO$_2$ 44, PaO$_2$ 55, bicarbonate 14 with a base deficit of –7. Yesterday, the CBG was pH 7.31, PaCO$_2$ 43, PaO$_2$ 60, bicarbonate 19 with a base deficit of –5. On examination, there is a 1 mL bilious residual. The nurse should consider which of the following as the most concerning finding as a precursor to the development of necrotizing enterocolitis?
    A. A 1 mL bilious residual
    B. Fluctuating oxygen requirement
    C. Persistent metabolic acidosis
    D. Two apneic events overnight

11. A 1205-g, 28-week-gestational-age infant is now postoperative day 2 from an ileal intestinal resection secondary to necrotizing enterocolitis. An orogastric (OG) tube is connected to low intermittent suction with 34 mL/kg/day of bilious-tinged output. The basic metabolic panel (serum chemistry) is sodium 129 mEq/L, potassium 3.2 mEq/L, chloride 91 mEq/L, bicarbonate 19 mEq/L, and calcium 8.5 mg/dL. The most appropriate action by the nurse should be to notify the provider and anticipate administration of which of the following?
    A. NS bolus of 20 mL/kg
    B. 1:1 replacement of OG output with 0.45 NS with potassium chloride every 8 hours via intravenous (IV)
    C. Potassium chloride bolus via IV
    D. Oral sodium supplements

12. A 2-week-old full-term infant with hypoplastic right lung and partial anomalous pulmonary venous return was started on a diuretic yesterday. The urinary output has been 7.5 mL/kg/h since initiating the diuretic. The current basic metabolic panel (serum chemistry) reports hemolyzed potassium. Which nursing action is the first priority?
    A. Redraw central potassium.
    B. Monitor for signs of hypokalemia.
    C. Obtain an electrocardiogram.
    D. Discuss the plan of care on rounds with the care team.

13. Which clinical presentation should the nurse find most indicative of fluid depletion?
    A. High urine output and high specific gravity
    B. Peripheral edema and weight gain
    C. Low urine output and high urine specific gravity
    D. Bradycardia and decreased pulses

14. Which of the following is the major extracellular cation that is most closely involved in water balance?
    A. Calcium
    B. Magnesium
    C. Potassium
    D. Sodium

15. A 3-kg full-term 4-day-old infant presents to the neonatal intensive care unit from home with serum sodium of 152 mEq/L. The infant has been feeding 20 mL of breast milk every 3 hours by bottle. Urinary output is 0.4 mL/kg/h. Vital signs: temperature 36.5°C (97.7°F), pulse 174, respiratory rate 36, blood pressure 69/45 mm Hg with a mean arterial pressure

of 55 mm Hg, and oxygen saturation (SpO_2) of 99% on room air. The nurse should consider these findings are most likely due to:
A. diabetes insipidus.
B. excessive insensible water loss.
C. increased free water intake.
D. insufficient enteral intake.

16. The basic metabolic panel (serum chemistry) of a term infant reveals low serum calcium at 24 hours of age. The most appropriate nursing action is to anticipate:
A. order for a calcium bolus.
B. administration of magnesium.
C. initiation of vitamin D supplements.
D. continued monitoring of the calcium level.

17. A full-term infant has a history of perinatal asphyxia and stress. A basic metabolic panel (serum chemistry) obtained at 24 hours of life shows serum calcium of 3.4 mg/dL. The nurse expects the etiology of this hypocalcemia to be the result of:
A. increased calcitonin release as a result of asphyxia and stress.
B. increased phosphorus levels secondary to an increased parathyroid hormone (PTH) response.
C. delay in the production of PTH due to asphyxia and stress.
D. reduction in calcium stores caused by asphyxia and stress.

18. The nurse should expect which type of infant to be at highest risk for metabolic bone disease?
A. Premature infant receiving thiazide diuretic
B. Infant of a diabetic mother
C. Infant with bronchopulmonary dysplasia receiving loop diuretics
D. Infant with a history of perinatal asphyxia

19. A 4-day-old full-term infant exhibits pedaling, sucking, and blinking movements. The nurse should expect which of the following electrolyte abnormalities as the most likely cause of these symptoms?
A. Hyponatremia
B. Hypernatremia
C. Hyperkalemia
D. Hypokalemia

20. A 24-hour-old, 32-week gestation, 1990-g infant is nothing-by-mouth and receiving IV fluids of D10W with 1:1 heparin at 5 mL/h via peripherally inserted central catheter. The glucose is 36 mg/dL via heel stick. The infant is irritable with a high-pitched cry. The nurse should perform which of the following as the initial response?
A. Initiate enteral feeding.
B. Repeat the glucose via venous draw.
C. Administer 2 mL/kg D10W bolus intravenously.
D. Repeat heel stick glucose in 30 minutes.

21. A 4-day-old, 26-week-gestation, 1200-g infant is exhibiting hyperkalemia with electrocardiogram changes. The heart rate is 186 beats per minute. Electrolytes are sodium 140 mEq/L, potassium 6.9 mEq/L, chloride 98 mEq/L, and bicarbonate 40 mEq/L. The nurse should expect which of the following as the most appropriate intervention?

A. Administration of sodium bicarbonate bolus
B. Administration of aerosolized albuterol
C. Calculation of sodium polystyrene (Kayexalate) dose
D. Initiation of insulin–glucose infusion

22. A 12-hour-old, 25-week-gestation, 800-g infant is nothing-by-mouth with IV fluids infusing at 100 mL/kg/day. The parents are concerned the infant has not voided. What is the most appropriate response by the nurse?
A. The infant needs a higher volume of IV fluid to void.
B. No urine output may be reflective of neurologic injury.
C. An infant may not urinate in the first 24 hours of life.
D. The infant will require bladder catheterization to facilitate urine drainage.

23. A nurse should understand that preterm infants experience insensible water loss primarily via:
A. skin and mucous membranes.
B. respiratory tract.
C. process of convection.
D. conductive currents.

24. A 4-week-old former preterm infant is on full feeds of maternal breast milk with caloric additives. Bowel sounds are hypotonic; abdominal examination is otherwise benign. A CBC and basic metabolic panel (serum chemistry) are obtained. The CBC is normal. Electrolytes are as follows: sodium 134 mEq/L, potassium 3.1 mEq/L, chloride 101 mEq/L, and bicarbonate 28 mEq/L. Nursing care of the infant should focus on which of the following as the most likely cause of the suspected intestinal ileus?
A. Early-onset bacterial sepsis
B. Intestinal ileus secondary to hypokalemia
C. Metabolic acidosis
D. Excessive sodium intake

25. A 4-day-old, 26-week-gestation infant presents with ionized calcium of 6.2 mg/dL. Other laboratory values reveal a high serum calcium, low phosphorus level, and high urinary calcium and phosphorus. The nurse should expect these laboratory findings to be indicative of:
A. maternal hypoparathyroidism.
B. low dietary intake of phosphorus.
C. inappropriate maternal intake of vitamin D.
D. excessive insensible water losses.

26. A 24-week gestation, 525-g infant has admission orders to run D10W with 1:1 heparin at 100 mL/kg/day. The nurse should calculate the IV infusion rate to deliver how many mL/h?
A. 4.3
B. 2.2
C. 3.1
D. 1.5

27. A 28-week-gestation infant is 4 hours postoperative from ileal resection and the removal of 20 cm of bowel. Physical examination: capillary refill >3 seconds, +1 pulses, and urinary output of 0.5 mL/kg/h. Vital signs: temperature 36.8°C (98.2°F), heart rate 178, respiratory rate 65, blood pressure 52/34 with a mean arterial pressure of 25, SpO_2 95% on 25% inspired oxygen. The infant is orally intubated and has an arterial blood gas: pH 7.25, $PaCO_2$ 45, PaO_2 54, and

bicarbonate 15 with base deficit of –6. The most appropriate initial action by the nurse is:

A. administration of sodium bicarbonate bolus.

B. administration of 10 mL/kg NS bolus.

C. increase the supplemental oxygen to 35%.

D. repeat the arterial blood gas within 30 minutes.

28. A 25-week-gestation, 645-g infant has D10W infusing at 1.6 mL/h via a peripheral IV. The blood glucose via heel stick was 36 mg/dL. What is the most appropriate initial nursing action?

A. Initiate a continuous insulin infusion.

B. Increase the IV glucose concentration to D15W.

C. Administer 10 mL/kg D10W bolus.

D. Increase the IV infusion rate to 2.6 mL/h and prepare a 2-mL/kg D10W bolus.

ANSWERS AND RATIONALES

1. **(B)** Hypocalcemia and palatal anomalies, a systolic murmur, and hypertelorism are seen collectively in DiGeorge syndrome and not typically in Treacher-Collins syndrome, trisomy 18, or Potter syndrome. Infants with DiGeorge syndrome (chromosomal deletion on chromosome 22 at q11.2 locus) present with hypocalcemia (<8.5–10.2 mg/dL) due to atresia or hypoplasia of the parathyroid gland. Infants with DiGeorge syndrome may have a systolic murmur related to associated cardiac defects (e.g., ventricular septal defect) and may also present with craniofacial anomalies (e.g., hypertelorism and cleft palate).

Reference: Lubbers LA. Congenital anomalies. In: Verklan M, Walden M, eds. *Core Curriculum for Neonatal Intensive Care Nursing.* 6th ed. St. Louis, MO: Elsevier; 2021:654-677.

2. **(D)** Perinatal asphyxia results in a metabolic acidosis due to hypoxia. The vast majority of potassium is found in the intracellular space. In the context of metabolic acidosis, a low serum PH shifts potassium from the intracellular space to the extracellular space. This results in a high serum potassium (>6.5 mEq/L) or hyperkalemia. By contrast, in metabolic alkalosis, the high serum pH shifts potassium from the extracellular space to the intracellular space; resulting in a serum hypokalemia (<3.5 mEq/L).

Reference: Bell SG. Fluid and electrolyte management. In: Verklan M, Walden M, eds. *Core Curriculum for Neonatal Intensive Care Nursing.* 6th ed. St. Louis, MO: Elsevier; 2021:131-143.

3. **(C)** Concurrent administration of phenytoin (Dilantin) and furosemide (Lasix) does not affect toxicity, serum calcium, or glucose levels. Concurrent administration of phenytoin (Dilantin) and furosemide (Lasix) reduces the diuretic response to Lasix by as much as 50%. It is essential to monitor for any diminished diuretic action when pairing Lasix and phenytoin together.

Reference: Preston CL. *Stockley's Drug Interactions Pocket Companion.* London: Pharmaceutical Press; 2016:347.

4. **(B)** Serum potassium of 6.5 mEq/L drawn by a venous or arterial puncture reflects high central potassium. Redrawing serum potassium using an arterial puncture would not be the most appropriate initial action. Hyperkalemia can be life-threatening due to possible cardiac arrest. The first, most appropriate action is to notify the provider for discontinuation of any potassium-containing fluids, nutritional supplements, and medications to reduce the amount of potassium being administered. An electrocardiogram can be considered in the context of hyperkalemia,

but it is not the initial action. The parents can be notified as soon as the treatment is initiated. It is not the most appropriate initial action.

Reference: Bell SG. Fluid and electrolyte management. In: Verklan M, Walden M, eds. *Core Curriculum for Neonatal Intensive Care Nursing.* 6th ed. St. Louis, MO: Elsevier; 2021:131-143.

5. **(A)** The serum sodium is low and the urinary output is high. Excessive administration of fluids can cause a dilutional hyponatremia, as evidenced by a high urinary output. Fluid restriction by decreasing the total fluid quantity will increase serum sodium. Initiation of sodium supplements or administering a normal saline bolus will increase the sodium but does not address the underlying volume overload. Sodium bicarbonate is not appropriate because it is used in the context of metabolic acidosis.

Reference: Gomella TL, Eyal FG, Bany-Mohammed F. *Neonatology: Management, Procedures, On-call Problems, Diseases, and Drugs.* 8th ed. New York: McGraw Hill Education; 2020.

6. **(B)** Potassium assists in regulating membrane potentials, so any disturbance in potassium can affect the muscle cells of the heart. Hypokalemia causes flattened T waves, whereas hyperkalemia causes peaked T waves and a widened QRS complex. Calcium abnormalities will not be reflective of this type of electrocardiogram pattern.

Reference: Bell SG. Fluid and electrolyte management. In: Verklan M, Walden M, eds. *Core Curriculum for Neonatal Intensive Care Nursing.* 6th ed. St. Louis, MO: Elsevier; 2021:131-143.

7. **(A)** Hypermagnesemia causes lethargy, hypotonia, flaccidity, and a poor suck due to the depressing effect on the central nervous system. Diarrhea is not related to magnesium abnormalities. Tremors, irritability, and seizures are symptoms associated with hypomagnesemia. Hyperreflexia progressing to seizures are symptoms associated with hypomagnesemia.

Reference: Bell SG. Fluid and electrolyte management. In: Verklan M, Walden M, eds. *Core Curriculum for Neonatal Intensive Care Nursing.* 5th ed. St. Louis, MO: Elsevier; 2021:131-143.

8. **(C)** The preterm infant lost 18% from birth weight in 4 days, which is greater than expected after the physiologic diuresis in the first week of life. Cold stress increases oxygen and glucose consumption, which can cause weight loss and hypoglycemia (glucose <50 mg/dL). If cold stress continues without intervention, such as placing the infant in an incubator to preserve a neutral thermal environment, progressive hypothermia will occur. If placing the infant in an incubator does not correct weight loss or glucose stability or other symptoms develop, sepsis can be considered. However, placing the infant in an incubator should be the first nursing intervention.

Reference: Brand MC, Shippey HA. Thermoregulation. In: Verklan M, Walden M, eds. *Core Curriculum for Neonatal Intensive Care Nursing.* 6th ed. St. Louis, MO: Elsevier; 2021:86-98.

9. **(B)** The total fluid goal and urinary output are appropriate, so volume overload is not the rationale for low-trending sodium. The sodium is on the low end of normal. Preterm infants have renal immaturity, so there is a tendency to excrete sodium. By increasing the sodium in the total parenteral nutrition, renal losses can therefore be compensated to maintain normal serum sodium.

Increasing the sodium will not eliminate free water. In the context of hyponatremia and volume overload, fluid restriction versus sodium supplement will correct the serum sodium.

Reference: Gomella TL, Eyal FG, Bany-Mohammed F. *Neonatology: Management Procedures, On-Call Problems, Diseases, and Drugs.* 8th ed. New York: McGraw Hill Education; 2020.

10. **(C)** A bilious residual, a fluctuating oxygen requirement, and two episodes of apnea overnight are concerning, but they are non-specific signs of neonatal sepsis. A persistent metabolic acidosis, as evidenced by the decrease in pH and decrease in bicarbonate, is most reflective of necrotizing enterocolitis (NEC). This is because NEC causes a lactic acidosis secondary to necrotic bowel.

Reference: Gomella TL, Eyal FG, Bany-Mohammed F. *Neonatology: Management Procedures, On-Call Problems, Diseases, and Drugs.* 8th ed. New York: McGraw Hill Education; 2020.

11. **(B)** Administering a one-time normal saline bolus will not address continuous gastric losses.

The serum chemistry reflects hyponatremia, hypokalemia, and hypochloremia due to increased electrolyte losses from gastric fluid via the orogastric tube. Replacing gastric losses with an intravenous (IV) fluid that contains sodium, chloride, and potassium will correct the serum sodium, chloride, and potassium slowly and will remedy continuous electrolyte losses. Administering a one-time potassium chloride bolus does not address sodium losses. Administering oral sodium supplements does not address sodium losses.

Reference: Arya S, Narendran V. Fluids, electrolytes and acid-base balance. In: Kenner C, Altimier BB, eds. *Comprehensive Neonatal Nursing Care.* 6th ed. New York: Springer Publishing Company; 2020:483.

12. **(A)** A normal potassium level is essential for appropriate cardiac function. As such, redrawing central potassium to appropriately monitor and treat a low potassium level is imperative. Discussing the plan of care with the medical team on rounds, monitoring for signs of hypokalemia, and obtaining an electrocardiogram will delay treatment and could be detrimental to the patient.

Reference: Bell SG. Fluid and electrolyte management. In: Verklan M, Walden M, eds. *Core Curriculum for Neonatal Intensive Care Nursing.* 6th ed. St. Louis, MO: Elsevier; 2021:131-146.

13. **(C)** High urine output is not associated with high urine specific gravity. Weight gain and peripheral edema suggest volume overload versus fluid depletion. A low urine output and a high urine specific gravity reflect an inadequate fluid status to perfuse the renal system. Although decreased pulses are a sign of fluid depletion, tachycardia as opposed to bradycardia is present in fluid depletion.

Reference: Bell SG. Fluid and electrolyte management. In: Verklan M, Walden M, eds. *Core Curriculum for Neonatal Intensive Care Nursing.* 6th ed. St. Louis, MO: Elsevier; 2021:131-146.

14. **(D)** Calcium is a cation mostly found in bone but also plays a role in blood clotting, cardiac function, neuromuscular excitability, nerve transmission, and cell membrane permeability. Magnesium is a catalyst for intracellular enzyme reactions such as muscle contraction and carbohydrate metabolism, and is critical for normal parathyroid function and bone-serum Ca homeostasis. Potassium is the major intracellular cation and plays a role in maintaining membrane potentials. It is well established that sodium is the major extracellular cation involved in water balance and regulation.

Reference: Bell SG. Fluid and electrolyte management. In: Verklan M, Walden M, eds. *Core Curriculum for Neonatal Intensive Care Nursing.* 6th ed. St. Louis, MO: Elsevier; 2021:131-146.

15. **(D)** Diabetes insipidus presents with hypernatremia, but with polyuria, not oliguria. Although excessive insensible water loss can also cause hypernatremia, this infant does not present with any risk factors for excessive insensible water losses to occur (e.g., prematurity, hyperthermia, and tachypnea). An increased free water intake would cause hyponatremia, not hypernatremia. A high serum sodium (>150 mEq/L), a low urinary output, tachycardia, and feeding volume of 53 mL/kg/day all suggest insufficient enteral intake to maintain hydration.

Reference: Bell SG. Fluid and electrolyte management. In: Verklan M, Walden M, eds. *Core Curriculum for Neonatal Intensive Care Nursing.* 6th ed. St. Louis, MO: Elsevier; 2021:131-146.

16. **(D)** Administering a calcium or magnesium bolus, as well as providing vitamin D supplementation, is not clinically warranted. Fetal calcium needs are met via active transport of calcium across the placenta. After birth, the calcium is sustained by stores and dietary provisions. The serum calcium will decrease in the first 24 hours of life to physiologic nadir because initially feeding volumes are low in the first 24 hours and parathyroid activity remains low. Monitoring is the most appropriate intervention as the calcium level should stabilize in 48–72 hours.

Reference: Bell SG. Fluid and electrolyte management. In: Verklan M, Walden M, eds. *Core Curriculum for Neonatal Intensive Care Nursing.* 6th ed. St. Louis, MO: Elsevier; 2021:131-146.

17. **(A)** Perinatal asphyxia and stress escalate calcitonin that suppresses calcium. Calcitonin is a counterregulatory hormone that is secreted from C cells of the thyroid gland and functions to decrease calcium levels by inhibiting bone-resorbing osteoclasts. In the context of perinatal asphyxia, tissue damage releases phosphorous into the circulation. As a result, there is a decrease in calcium uptake and subsequent hypocalcemia. Parathyroid hormone production is delayed in the context of infants of a diabetic mother. Calcium stores are decreased secondary to prematurity.

Reference: Bell SG. Fluid and electrolyte management. In: Verklan M, Walden M, eds. *Core Curriculum for Neonatal Intensive Care Nursing.* 6th ed. St. Louis, MO: Elsevier; 2021:131-146.

18. **(C)** Infants on thiazide diuretics have calcium reabsorption and therefore decreased urinary excretion. Although infants of a diabetic mother can have hypocalcemia due to a delay in parathyroid hormone (PTH) production, it typically does not cause metabolic bone disease. In utero, calcium and phosphorous are transferred to the fetus between 32 and 36 weeks' gestation. Inadequate intake of calcium and phosphorus results in metabolic bone disease. Risk factors include prematurity, chronic medical issues such as bronchopulmonary dysplasia, and chronic diuretic therapy especially with furosemide. Perinatal asphyxia is a not a major contributor to metabolic bone disease.

Reference: Admakin DH, Radmacher PG. Nutrition and selected disorder of the gastrointestinal tract. In: *Klaus & Fanaroff's Care of the High-Risk Neonate.* 7th ed. St. Louis, MO: Saunders Elsevier; 2020:80-120.e6.

19. **(A)** Hyponatremia is the electrolyte abnormality that would most likely cause seizure activity (i.e., pedaling, sucking, and blinking movements). This is because hyponatremia disrupts brain volume, particularly the equal osmolality of extracellular and intracellular fluid. When there is a decreasing cellular osmolality, water influx and subsequent cerebral edema occur. Cerebral edema is the major factor that causes symptoms such as seizures. Hypernatremia can cause seizures if severe, but hyponatremia is more often the cause. Potassium abnormalities are most commonly reflected via electrocardiogram rhythm disturbances versus seizure activity.

Reference: Vellaichamy M. Pediatric hyponatremia. In: Windle M, Evans B, Corden T, Cantwell G, eds. *Medscape.* Available at: https://emedicine.medscape.com/article/907841-overview. Updated December 21, 2020; Accessed April 13, 2022.

20. **(C)** The infant is nothing-by-mouth and 32 weeks' gestation. The infant may not tolerate enteral feedings, as oromotor coordination is not well established in the preterm infant. Repeating a central glucose or continuing to monitor will delay treatment of a symptomatic infant. The most appropriate action is to administer a D10W bolus of 2 mL/kg. Repeating a heel stick glucose on a symptomatic infant delays care.

Reference: Gomella TL, Eyal FG, Bany-Mohammed F. *Neonatology: Management, Procedures, On-Call Problems, Diseases, and Drugs.* 8th ed. New York: McGraw Hill Education; 2020.

21. **(D)** Although sodium bicarbonate, albuterol, and sodium polystyrene sulfonate (Kayexalate) can also drive potassium into the cell, they have been associated with other risks and are not first-line therapies. Albuterol's mechanism of action for treating hyperkalemia is not well understood, therefore the use is controversial. Kayexalate exchanges sodium for potassium in the gut, but the onset of action may not be appropriate to rapidly correct symptomatic hyperkalemia. Kayexalate may be associated with irritation, colitis, or NEC in preterm infants. An insulin–glucose infusion is the first-line therapy in preterm infants. Insulin causes cellular intake of potassium, thus decreasing serum potassium levels without depleting total body stores.

Reference: Gomella TL, Eyal FG, Bany-Mohammed F. *Neonatology: Management, Procedures, On-Call Problems, Diseases, and Drugs.* 8th ed. New York: McGraw Hill Education; 2020.

22. **(C)** Increasing the IV fluids at 12 hours of life may interfere with the physiologic diuresis. There is no indication that the infant experienced neurologic injury. Most healthy premature, full-term, and post-term infants void by 24 hours of life. This is because at birth renal blood flow may not increase initially but will increase by 24 hours once the renal vascular resistance falls. It is appropriate that the infant at 12 hours of life has not voided. Although inserting a bladder catheter can determine whether urine is present, this invasive procedure is not indicated.

Reference: Gomella TL, Eyal FG, Bany-Mohammed F. *Neonatology: Management, Procedures, On-Call Problems, Diseases, and Drugs.* 8th ed. New York: McGraw Hill Education; 2020.

23. **(A)** Approximately two-thirds of insensible water loss occurs via evaporation of body water from the skin and mucus membranes. The respiratory tract only accounts for about one-third of insensible water losses. Convection refers to the transfer of heat through surrounding air (i.e., drafts) and is not involved in insensible water loss. Conduction refers to the transfer of heat through direct contact with objects, such as scales, mattresses, or x-ray plates, and does not account for insensible water loss.

Reference: Blackburn ST. *Maternal, Fetal & Neonatal Physiology: A Clinical Perspective.* 5th ed. St. Louis, MO: Elsevier; 2018.

24. **(B)** The abdominal examination and complete blood count are within normal limits, so early-onset bacterial sepsis is not the most likely cause. Potassium is essential for appropriate function of the muscle cells of the gastrointestinal system. Hypokalemia (<3.5 mEq/L) can cause an intestinal ileus. Hypernatremia and metabolic acidosis are not causes of an intestinal ileus.

Reference: Bell SG. Fluid and electrolyte management. In: Verklan M, Walden M, eds. *Core Curriculum for Neonatal Intensive Care Nursing.* 6th ed. St. Louis, MO: Elsevier; 2021:131-146.

25. **(A)** Maternal hypoparathyroidism chronically stimulates the fetal parathyroid gland with a subsequent increase in PTH activity. Neonatal hyperparathyroidism occurs as evidenced by a high serum calcium, low phosphorous level, and high urinary calcium and phosphorous. The PTH acts by increasing renal tubular reabsorption of calcium, causing high serum calcium. PTH will decrease renal tubular reabsorption of phosphate, causing a low serum phosphorous. Neonatal hyperparathyroidism can also be diagnosed by high urinary calcium and phosphorus levels due to increased excretion in the urine. Low dietary intake of phosphorous, inappropriate vitamin D intake, and prematurity alone do not adequately explain the laboratory values.

Reference: Gomella TL, Eyal FG, Bany-Mohammed F. *Neonatology: Management, Procedures, On-call Problems, Diseases, and Drugs.* 8th ed. New York: McGraw Hill Education; 2020.

26. **(B)** 100 mL/kg/day multiplied by 0.525 kg = 52.5 mL/day; 52.5 mL/day divided by 24 hours = 2.2 mL/h.

Reference: Kleinman K, McDaniel L, Molloy M. *The Harriet Lane Handbook.* 22nd ed. Philadelphia, PA: Saunders Elsevier; 2021.

27. **(B)** Sodium bicarbonate does not address the underlying issue and is controversial due to the risk of intraventricular hemorrhage. Poor capillary refill (>3 seconds), weak pulses, low urine output, tachycardia, and low blood pressure all indicate poor perfusion. The arterial blood gas reveals an underlying metabolic acidosis secondary to inadequate volume. Increasing the oxygen to 35% does not treat metabolic acidosis. It would be appropriate to repeat the arterial blood gas after the normal saline bolus is administered to correct the volume depletion.

Reference: Gomella TL, Eyal FG, Bany-Mohammed F. *Neonatology: Management, Procedures, On-Call Problems, Diseases, and Drugs.* 8th ed. New York: McGraw Hill Education; 2020.

28. **(D)** Initiating an insulin drip will further lower the glucose level versus raising the level. Starting a D15W infusion to maintain a glucose infusion rate (GIR) will eventually treat the hypoglycemia and will allow for the maintenance of the same total fluid goal but does not treat current hypoglycemia. Additionally, the highest level of dextrose allowed in a peripheral IV is D12.5W. Simply administering a glucose bolus will not achieve a sufficient constant level of glucose. A normal GIR is 6–8 mcg/kg/min. The current GIR (4 mcg/kg/min) is insufficient to maintain euglycemia; increasing the GIR to approximately 6 mcg/kg/min will promote euglycemia. In addition, a 2-mL/kg D10W bolus is the most appropriate intervention to rapidly raise the blood glucose level.

Reference: Gomella TL, Eyal FG, Bany-Mohammed F. *Neonatology: Management, Procedures, On-Call Problems, Diseases, and Drugs.* 8th ed. New York: McGraw Hill Education; 2020.

Chapter 8

Nutrition and Feeding

1. The primary goal of delivering parenteral and enteral nutrition to the preterm infant is to:
   A. achieve the rate and composition of weight gain of a fetus at the same postmenstrual age.
   B. increase protein and energy deficits during the early neonatal period.
   C. enhance postnatal growth failure and suboptimal neurodevelopmental outcomes.
   D. meet total energy requirements for growing preterm infants of 80 kcal/kg/day.

2. Which of the following substrates is most influential to achieve optimal weight gain for the premature infant?
   A. Carbohydrate
   B. Fat
   C. Protein
   D. Sodium

3. The proteins whey and casein exist in a ratio of 80 (whey) to 20 (casein) in which of the following?
   A. Mature breast milk
   B. Colostrum
   C. Cow milk–based formula
   D. Soy-based formula

4. The nurse should anticipate the tapering of parenteral amino acid intake in the extremely low-birth-weight infant when enteral nutrition reaches how many milliliters per kilogram per day?
   A. 20
   B. 40
   C. 75
   D. 140

5. In extremely premature infants, initial enteral feedings of colostrum will result in which of the following?
   A. Delay induction of many digestive enzymes.
   B. Prohibit the endocytosis of proteins.
   C. Deliver low concentrations of secretory IgA.
   D. Facilitate rapid growth of the intestinal mucosal surface.

6. The predominant disaccharide in human milk is:
   A. sucrose.
   B. lactose.
   C. fructose.
   D. glucose.

7. The nursing plan of care for the growing preterm infant includes approximately how many calories per kilogram per day to sustain adequate energy intake?
   A. 40
   B. 80
   C. 120
   D. 150

8. Carbohydrates should supply what percent of an infant's total caloric intake?
   A. 7–16
   B. 25–35
   C. 40–50
   D. 80–90

9. When educating parents on optimal growth in their premature infant, the nurse should explain that they gain an average of how many grams per kg per day to achieve adequate growth?
   A. 5
   B. 15
   C. 50
   D. 100

10. The purpose of adding carnitine to total parenteral nutrition solutions for preterm infants who are not being enterally feed and receiving intravenous lipids is to:

A. facilitate digestion of lactose.
B. transport long-chain fatty acids.
C. synthesize bile acids.
D. support gut integrity.

11. The nurse recognizes that minimal enteral (trophic) feedings with expressed human milk should be initiated at a rate of:
    A. 2–5 mL/kg/day.
    B. 6–9 mL/kg/day.
    C. 10–20 mL/kg/day.
    D. 30–40 mL/kg/day.

12. The nurse should recognize that hypocaloric (trophic) enteral feedings benefit the preterm infant in which way?
    A. Sufficient calories to sustain somatic growth.
    B. Promote intestinal maturation with small volumes.
    C. Enhance villous atrophy.
    D. Replace the need for parenteral nutrition.

13. The principal parenteral energy source for neural tissue and metabolic processes in an infant weighing less than 1000 g is intravenous:
    A. fat emulsion.
    B. amino acids.
    C. sodium.
    D. glucose.

14. The nurse explains to the parents of a premature infant that maternal breast milk is the optimal primary nutritional source due to which of the following?
    A. Reduces the risk of necrotizing enterocolitis (NEC).
    B. Meets all nutritional requirements of premature infant.
    C. Increases rate of growth compared with formula-fed infants.
    D. Does not contain bacteria or viruses that could cause illness.

15. Which of the following statements by the nurse to a parent most accurately describes the protein content of preterm human milk?
    A. Less than term human milk
    B. Equal to term human milk and increases over the first few weeks of lactation
    C. Equal to term human milk throughout lactation
    D. Greater than term human milk

16. The nurse recognizes the importance of a standardized feeding protocol because it leads to which of the following?
    A. Increased incidence of NEC
    B. Improved rates of growth
    C. Higher rates of practice variation within a facility
    D. Increased amount of time to reach full enteral feeds

17. Neonates need a variety of different vitamins, minerals, and micronutrients to support growth and development. Which essential cofactor(s) is (are) required for neonatal immune maturation and function?
    A. Zinc
    B. Vitamin D
    C. Arachidonic acid and docosahexaenoic acid
    D. Copper

18. The potential adverse effect(s) of lipid emulsions for the preterm infant is(are):
    A. impaired pulmonary gas exchange and bilirubin toxicity.
    B. hypolipidemia.
    C. hypernatremia and hyperkalemia.
    D. hypoglycemia.

19. Which of the following element(s) may not be a necessary additive to the total parenteral nutrition solution for the first several days of life secondary to diuresis and the establishment of renal function in the extremely low-birth-weight infant not exposed to maternal magnesium sulfate therapy?
    A. Sodium and potassium
    B. Magnesium
    C. Amino acids
    D. Calcium

20. Iron deficiency in preterm infants can lead to which of the following?
    A. Suboptimal bone mineralization
    B. Oxidative red blood cell injury and hemolysis
    C. Poor repair and growth of epithelial tissue
    D. Anemia leading to adverse effects on brain development and function

21. A preterm infant is receiving enteral feedings with iron supplementation of 2 mg/kg/day. Enteral feedings were resumed after a packed red blood cell transfusion. The nurse should be aware that iron supplementation was discontinued for which of the following reasons?
    A. Avoid excessive serum ferritin levels
    B. Provide for normalization of serum hemoglobin levels
    C. Permit normalization of serum sodium levels
    D. Avoid accumulation of methemoglobin in the blood

22. The mother of an extremely low-birth-weight infant reports that she is pumping very small amounts of breast milk and asks the nurse about alternative options for maternal breast milk. Which of the following statements is most appropriate for the nurse to share with the mother?
    A. Human donor milk has the same nutritional properties as maternal breast milk.
    B. Formula is an option because donor human milk may put the infant at risk for HIV or cytomegalovirus.
    C. Formula is an option and may decrease the incidence of NEC.
    D. Donor human milk may decrease the incidence of NEC.

23. When caring for an appropriate-for-gestational-age preterm infant, the nurse would expect the neonate to regain birth weight within how many days?
    A. 7–10 days
    B. 10–15 days
    C. 30 days
    D. 3–5 days

24. A very low-birth-weight (VLBW) infant has received several weeks of parenteral nutrition. Laboratory studies reveal a conjugated (direct) bilirubin level of 2 mg/dL. The infant should be evaluated for which of the following?
    A. Cholestatic jaundice
    B. Pneumatosis

C. Glucose-6-phosphate dehydrogenase deficiency
D. Intraventricular hemorrhage

25. Which of the following nutritional deficiencies is associated with poor weight gain, scaling rash, sparse hair growth, thrombocytopenia, and decreased platelet aggregation?
    A. Zinc deficiency
    B. Copper deficiency
    C. Iodine deficiency
    D. Essential fatty acid deficiency

26. The optimal ratio of calcium to phosphorus to meet recommended dietary daily requirements and enhance growth for the premature infant is:
    A. 1:1.
    B. 1:2.
    C. 1:4.
    D. 2:1.

27. An early cause of hypocalcemia in the neonate is:
    A. hypophosphatemia.
    B. maternal diabetes.
    C. maternal hypermagnesemia.
    D. thiazide diuretics.

28. Which of the following presents the highest degree of nutritional challenge for the VLBW infant?
    A. Low ratio of body surface area compared to weight
    B. Limited ability to digest and absorb fats, carbohydrates, and macro-/micronutrients
    C. Decreased energy needs related to body composition
    D. Decreased water requirements

ANSWERS AND RATIONALES

1. **(A)** The current goal of parenteral and enteral nutrition is to attain approximately the same rate and composition of weight gain as a normal fetus at the same postmenstrual age. Any increase in protein and energy deficits should be avoided during the neonatal period. A large percentage of very low-birth-weight (VLBW) infants will experience inadequate growth and weigh less than the 10th percentile at 36 weeks' postmenstrual age. Poor postnatal growth has been associated with suboptimal neurodevelopmental outcomes. The total estimated energy requirement for maturing premature infants is 90–120 kcal/kg/day.

References: Brown L, Hendrickson K, Evans R, Davis J, Hay Jr WW. Enteral nutrition. In: Gardner S, Carter B, Enzman-Hines M, Hernandez J, eds. *Merenstein & Gardner's Handbook of Neonatal Intensive Care.* 9th ed. St. Louis, MO: Elsevier; 2021:480-533.

Poindexter BB, Martin CR. Nutrient requirements and provision of nutritional support in the premature neonate. In: Martin R, Fanaroff A, Walsh M, eds. *Fanaroff and Martin's Neonatal-Perinatal Medicine: Diseases of the Fetus and Infant.* 11th ed. Philadelphia, PA: Elsevier; 2020:670-689.

2. **(C)** Carbohydrates have been used to augment energy nutrition; however, their benefits do not appear to be independent of protein supply. Additionally, if carbohydrates exceed desirable amounts, glucose polymers can lead to hyperosmolality in the gut lumen, resulting in diarrhea. Fat provides the major source of energy for growing preterm infants; however, the nutritional value of human milk fat may vary with time and does not always provide a complete source of nutrients for premature infants. Proteins

are the driving source for weight gain in the premature infant as the major functional and structural components of all human cells. Sodium is an important electrolyte for cell metabolism but is not as imperative to growth as protein.

References: Blackburn S. Gastrointestinal and hepatic systems and perinatal nutrition. In: Blackburn S, ed. *Maternal, Fetal, & Neonatal Physiology: A Clinical Perspective.* 5th ed. St. Louis, MO: Elsevier; 2018:387-434.

Brown L, Hendrickson K, Evans R, Davis J, Hay Jr WW. Enteral nutrition. In: Gardner S, Carter B, Enzman-Hines M, Hernandez J, eds. *Merenstein & Gardner's Handbook of Neonatal Intensive Care.* 9th ed. St. Louis, MO: Elsevier; 2021:480-533.

Gomella TL, Eyal FG, Bany-Mohammed F. Nutritional management. In: Gomella TL, Eyal FG, Bany-Mohammed F, eds. *Gomella's Neonatology: Management, Procedures, On-Call Problems, and Drugs.* 8th ed. New York: McGraw Hill; 2020:125-165.

Poindexter BB, Martin CR. Nutrient requirements and provision of nutritional support in the premature neonate. In: Martin R, Fanaroff A, Walsh M, eds. *Fanaroff and Martin's Neonatal-Perinatal Medicine: Diseases of the Fetus and Infant.* 11th ed. Philadelphia, PA: Elsevier; 2020:670-689.

3. **(B)** Mature breast milk has a whey:casein ratio of 55:45. Colostrum has a whey:casein ratio of 80:20. Cow milk–based infant formula has a whey:casein ratio of 60:40. Soy-based infant formula does not contain whey and casein proteins.

References: Blackburn S. Gastrointestinal and hepatic systems and perinatal nutrition. In: Blackburn S, ed. *Maternal, Fetal, & Neonatal Physiology: A Clinical Perspective.* 5th ed. St. Louis, MO: Elsevier; 2018:387-434.

Brown L, Hendrickson K, Evans R, Davis J, Hay Jr WW. Enteral nutrition. In: Gardner S, Carter B, Enzman-Hines M, Hernandez J, eds. *Merenstein & Gardner's Handbook of Neonatal Intensive Care.* 9th ed. St. Louis, MO: Elsevier; 2021:480-533.

4. **(C)** Enteral intake of 20 mL/kg/day involves hypocaloric low-volume feeds and does not supply enough enteral protein to warrant parenteral amino acid tapering. A significant part of the enteral protein intake does not reach the systemic circulation and is not immediately available for the growth of other tissues. Enteral intake of 40 mL/kg/day, although greater in volume than trophic feeds, still does not supply enough enteral protein to warrant parenteral amino acid tapering. A minimum of 75 mL/kg/day of enteral nutrition should be achieved before parenteral amino acids are tapered in extremely low–birth-weight and VLBW infants. Protein malnutrition can easily develop in this patient population during the transition from parenteral to enteral nutrition. Enteral intake of 140 mL/kg/day is approaching a full enteral feeding volume, and the infant most likely will not require parenteral nutrition.

Reference: Poindexter BB, Martin CR. Nutrient requirements and provision of nutritional support in the premature neonate. In: Martin R, Fanaroff A, Walsh M, eds. *Fanaroff and Martin's Neonatal-Perinatal Medicine: Diseases of the Fetus and Infant.* 11th ed. Philadelphia, PA: Elsevier; 2020:670-689.

5. **(D)** Colostrum contains growth factors, and initial enteral feedings of colostrum in the premature infant stimulate rapid growth in the intestinal mucosal surface area and propagation of many digestive enzymes. It also promotes endocytosis of proteins and delivers high concentrations of secretory IgA.

Reference: Benjamin JT, Mezu-Ndubuisi OJ, Maheshwari A. Developmental immunology. In: Martin RJ, Fanaroff AA, Walsh MC, eds. *Fanaroff & Martin's Neonatal-Perinatal Medicine: Diseases of the Fetus and Infant.* 11th ed. Philadelphia, PA: Elsevier Saunders; 2020:752-788.

6. **(B)** Sucrose is a disaccharide and is hydrolyzed into glucose and fructose in the small intestine. Lactose is the main disaccharide in human milk and is hydrolyzed into glucose and galactose in the small intestine by the enzyme lactase. Fructose is a monosaccharide that is predominantly found in plants. Glucose is a monosaccharide that is predominantly found in food as a building block in complex carbohydrates. It is quickly absorbed from the lumen of the small intestine, across the epithelium, and into the bloodstream.

References: Blackburn S. Gastrointestinal and hepatic systems and perinatal nutrition. In: Blackburn S, ed. *Maternal, Fetal, & Neonatal Physiology: A Clinical Perspective.* 5th ed. St. Louis, MO: Elsevier; 2018:387-434.

Poindexter BB, Martin CR. Nutrient requirements and provision of nutritional support in the premature neonate. In: Martin R, Fanaroff A, Walsh M, eds. *Fanaroff and Martin's Neonatal-Perinatal Medicine: Diseases of the Fetus and Infant.* 11th ed. Philadelphia, PA: Elsevier; 2020:670-689.

7. **(C)** Forty to eighty kcal/kg per day are both lower energy intakes and may not be adequate to support basal metabolism and net protein/fat balance. The average energy intake for preterm infants to support weight gain is 105–130 kcal/kg per day. One hundred fifty kcal/kg per day is a higher energy intake and can result in greater fat accumulations and does not enhance neurologic development or achieve proper growth and body composition in comparison to their normal fetal equivalents.

References: Blackburn S. Gastrointestinal and hepatic systems and perinatal nutrition. In: Blackburn S, ed. *Maternal, Fetal, & Neonatal Physiology: A Clinical Perspective.* 5th ed. St. Louis, MO: Elsevier; 2018:387-434.

Gomella TL, Eyal FG, Bany-Mohammed F. Nutritional management. In: Gomella TL, Eyal FG, Bany-Mohammed F, eds. *Gomella's Neonatology: Management, Procedures, On-Call Problems, and Drugs.* 8th ed. New York: McGraw Hill; 2020:125-165.

Poindexter BB, Martin CR. Nutrient requirements and provision of nutritional support in the premature neonate. In: Martin R, Fanaroff A, Walsh M, eds. *Fanaroff and Martin's Neonatal-Perinatal Medicine: Diseases of the Fetus and Infant.* 11th ed. Philadelphia, PA: Elsevier; 2020:670-689.

8. **(C)** Carbohydrates are the principal source of energy for the brain and heart and should supply 40–50% of an infant's total caloric intake. Values less than the recommended amount may result in hypoglycemia. Values higher than the recommended amount may lead to diarrhea and are associated with high-energy diets. Increasing evidence suggests that high-energy diets in the neonatal period have the potential to result in rapid adipose gains and may contribute to obesity, insulin resistance, and type 2 diabetes later in life.

References: Blackburn S. Gastrointestinal and hepatic systems and perinatal nutrition. In: Blackburn S, ed. *Maternal, Fetal, & Neonatal Physiology: A Clinical Perspective.* 5th ed. St. Louis, MO: Elsevier; 2018:387-434.

Gomella TL, Eyal FG, Bany-Mohammed F. Nutritional management. In: Gomella TL, Eyal FG, Bany-Mohammed F, eds. *Gomella's Neonatology: Management, Procedures, On-Call Problems, and Drugs.* 8th ed. New York: McGraw Hill; 2020:125-165.

Poindexter BB, Martin CR. Nutrient requirements and provision of nutritional support in the premature neonate. In: Martin R, Fanaroff A, Walsh M, eds. *Fanaroff and Martin's Neonatal-Perinatal Medicine: Diseases of the Fetus and Infant.* 11th ed. Philadelphia, PA: Elsevier; 2020:670-689.

9. **(B)** The infant needs to gain approximately 15 g/kg/day for optimal weight gain. Infants that do not grow at intrauterine growth rates are vulnerable for energy and protein deficits in addition to postnatal growth restriction. Infants that grow more than intrauterine growth rates may be vulnerable to later risks of adult chronic diseases such as diabetes, hypertension, dyslipidemia, and cardiovascular disease.

References: Blackburn S. Gastrointestinal and hepatic systems and perinatal nutrition. In: Blackburn S, ed. *Maternal, Fetal, & Neonatal Physiology: A Clinical Perspective.* 5th ed. St. Louis, MO: Elsevier; 2018:387-434.

Brown L, Hendrickson K, Evans R, Davis J, Hay Jr WW. Enteral nutrition. In: Gardner S, Carter B, Enzman-Hines M, Hernandez J, eds. *Merenstein & Gardner's Handbook of Neonatal Intensive Care.* 9th ed. St. Louis, MO: Elsevier; 2021:480-533.

Gomella TL, Eyal FG, Bany-Mohammed F. Nutritional management. In: Gomella TL, Eyal FG, Bany-Mohammed F, eds. *Gomella's Neonatology: Management, Procedures, On-Call Problems, and Drugs.* 8th ed. New York: McGraw Hill; 2020:125-165.

Poindexter BB, Martin CR. Nutrient requirements and provision of nutritional support in the premature neonate. In: Martin R, Fanaroff A, Walsh M, eds. *Fanaroff and Martin's Neonatal-Perinatal Medicine: Diseases of the Fetus and Infant*. 11th ed. Philadelphia, PA: Elsevier; 2020:670-689.

10. **(B)** Lactase is the enzyme necessary for the digestion of lactose. Carnitine is a carrier molecule needed to transport long-chain fatty acids into mitochondria for oxidation. Preterm infants less than 34 weeks' gestation are usually dependent on lipids as an energy source and are at risk of not being able to appropriately store and synthesize carnitine, therefore, requiring supplementation in total parenteral nutrition solutions. Cholesterol is a major component of cell membranes and synthesizes bile acids. Glutamine is a key amino acid, which may play an important role in supporting gut integrity and acts as a substrate for small intestinal mucosa.

References: Blackburn S. Gastrointestinal and hepatic systems and perinatal nutrition. In: Blackburn S, ed. *Maternal, Fetal, & Neonatal Physiology: A Clinical Perspective*. 5th ed. St. Louis, MO: Elsevier; 2018:387-434.

Gomella TL, Eyal FG, Bany-Mohammed F. Nutritional management. In: Gomella TL, Eyal FG, Bany-Mohammed F, eds. *Gomella's Neonatology: Management, Procedures, On-Call Problems, and Drugs*. 8th ed. New York: McGraw Hill; 2020:125-165.

Poindexter BB, Martin CR. Nutrient requirements and provision of nutritional support in the premature neonate. In: Martin R, Fanaroff A, Walsh M, eds. *Fanaroff and Martin's Neonatal-Perinatal Medicine: Diseases of the Fetus and Infant*. 11th ed. Philadelphia, PA: Elsevier; 2020:670-689.

11. **(C)** Two to nine mL/kg/day would be an inappropriate volume for minimal enteral feedings. Minimal enteral feedings should be initiated at a rate of 10–20 mL/kg/day to facilitate postnatal gastrointestinal maturation and to minimize mucosal atrophy. A feeding volume of 30–40 mL/kg/day would be representative of advancing enteral nutrition.

References: Blackburn S. Gastrointestinal and hepatic systems and perinatal nutrition. In: Blackburn S, ed. *Maternal, Fetal, & Neonatal Physiology: A Clinical Perspective*. 5th ed. St. Louis, MO: Elsevier; 2018:387-434.

Gomella TL, Eyal FG, Bany-Mohammed F. Nutritional management. In: Gomella TL, Eyal FG, Bany-Mohammed F, eds. *Gomella's Neonatology: Management, Procedures, On-Call Problems, and Drugs*. 8th ed. New York: McGraw Hill; 2020:125-165.

Poindexter BB, Martin CR. Nutrient requirements and provision of nutritional support in the premature neonate. In: Martin R, Fanaroff A, Walsh M, eds. *Fanaroff and Martin's Neonatal-Perinatal Medicine: Diseases of the Fetus and Infant*. 11th ed. Philadelphia, PA: Elsevier; 2020:670-689.

12. **(B)** Minimal enteral or trophic feedings are hypocaloric and do not contain sufficient calories to sustain somatic growth. Minimal enteral or trophic feedings facilitate intestinal maturation with small volumes (typically less than 24 mL/kg/day). Minimal enteral or trophic feedings facilitate intestinal maturation, and the lack of any enteral feedings may lead to intestinal villous atrophy. Minimal enteral or trophic feedings are hypocaloric, low-volume feeds and do not replace the need for parenteral nutrition.

References: Blackburn S. Gastrointestinal and hepatic systems and perinatal nutrition. In: Blackburn S, ed. *Maternal, Fetal, & Neonatal Physiology: A Clinical Perspective*. 5th ed. St. Louis, MO: Elsevier; 2018:387-434.

Gomella TL, Eyal FG, Bany-Mohammed F. Nutritional management. In: Gomella TL, Eyal FG, Bany-Mohammed F, eds. *Gomella's Neonatology: Management, Procedures, On-Call Problems, and Drugs*. 8th ed. New York: McGraw Hill; 2020:125-165.

Poindexter BB, Martin CR. Nutrient requirements and provision of nutritional support in the premature neonate. In: Martin R, Fanaroff A, Walsh M, eds. *Fanaroff and Martin's Neonatal-Perinatal Medicine: Diseases of the Fetus and Infant*. 11th ed. Philadelphia, PA: Elsevier; 2020:670-689.

13. **(D)** Intravenous fat emulsions or lipids are important to prevent essential fatty acid deficiency. Intravenous amino acids are important to achieve protein balance and preserve endogenous protein stores in premature infants. Intravenous sodium is an electrolyte, not a source of energy. The main intravenous energy source for neural tissue and metabolic processes is glucose. The rate of glucose production in neonates weighting less than 1000 g is approximately 8–9 mg/kg/min.

References: Blackburn S. Gastrointestinal and hepatic systems and perinatal nutrition. In: Blackburn S, ed. *Maternal, Fetal, & Neonatal Physiology: A Clinical Perspective*. 5th ed. St. Louis, MO: Elsevier; 2018:387-434.

Gomella TL, Eyal FG, Bany-Mohammed F. Nutritional management. In: Gomella TL, Eyal FG, Bany-Mohammed F, eds. *Gomella's Neonatology: Management, Procedures, On-Call Problems, and Drugs*. 8th ed. New York: McGraw Hill; 2020:125-165.

Poindexter BB, Martin CR. Nutrient requirements and provision of nutritional support in the premature neonate. In: Martin R, Fanaroff A, Walsh M, eds. *Fanaroff and Martin's Neonatal-Perinatal Medicine: Diseases of the Fetus and Infant*. 11th ed. Philadelphia, PA: Elsevier; 2020:670-689.

14. **(A)** Maternal breast milk is the optimal primary nutritional source for premature neonates; evidence has shown that it reduces the incidence of necrotizing enterocolitis. Maternal breast milk does not completely meet all the nutritional needs of premature infants. Premature infants fed human milk may have slower growth rates compared with infants fed formula. Maternal breast milk does contain bacteria and viruses.

References: Blackburn S. Gastrointestinal and hepatic systems and perinatal nutrition. In: Blackburn S, ed. *Maternal, Fetal, & Neonatal Physiology: A Clinical Perspective*. 5th ed. St. Louis, MO: Elsevier; 2018:387-434.

Gomella TL, Eyal FG, Bany-Mohammed F. Nutritional management. In: Gomella TL, Eyal FG, Bany-Mohammed F, eds. *Gomella's Neonatology: Management, Procedures, On-Call Problems, and Drugs*. 8th ed. New York: McGraw Hill; 2020:125-165.

Poindexter BB, Martin CR. Nutrient requirements and provision of nutritional support in the premature neonate. In: Martin R, Fanaroff A, Walsh M, eds. *Fanaroff and Martin's Neonatal-Perinatal Medicine: Diseases of the Fetus and Infant*. 11th ed. Philadelphia, PA: Elsevier; 2020:670-689.

15. **(D)** The protein content of preterm human milk is greater than term human milk; however, the protein content decreases over the first few weeks of lactation.

References: Blackburn S. Gastrointestinal and hepatic systems and perinatal nutrition. In: Blackburn S, ed. *Maternal, Fetal, & Neonatal Physiology: A Clinical Perspective*. 5th ed. St. Louis, MO: Elsevier; 2018:387-434.

Brown L, Hendrickson K, Evans R, Davis J, Hay Jr WW. Enteral nutrition. In: Gardner S, Carter B, Enzman-Hines M, Hernandez J, eds. *Merenstein & Gardner's Handbook of Neonatal Intensive Care*. 9th ed. St. Louis, MO: Elsevier; 2021:480-533.

Gomella TL, Eyal FG, Bany-Mohammed F. Nutritional management. In: Gomella TL, Eyal FG, Bany-Mohammed F, eds. *Gomella's Neonatology: Management, Procedures, On-Call Problems, and Drugs*. 8th ed. New York: McGraw Hill; 2020:125-165.

Poindexter BB, Martin CR. Nutrient requirements and provision of nutritional support in the premature neonate. In: Martin R, Fanaroff A, Walsh M, eds. *Fanaroff and Martin's Neonatal-Perinatal Medicine: Diseases of the Fetus and Infant*. 11th ed. Philadelphia, PA: Elsevier; 2020:670-689.

16. **(B)** Implementing evidence-based standardized feeding guidelines can decrease rates of practice variation and lead to improved rates of growth velocity and improved clinical outcomes. These include decreasing the duration of parenteral nutrition, decreasing the time to reach full enteral feeds, and minimizing incidence of necrotizing enterocolitis.

References: Blackburn S. Gastrointestinal and hepatic systems and perinatal nutrition. In: Blackburn S, ed. *Maternal, Fetal, & Neonatal Physiology: A Clinical Perspective*. 5th ed. St. Louis, MO: Elsevier; 2018:387-434.

Brown L, Hendrickson K, Evans R, Davis J, Hay Jr WW. Enteral nutrition. In: Gardner S, Carter B, Enzman-Hines M, Hernandez J, eds. *Merenstein & Gardner's Handbook of Neonatal Intensive Care*. 9th ed. St. Louis, MO: Elsevier; 2021:480-533.

Gomella TL, Eyal FG, Bany-Mohammed F. Nutritional management. In: Gomella TL, Eyal FG, Bany-Mohammed F, eds. *Gomella's Neonatology: Management, Procedures, On-Call Problems, and Drugs*. 8th ed. New York: McGraw Hill; 2020:125-165.

17. **(A)** Zinc is an essential micronutrient needed for protein and nucleic acid synthesis and to enhance maturation and function of the immune system. Vitamin D promotes bone mineralization, intestinal calcium, phosphorus absorption, and calcium reabsorption from bone. Arachidonic acid and docosahexaenoic acid are considered conditional essential nutrients in preterm infants and should be provided during enteral feedings to improve neurologic and visual development and modulate immune functions. Copper is an essential micronutrient needed for hemoglobin synthesis.

References: Blackburn S. Gastrointestinal and hepatic systems and perinatal nutrition. In: Blackburn S, ed. *Maternal, Fetal, & Neonatal Physiology: A Clinical Perspective*. 5th ed. St. Louis, MO: Elsevier; 2018:387-434.

Brown L, Hendrickson K, Evans R, Davis J, Hay Jr WW. Enteral nutrition. In: Gardner S, Carter B, Enzman-Hines M, Hernandez J, eds. *Merenstein & Gardner's Handbook of Neonatal Intensive Care*. 9th ed. St. Louis, MO: Elsevier; 2021:480-533.

Gomella TL, Eyal FG, Bany-Mohammed F. Nutritional management. In: Gomella TL, Eyal FG, Bany-Mohammed F, eds. *Gomella's Neonatology: Management, Procedures, On-Call Problems, and Drugs*. 8th ed. New York: McGraw Hill; 2020:125-165.

18. **(A)** High lipid infusion rates can be associated with decreases in oxygenation and the displacement of bilirubin from albumin-binding sites. Premature infants less than 28 weeks' gestation are vulnerable to hyperlipidemia via lipid emulsion infusions due to reduced lipoprotein lipase activity and triglyceride clearance. Lipid emulsions should not directly lead to hypernatremia and hyperkalemia. Lipid emulsions can cause hyperglycemia, especially with rates greater than 6 g/kg/day.

References: Blackburn S. Gastrointestinal and hepatic systems and perinatal nutrition. In: Blackburn S, ed. *Maternal, Fetal, & Neonatal Physiology: A Clinical Perspective*. 5th ed. St. Louis, MO: Elsevier; 2018:387-434.

Brown L, Hendrickson K, Evans R, Davis J, Hay Jr WW. Enteral nutrition. In: Gardner S, Carter B, Enzman-Hines M, Hernandez J, eds. *Merenstein & Gardner's Handbook of Neonatal Intensive Care*. 9th ed. St. Louis, MO: Elsevier; 2021:480-533.

Gomella TL, Eyal FG, Bany-Mohammed F. Nutritional management. In: Gomella TL, Eyal FG, Bany-Mohammed F, eds. *Gomella's Neonatology: Management, Procedures, On-Call Problems, and Drugs*. 8th ed. New York: McGraw Hill; 2020:125-165.

19. **(A)** The addition of sodium and potassium to parenteral nutrition may not be necessary for the first several days in extremely low-birth-weight infants because of the expected free water diuresis during the first week of life and their immature renal function. Magnesium is an essential mineral, and parenteral supplementation should commence on the first day of life for stabilization of serum calcium values and bone mineralization and growth. Parenteral amino acid supplementation should begin immediately after the birth to promote growth. Calcium is an essential mineral, and adequate supply of parenteral calcium immediately after birth is crucial to reduce the risk of early hypocalcemia.

References: Blackburn S. Gastrointestinal and hepatic systems and perinatal nutrition. In: Blackburn S, ed. *Maternal, Fetal, & Neonatal Physiology: A Clinical Perspective*. 5th ed. St. Louis, MO: Elsevier; 2018:387-434.

Gomella TL, Eyal FG, Bany-Mohammed F. Nutritional management. In: Gomella TL, Eyal FG, Bany-Mohammed F, eds. *Gomella's Neonatology: Management, Procedures, On-Call Problems, and Drugs*. 8th ed. New York: McGraw Hill; 2020:125-165.

Poindexter BB, Martin CR. Nutrient requirements and provision of nutritional support in the premature neonate. In: Martin R, Fanaroff A, Walsh M, eds. *Fanaroff and Martin's Neonatal-Perinatal Medicine: Diseases of the Fetus and Infant*. 11th ed. Philadelphia, PA: Elsevier; 2020:670-689.

20. **(D)** Vitamin D is a fat-soluble vitamin that supports bone mineralization, intestinal calcium, phosphorus absorption, and calcium reabsorption from bone. Vitamin E aids in protecting the red blood cells from oxidative injury and hemolysis. Vitamin A is a fat-soluble vitamin that is needed for repair and growth of epithelial tissue. If iron stores are depleted and not available from dietary sources, the infant's hemoglobin will decline and potentially lead to an anemic state. Iron deficiency in preterm infants can also lead to adverse effects on brain development and function.

References: Blackburn S. Gastrointestinal and hepatic systems and perinatal nutrition. In: Blackburn S, ed. *Maternal, Fetal, & Neonatal Physiology: A Clinical Perspective*. 5th ed. St. Louis, MO: Elsevier; 2018:387-434.

Gomella TL, Eyal FG, Bany-Mohammed F. Nutritional management. In: Gomella TL, Eyal FG, Bany-Mohammed F, eds. *Gomella's Neonatology: Management, Procedures, On-Call Problems, and Drugs*. 8th ed. New York: McGraw Hill; 2020:125-165.

Poindexter BB, Martin CR. Nutrient requirements and provision of nutritional support in the premature neonate. In: Martin R, Fanaroff A, Walsh M, eds. *Fanaroff and Martin's Neonatal-Perinatal Medicine: Diseases of the Fetus and Infant*. 11th ed. Philadelphia, PA: Elsevier; 2020:670-689.

21. **(A)** Iron supplements were discontinued after the blood transfusion to minimize the risk of excessive serum ferritin levels. High ferritin levels can lead to an increased risk of infection, impaired growth, and formation of reactive oxygen species. Hemoglobin levels are maintained in the presence of physiologic erythropoiesis and through the use of red blood cell transfusions and recombinant human erythropoietin. Serum sodium levels are influenced by many factors, including aldosterone production, kidney function, ability or inability to excrete water, excessive sodium losses, excessive or inadequate sodium intake, inadequate water intake, medications, disease processes, and inherited disorders. Methemoglobinemia occurs when methemoglobin production is increased or the capacity to reduce methemoglobin is decreased. Acquired methemoglobinemia in infants usually occurs from inhalation of nitrates.

References: Blackburn S. Gastrointestinal and hepatic systems and perinatal nutrition. In: Blackburn S, ed. *Maternal, Fetal, & Neonatal Physiology: A Clinical Perspective*. 5th ed. St. Louis, MO: Elsevier; 2018:387-434.

Letterio J, Pateva I, Petrosiute A, Ahuja S. Hematologic and oncologic problems in the fetus and neonate. In: Martin RJ, Fanaroff AA, Walsh MC, eds. *Fanaroff & Martin's Neonatal-Perinatal Medicine: Diseases of the Fetus and Infant*. 11th ed. Philadelphia, PA: Elsevier Saunders; 2020:1416-1475.

Poindexter BB, Martin CR. Nutrient requirements and provision of nutritional support in the premature neonate. In: Martin R, Fanaroff A, Walsh M, eds. *Fanaroff and Martin's Neonatal-Perinatal Medicine: Diseases of the Fetus and Infant*. 11th ed. Philadelphia, PA: Elsevier; 2020:670-689.

22. **(D)** Donor human milk is pasteurized to prevent bacterial and viral contamination; however, pasteurization does change the nutritional and biologic quality of donor human milk compared with fresh mother's breast milk. Currently, donors are screened to prevent the risk of infection or toxic contamination, and donor human milk is pasteurized to provide microbiologic safety. Formula is not a better alternative because evidence suggests that avoiding formula may reduce the incidence of NEC. An important advantage to using donor human milk instead of formula is to predominantly decrease the incidence of necrotizing enterocolitis (NEC) in premature infants.

References: Blackburn S. Gastrointestinal and hepatic systems and perinatal nutrition. In: Blackburn S, ed. *Maternal, Fetal, & Neonatal Physiology: A Clinical Perspective*. 5th ed. St. Louis, MO: Elsevier; 2018:387-434.

Gomella TL, Eyal FG, Bany-Mohammed F. Nutritional management. In: Gomella TL, Eyal FG, Bany-Mohammed F, eds. *Gomella's Neonatology: Management, Procedures, On-Call Problems, and Drugs*. 8th ed. New York: McGraw Hill; 2020:125-165.

Poindexter BB, Martin CR. Nutrient requirements and provision of nutritional support in the premature neonate. In: Martin R, Fanaroff A, Walsh M, eds. *Fanaroff and Martin's Neonatal-Perinatal Medicine: Diseases of the Fetus and Infant*. 11th ed. Philadelphia, PA: Elsevier; 2020:670-689.

23. **(B)** Term and preterm infants lose weight after birth secondary to the loss of extracellular free water. Term infants typically regain birth weight by 7–10 days. Preterm infants typically regain birth weight by 10–15 days. Growth rates are more rapid during the neonatal period than any other time. Recommendations have been that postnatal growth of preterm infants follow the same pattern as intrauterine growth of the fetus at the same gestation. During the first week of life lower than optimal nutritional intake may result in significant energy and protein deficits. Many times, very low-birth-weight infants and extremely low-birth-weight infants do not grow at intrauterine rates, which delays the regaining of birth weight.

References: Gomella TL, Eyal FG, Bany-Mohammed F. Nutritional management. In: Gomella TL, Eyal FG, Bany-Mohammed F, eds. *Gomella's Neonatology: Management, Procedures, On-Call Problems, and Drugs.* 8th ed. New York: McGraw Hill; 2020:125-165.

Blackburn S. Gastrointestinal and hepatic systems and perinatal nutrition. In: Blackburn S, ed. *Maternal, Fetal, & Neonatal Physiology: A Clinical Perspective.* 5th ed. St. Louis, MO: Elsevier; 2018:387-434.

Poindexter BB, Martin CR. Nutrient requirements and provision of nutritional support in the premature neonate. In: Martin R, Fanaroff A, Walsh M, eds. *Fanaroff and Martin's Neonatal-Perinatal Medicine: Diseases of the Fetus and Infant.* 11th ed. Philadelphia, PA: Elsevier; 2020:670-689.

24. **(A)** The primary complication of prolonged parenteral nutrition is cholestatic jaundice, because total parental nutrition has been recognized as an important cause of intracellular and intracanalicular cholestasis. Conjugated hyperbilirubinemia is never normal and should always be evaluated. Pneumatosis is a radiographic finding caused by gas within the bowel wall and is a pathologic sign of necrotizing enterocolitis and is not a primary complication of parenteral nutrition. Glucose-6-phosphate dehydrogenase deficiency is an X-linked genetic condition that is associated with severe hemolytic jaundice and anemia after exposure to certain triggers. Intraventricular hemorrhage occurs in the germinal matrix, ruptures into the lateral ventricle, and can lead to acute enlargement of the lateral ventricle. It is not a primary complication of parenteral nutrition.

References: Gomella TL, Eyal FG, Bany-Mohammed F. Nutritional management. In: Gomella TL, Eyal FG, Bany-Mohammed F, eds. *Gomella's Neonatology: Management, Procedures, On-Call Problems, and Drugs.* 8th ed. New York: McGraw Hill; 2020:125-165.

Kaplan M, Wong RJ, Burgis JC, Sibley E, Stevenson DK. Neonatal jaundice and liver diseases. In: Martin RJ, Fanaroff AA, Walsh MC, eds. *Fanaroff & Martin's Neonatal-Perinatal Medicine: Diseases of the Fetus and Infant Diseases of the Fetus and Infant.* 11th ed. Philadelphia, PA: Elsevier; 2020:1788-1852.

Poindexter BB, Martin CR. Nutrient requirements and provision of nutritional support in the premature neonate. In: Martin R, Fanaroff A, Walsh M, eds. *Fanaroff and Martin's Neonatal-Perinatal Medicine: Diseases of the Fetus and Infant.* 11th ed. Philadelphia, PA: Elsevier; 2020:670-689.

25. **(D)** Zinc deficiencies can be associated with stunted growth, erythematous skin rash, and increased risk for infections in preterm infants. Copper deficiencies can be associated with poor growth, osteopenia, neutropenia, iron-resistant anemia, pallor, edema, hypotonia, and seborrheic dermatitis. Iodine deficiencies are associated with hypothyroidism, thyroid enlargement, cretinism, poor growth, and increased neonatal and infant mortality. Essential fatty acid deficiency is associated with poor weight gain, scaling rash, sparse hair growth, thrombocytopenia, and decreased platelet aggregation and can be prevented by supplementing exogenous intravenous fat emulsions within 72 hours.

References: Blackburn S. Gastrointestinal and hepatic systems and perinatal nutrition. In: Blackburn S, ed. *Maternal, Fetal, & Neonatal Physiology: A Clinical Perspective.* 5th ed. St. Louis, MO: Elsevier; 2018:387-434.

Poindexter BB, Martin CR. Nutrient requirements and provision of nutritional support in the premature neonate. In: Martin R, Fanaroff A, Walsh M, eds. *Fanaroff and Martin's Neonatal-Perinatal Medicine: Diseases of the Fetus and Infant.* 11th ed. Philadelphia, PA: Elsevier; 2020:670-689.

26. **(D)** The ratio of calcium to phosphorus should be approximately 2:1 to enhance growth and meet recommended daily requirements based upon rates of fetal accretion and an estimate of 50–70% intestinal absorption. In human milk the ratio of calcium to phosphorus is also 2:1. Ratios outside the recommended daily requirements may lead to inappropriate serum levels of calcium and phosphorus, and further lead to unsuitable accretion rates of minerals by the skeleton and absorption of minerals by the preterm intestine.

References: Abrams SA, Tiosano D. Disorders of calcium, phosphorus, and magnesium metabolism in the neonate. In: Martin R, Fanaroff A, Walsh M, eds. *Fanaroff and Martin's Neonatal-Perinatal Medicine: Diseases of the Fetus and Infant.* 11th ed. Philadelphia, PA: Elsevier; 2020:1611-1642.

Blackburn S. Gastrointestinal and hepatic systems and perinatal nutrition. In: Blackburn S, ed. *Maternal, Fetal, & Neonatal Physiology: A Clinical Perspective.* 5th ed. St. Louis, MO: Elsevier; 2018:387-434.

Poindexter BB, Martin CR. Nutrient requirements and provision of nutritional support in the premature neonate. In: Martin R, Fanaroff A, Walsh M, eds. *Fanaroff and Martin's Neonatal-Perinatal Medicine: Diseases of the Fetus and Infant.* 11th ed. Philadelphia, PA: Elsevier; 2020:670-689.

27. **(B)** Hypophosphatemia causes insufficient deposition of calcium and can lead to hypercalcemia. Infants of diabetic mothers are at risk of developing early hypocalcemia that can persist for several days due to maternal magnesium losses and can lead to fetal magnesium deficiency and secondary functional hypoparathyroidism in the newborn. The severity of the maternal diabetes is associated with the degree of hypocalcemia observed in the neonate. Thiazide diuretics can contribute to hypercalcemia by decreasing the renal excretion of calcium.

References: Abrams SA, Tiosano D. Disorders of calcium, phosphorus, and magnesium metabolism in the neonate. In: Martin R, Fanaroff A, Walsh M, eds. *Fanaroff and Martin's Neonatal-Perinatal Medicine: Diseases of the Fetus and Infant.* 11th ed. Philadelphia, PA: Elsevier; 2020:1611-1642.

Blackburn S. Gastrointestinal and hepatic systems and perinatal nutrition. In: Blackburn S, ed. *Maternal, Fetal, & Neonatal Physiology: A Clinical Perspective.* 5th ed. St. Louis, MO: Elsevier; 2018:387-434.

28. **(B)** VLBW infants have an increased ratio of surface area to body weight and, due to their limited protein and fat stores, have exaggerated energy needs that are specific to their clinical condition, body composition, environmental temperatures, and stressors of the neonatal intensive care environment. VLBW infants have an immature gastrointestinal system, which limits their ability to digest and absorb fats, carbohydrates, macronutrients, and micronutrients. They have increased water requirements due to high rates of insensible water losses and their immature renal function.

References: Blackburn S. Gastrointestinal and hepatic systems and perinatal nutrition. In: Blackburn S, ed. *Maternal, Fetal, & Neonatal Physiology: A Clinical Perspective.* 5th ed. St. Louis, MO: Elsevier; 2018:387-434.

Brown L, Hendrickson K, Evans R, Davis J, Hay Jr WW. Enteral nutrition. In: Gardner S, Carter B, Enzman-Hines M, Hernandez J, eds. *Merenstein & Gardner's Handbook of Neonatal Intensive Care.* 9th ed. St. Louis, MO: Elsevier; 2021:480-533.

Chapter 9

Developmentally Supportive Care

1. A nurse is teaching a mother to feed her preterm infant by keeping the nipple in the infant's mouth and regularly tilting the bottle slightly to stop the flow of expressed mother's milk. This method of shortened sucking bursts that lets the infant pause, swallow, and breathe is referred to as:
   A. paced feeding.
   B. synactive feeding.
   C. infant-driven feeding.
   D. interactive feeding.

2. Repetitive noxious stimuli to the mouth, such as suctioning, can result in which developmental disorder?
   A. Oral aversion
   B. Feeding strike
   C. Feeding opposition
   D. Feeding intolerance

3. Which is true of noise exposure for premature infants in neonatal intensive care units (NICUs)?
   A. A safe range to decrease physiologic stress is 100–110 dB.
   B. The human voice does not generally exceed the recommended decibel level.
   C. Increased environmental noise levels are a stressor to all infants, including preterm, term, ill, and well.
   D. Being inside an incubator sufficiently protects the infant from excessive decibel levels.

4. Effects and benefits of kangaroo (skin-on-skin) care have been reported with as little as 10 minutes of kangaroo care. Which statement best describes the research findings on kangaroo care?
   A. Kangaroo care has positive effects on breast-feeding, sleep, and infection rates.
   B. Kangaroo care interval is best described as one sleep cycle—approximately 2 hours.
   C. Kangaroo care increases anxiety in parents due to worry about monitoring of their infant.
   D. Kangaroo care is embraced uniformly by all staff members, and there are no barriers to its use.

5. Contraindications to kangaroo care include:
   A. paternal hair on chest.
   B. mechanical ventilation.
   C. maternal preeclampsia requiring magnesium sulfate therapy.
   D. infection of the skin of the chest of the kangaroo care provider.

6. Maturational hypotonia can lead to acquired positioning malformations in preterm infants, which include abnormal head molding, hip adduction, external rotation, and:
   A. arching posture.
   B. fixed neck flexion.
   C. wrist and ankle torsion.
   D. scapular abduction and shoulder extension.

7. Best practices for a developmentally supportive NICU environment include:
   A. windows that allow daylight in and use of auditory alarms.
   B. continuous fluorescent lighting and placement of pagers on vibrate mode.
   C. day–night cycling of light and rigid timing of nursing care.
   D. use of a procedure light and assessment of stress signals when providing nursing care.

8. Feeding success has implications for mother–infant bonding, as well as decreasing length of NICU stay. Interventions that facilitate feeding success include:
   A. paced feeding, kangaroo care before feedings, and provision of nonnutritive sucking.
   B. continuous drip feedings, appropriate type of nipple, and increasing environmental stimuli at feeding time.
   C. appropriate temperature of feedings, vigorous patting to encourage adequate burping, and use of a high-flow nipple.
   D. clustering of care, playing of music in the incubator for 6–12 hours a day, and use of a rocking mattress.

9. A 30-week-gestation infant who is not physiologically stable will be undergoing a painful procedure. Which of the following techniques can be taught to parents so that they can provide developmental support to their infant to reduce pain response behaviors?
   A. Singing to the infant during the procedure
   B. Rapid stroking of the extremities
   C. Using their hands to provide flexed containment of the extremities
   D. Using a soft blanket to maintain gentle extension of the extremities

10. A parent begins tapping on the incubator to wake up a sleeping infant for a visit. The most appropriate intervention at this time is to:
    A. suggest the parent wait until the infant is awake.
    B. identify a state-appropriate activity that the parent can do.
    C. encourage the parent's interactions with the infant.
    D. gently discourage the parent by stating, "The baby doesn't like that."

11. An appropriate nursing intervention to provide developmental support to an infant during gavage feeding is to:
    A. feed on a strictly routine schedule.
    B. provide nonnutritive sucking before, during, and after the procedure.
    C. use a bright light to allow visualization of the correct placement of the tube.
    D. restrain the infant's body in an extended, supine posture with a soft fabric restraint to prevent the tube from being dislodged.

12. Signs of sensory overstimulation in neonates include finger and toe splaying, gaze aversion, and hiccups. The most appropriate nursing intervention to provide neurodevelopmental support to an infant exhibiting one or more of these behaviors during nursing care is to:
    A. swaddle the infant and provide a time-out for rest and recovery.
    B. dim the lights to decrease stimulation and continue with the care.
    C. play music during care to provide auditory distraction and calm the infant.
    D. hurry and finish the care being provided to shorten the noxious exposure.

13. The father of an infant in the NICU is worried because his infant's incubator is covered and he is concerned that no one will notice if the infant's condition deteriorates or the infant needs attention. Which is the best explanation to provide?
    A. Looking at the fabric cover of the incubator stimulates the infant's retina to mature.
    B. Covered incubators allow decreased light so that the infant can rest but also immediate visualization if needed.
    C. NICU monitors detect adverse events and track the time of the event.
    D. Constant darkness will help the infant adjust to normal sleep patterns after discharge from the NICU.

14. Which of the following is true of kangaroo care?
    A. Olfactory sensations occur with the rise and fall of the parent's chest.
    B. Documentation of length of kangaroo care time is not needed, because it is universally well tolerated.
    C. The practice of standing transfer may increase stress during movement from the incubator to the parent's chest.
    D. Skin-to-skin contact provides tactile stimulation, promotes physiologic stability, and improves maternal milk production.

15. Which of the following is true of newborn sleep states?
    A. Oxygen consumption is lowest during rapid eye movement (REM) sleep.
    B. The best state for interaction with parents is the active alert state.
    C. Early dominant sleep states are light/active (REM) sleep and deep/quiet (non-REM) sleep.
    D. As the infant matures, less time is spent in the quiet alert state.

16. Developmental care supports sensory integration. Infants born preterm and/or critically ill are at high risk for sensory integration dysfunction due to the presence of sensory stimulation outside the normal sequence, brain injury, and environmental excesses. An example of appropriate sensory developmental care is:
    A. introduction of music at 28 weeks' gestation.
    B. mixing medications with a small amount of feedings before the main feeding.
    C. having parents implement infant massage as soon as possible in order to have them make a "connection" with their infant.
    D. using covers on incubators and/or decreasing ambient light at night to support sleep–wake cycles.

17. Which statement about the development of the human brain is the most accurate?
    A. The newborn brain is largely formed by term and is completely developed by 2 years of age.
    B. Developmental outcome is influenced almost entirely by genetic history, and environmental events have a minimal effect.
    C. The brain is a chain of communicating cells, and every touch, movement, and emotion affects its wiring and development.
    D. The brain of a preterm infant at 24 weeks' gestation has many cortical sulci, and these involutions can be harmed by inappropriate stimulation, excessive noise, and repetitive painful stimuli.

18. A mother is caring for her infant daughter who is now 31 weeks adjusted age. The mother tells the nurse that she was reading about sleeping in preterm infants and would like to understand more about transitional sleep in preterms. The nurse explains that transitional sleep:
    A. is the predominate sleep state for infants under 36 weeks' gestation.
    B. helps a preterm infant transition from REM to non-REM sleep.
    C. is a more active form of quiet sleep.
    D. helps preterm infants learn to decrease their sleep time.

19. The five constructs of developmental care are a method to operationalize developmental principles into practical applications for each individual infant. The constructs include cues, clues, consider, connect, and communicate. An example of *consider* would be to:
    A. observe the infant and determine whether the behaviors the nurse sees indicate stability or stress.
    B. check the situation and the environment for reasons for the observed behavior.
    C. decide what would be the best response based on the knowledge of the infant and the infant's reaction.
    D. see if it is possible to determine what events trigger infant stressors.

20. The nurse admitting a 26-week infant who is on high-frequency ventilation and vasopressors is talking with the parents of the infant. The parents would like to start infant massage on their son now. The most appropriate response by the nurse to this request is:
    A. "Infant massage has shown to have positive effects for preterm infants."
    B. "Your son is too sick to be touched at this time."
    C. "Touch is important, and your son needs you to make contact with him, but massage may be too much stimulation for him at this time."
    D. "Massage can only be done by a certified infant massage therapist."

21. A nurse is floating to the NICU and caring for infants in the feeder–grower area of the unit. After feeding she swaddles the infant tightly with the arms down at the sides and places the infant in a Safe Sleep position. Her NICU "buddy" discusses with her the NICU Safe Sleep program and some other elements of developmental care. One item the NICU buddy highlights is:

A. the best time to initiate Safe Sleep is 2 days before an infant goes home.

B. infants need to have access to their hands for self-consoling behaviors.

C. after feeding, infants are placed prone for 30 minutes and then put on their back.

D. completely swaddling a Safe Sleep infant helps the infant feel more secure when learning to sleep on the back.

22. Care in the NICU focuses on ways to foster the parent/family as the expert in the relationship with their infant. An example of this fostering would be the nurse:

A. telling the parent how to feed their infant.

B. having the mother watch the nurse give the first bath.

C. making sure the parents are informed of the specific feeding times.

D. identifying cues that the parent can use to calm the infant.

23. Core measures for developmental care have been identified and include (1) protected sleep, (2) pain and stress assessment and management, (3) developmentally supportive activities of daily living, (4) family-centered care, and (5) the healing environment. What is an example of a criterion for the core measure developmentally supportive activities of daily living?

A. All caregiving activities are modified according to the infant's state.

B. Physical and auditory privacy is offered at each patient bed space.

C. Resources are available 24/7 to support implementation of developmental care.

D. Skin assessment is done once per shift and documented.

24. An example of how an individual nurse may foster developmental care when doing direct care for an individual infant is:

A. teaching the family the quickest way to complete a bath.

B. alerting the infant to any care activity by speaking softly to him or her and making gentle physical contact with them.

C. allowing the infant to cry and learn self-consoling as he or she matures.

D. educating the parents on the unit times for caregiving.

25. NICUs are lit with bright light 24 hours a day. The light that a preterm or sick infant is exposed to will vary by their location in the NICU, regional variations caused by climate and/or season, the use of lights such as phototherapy and procedure, or retinopathy of prematurity (ROP) examinations, and infant factors such as eye shielding or head position. Exposure to light has been shown to impact a variety of factors such as altering state organization and nutrients in formula, breast milk, and parenteral nutrition. Which of the following is the most accurate statement about light use and outcome?

A. Cycled lighting for preterm infants for 2 weeks prior to discharge promotes the achievement of circadian entrainment within 1 week post discharge.

B. Low-level uncycled lighting for preterm infants for 2 weeks prior to discharge promotes the achievement of circadian entrainment within 1 week post discharge.

C. Cycled lighting has been shown to improve weight gain and feeding efficiency but not the progression to oral feeding.

D. Decreased lighting has been shown to improve ROP rate.

26. Which statement about the responsibility of the NICU care team for creating a healthy physical environment for the neonate in the NICU is most true?

A. NICUs need to be aware of the environmental exposure to the infant, as previously the infant was protected by the mother and the placenta.

B. Hospitals must now qualify as meeting Leadership in Energy and Environmental Design (LEED) standards.

C. Assessment of all the NICU physical structures such as flooring, tiles, countertops, and paint should be done on a routine basis in order to improve the environment the infant is exposed to while in the NICU.

D. Toxic cleaning chemicals, while unavoidable, should be minimized.

27. Which of the following is the **best** statement about the epigenetics of the NICU infant?

A. Early adverse NICU life experiences are overcome by the plasticity of the NICU infant's brain and have no lasting epigenetic effects.

B. Developmental care interventions such as positioning and light modification improve an infant's epigenetics.

C. NICU caregivers can create positive early life experiences by supporting developmental care practices and early parental nurturing opportunities to help protect against epigenetic factors.

D. Epigenetics are preset in utero and will define the infant's reactions to stress in the NICU.

28. The mother of an infant who was born at 26 weeks gestation and who is now 31 weeks adjusted age is doing skin-to-skin care with her infant. When the nurse enters the room, the mother tells her that the infant was sleeping but woke up and was crying but quickly settled down and is now looking at her while grasping the blanket edge and touching mother's skin. The mother asks the nurse what she should do, since previously the infant always slept. The nurse explains that:

A. while the infant is in this awake alert state, the mother should not touch the infant but just be quiet and keep holding the infant in the kangaroo position.

B. her infant is exhibiting a stable awake state and is ready for some interaction with the mother such as talking or singing softly or touch such as kissing or stroking.

C. her infant is ready for infant massage as she is able to self-calm, as demonstrated by her clasping the blanket.

D. since the infant is showing some self-regulation strategies by grasping the blanket, the mother can make continuous eye contact with the infant until the infant closes their eyes.

ANSWERS AND RATIONALES

1. **(A)** Paced feeding supports feeding success by coordinating sucking, promoting swallowing, regulating breathing breaks, and increasing stability. The synactive model of infant behavior is a major theoretical framework for establishing physiologic stability as the foundation for the organization of motor, state, and attentive–interactive behaviors. In infant-driven feeding, the infant determines when to be fed. Interactive feeding is a nonexistent term.

Reference: Spruill CT. Developmental support. In: Verklan M, Walden M, Forest S, eds. Core Curriculum for Neonatal Intensive Care Nursing. 6th ed. St. Louis, MO: Elsevier; 2021:185.

2. **(A)** Oral aversion can develop in response to repetitive invasive procedures, feeding on a schedule instead of on demand, and having multiple caregivers. Feeding strike occurs when an infant refuses to breastfeed and is not in the process of being weaned. Feeding opposition is a nonexistent term. Signs of feeding intolerance are abdominal distention, emesis, residuals, and blood in the stool.

Reference: Gardner SL, Goldson E. The neonate and the environment: impact on development. In: Gardner SL, Carter, BS, Enzman-Hines M, Niermeyer S, eds. Merenstein & Gardner's Handbook of Neonatal Intensive Care: An Interprofessional Approach. 9th ed. St. Louis, MO: Elsevier; 2021:386-389.

3. **(C)** Recommended noise levels are below 45 dB. Hearing damage is possible in adults at 85 dB. Loud noise affects all infants. Noise increases avoidance behaviors, disturbs sleep, increases cerebral blood flow and intraventricular hemorrhage, increases cardiorespiratory instability, and increases sensorineural hearing loss. The human voice is the greatest contributor to excessive noise in the neonatal intensive care unit (NICU). Incubators produce internal noise, and the sound of the doors closing is louder on the inside of an incubator.

Reference: Gardner SL, Goldson E. The neonate and the environment: impact on development. In: Gardner SL, Carter BS, Enzman-Hines M, Niermeyer S, eds. Merenstein & Gardner's Handbook of Neonatal Intensive Care: An Interprofessional Approach. 9th ed. St. Louis, MO: Elsevier; 2021:375-381 [Table 13.10 and Box 13.12].

4. **(A)** Kangaroo care has been reported to enhance parental bonding and increase confidence. Other beneficial effects are improved breastfeeding, improved sleep patterns, and lower infection rates. One dose is best described as one sleep–wake cycle, which is 65 minutes in preterm infants. Barriers remain to full implementation of kangaroo care due to issues of perceptions of infant and parent readiness, as well as staff time.

References: Gardner SL, Goldson E. The neonate and the environment: impact on development. In: Gardner SL, Carter BS, Enzman-Hines M, Niermeyer S, eds. Merenstein & Gardner's Handbook of Neonatal Intensive Care: An Interprofessional Approach. 9th ed. St. Louis, MO: Elsevier; 2021:362-363.

Spruill CT. Developmental support. In: Verklan MT, Walden M, Forest S, eds. Core Curriculum for Neonatal Intensive Care Nursing. 6th ed. St. Louis, MO: Elsevier; 2021:186.

5. **(D)** Skin infection on the chest of the kangaroo care provider could potentially be transmitted to the infant, so kangaroo care should be avoided until the skin is clear. There is no evidence that hairy chests cause overheating or infection. All infants should be monitored during kangaroo care, which allows safe administration of conventional mechanical ventilation and/or nasal continuous positive airway pressure during kangaroo care. A staff member is needed to attend to the ventilator tubing during transfer to the chest to prevent accidental extubation. Unless the mother is too groggy to feel safe during kangaroo care, maternal preeclampsia requiring magnesium sulfate therapy is not a contraindication.

Reference: Gardner SL, Goldson E. The neonate and the environment: impact on development. In: Gardner SL, Carter BS, Enzman-Hines M, Niermeyer S, eds. Merenstein & Gardner's Handbook of Neonatal Intensive Care: An Interprofessional Approach. 9th ed. St. Louis, MO: Elsevier; 2021:361-366.

6. **(A)** Abnormal head molding, hip adduction and external rotation, and arching posture are prevented by correct neurodevelopmental positioning. Fixed neck extension, not flexion, is an acquired positioning malformation that can be prevented by appropriate positioning. Wrist and ankle torsion are not acquired positioning malformations. Scapular adduction and shoulder retraction are acquired positioning malformations that can be prevented by appropriate positioning.

References: Spruill CT. Developmental support. In: Verklan MT, Walden M, Forest S, eds. Core Curriculum for Neonatal Intensive Care Nursing. 6th ed. St. Louis, MO: Elsevier; 2021:184-185.

Gardner SL, Goldson E. The neonate and the environment: impact on development. In: Gardner SL, Carter, BS, Enzman-Hines M, Niermeyer S, eds. Merenstein & Gardner's Handbook of Neonatal Intensive Care: An Interprofessional Approach. 9th ed. St. Louis, MO: Elsevier; 2021:368-373.

7. **(D)** Best practices include the use of a procedure light to allow for a focused source instead of overhead lighting, and assessment of stress signals when providing nursing care so that the nurse can determine when to stop providing care and let the infant recover, also known as cue-based care timing. Additionally, avoidance of overhead paging promotes a developmentally supportive environment. Windows that allow daylight in are helpful for staff and family well-being but auditory alarms should be avoided, as they increase ambient noise and disrupt sleep. Continuous fluorescent lighting can disrupt sleep–wake states. Day–night cycling of light can help decrease levels of stress hormones such as cortisol but rigid timing of nursing care is not recognizing the individual needs of each infant.

Reference: Gardner SL, Goldson E. The neonate and the environment: impact on development. In: Gardner SL, Carter BS, Enzman-Hines M, Niermeyer S, eds. Merenstein & Gardner's Handbook of Neonatal Intensive Care: An Interprofessional Approach. 9th ed. St. Louis, MO: Elsevier; 2021:335-406.

8. **(A)** Feeding success can be facilitated by decreasing environmental stimuli to allow the infant to focus on the feeding and avoid overstimulating and overwhelming the infant; reducing the stress of burping by positioning and gentle handling; using paced feedings to allow for reorganization of suck, swallowing, and breath coordination; providing kangaroo care before feedings; and providing nonnutritive sucking. Nipple type needs to be continuously evaluated and individualized. There is no consensus on the warming of feedings, but extremes in temperature should be avoided. Use of a high-flow nipple can lead to coughing and choking. Clustering of care may not allow for sufficient time for the infant to rest between care intervals; hours of music playing increases ambient noise levels; rocking mattresses may be overstimulating.

References: Gardner SL, Goldson E. The neonate and the environment: impact on development. In: Gardner SL, Carter BS, Enzman-Hines M, Niermeyer S, eds. Merenstein & Gardner's Handbook of Neonatal Intensive Care: An Interprofessional Approach. 9th ed. St. Louis, MO: Elsevier; 2021:384-392.

Spruill CT. Developmental support. In: Verklan MT, Walden M, Forest S, eds. Core Curriculum for Neonatal Intensive Care Nursing. 6th ed. St. Louis, MO: Elsevier; 2021:184-185.

9. **(C)** Gentle human touch to provide flexion and containment has a soothing effect. Additional auditory stimulation may be overwhelming. Stroking can result in decreased oxygen saturation and behavioral stress in preterm infants in unstable condition. Human touch is preferable to cloth, and flexion simulates the in utero position.

References: Gardner SL, Goldson E. The neonate and the environment: impact on development. In: Gardner SL, Carter BS, Enzman-Hines M, Niermeyer S, eds. Merenstein & Gardner's Handbook of Neonatal Intensive Care: An Interprofessional Approach. 9th ed. St. Louis, MO: Elsevier; 2021:357-372.

Spruill CT. Developmental support. In: Verklan MT, Walden M, eds. Core Curriculum for Neonatal Intensive Care Nursing. 6th ed. St. Louis, MO: Elsevier; 2021:186.

10. **(B)** If at all possible, a sleeping infant should not be awakened. If it is necessary to awaken the infant, as gentle a method as possible should be used. Nurses should educate parents on their infant's behavioral states and cues. Parental involvement should never be discouraged, but if the interaction is inappropriate, parents should be given alternatives. Because infants spend so much time asleep, parents need to be taught activities that they can do even while their infant is asleep. A goal of developmentally

supportive care is to minimize external auditory stimuli. Tapping on the incubator should be avoided.

References: Spruill CT. Developmental support. In: Verklan MT, Walden M, Forest S, eds. Core Curriculum for Neonatal Intensive Care Nursing. 6th ed. St. Louis, MO: Elsevier; 2021:177-178.

Gardner SL, Goldson E. The neonate and the environment: impact on development. In: Gardner SL, Carter BS, Enzman-Hines M, Niermeyer S, eds. Merenstein & Gardner's Handbook of Neonatal Intensive Care: An Interprofessional Approach. 9th ed. St. Louis, MO: Elsevier; 2021:342.

11. **(B)** Nonnutritive sucking accelerates maturation of the sucking reflex and improves weight gain. Feeding should be infant driven rather than on a routine schedule, based on infant readiness to feed and indicators of feeding fullness. Use of noxious stimuli such as a bright light will cause the infant to close their eyes and disengage in the activity. Prone or side-lying positioning improves gastric emptying and decreases regurgitation.

References: Gardner SL, Goldson E. The neonate and the environment: impact on development. In: Gardner SL, Carter BS, Enzman-Hines M, Niermeyer S, eds. Merenstein & Gardner's Handbook of Neonatal Intensive Care: An Interprofessional Approach. 9th ed. St. Louis, MO: Elsevier; 2021:384-387 [Boxes 13.15–13.17].

Spruill CT. Developmental support. In: Verklan MT, Walden M, Forest S, eds. Core Curriculum for Neonatal Intensive Care Nursing. 6th ed. St. Louis, MO: Elsevier; 2021:180.

12. **(A)** Swaddling the infant and implementing a time-out for rest and recovery provide neurodevelopmental support, promote self-regulatory behavior, and allow return to physiologic homeostasis. Just dimming the lights may not decrease stimulation enough to allow for recovery of physiologic stability. Playing music during care to provide auditory distraction is not recommended because the noise may add to the overstimulation and decompensation. If signs of stress are exhibited, care activities should be stopped and the infant allowed to recover physiologic stability. Continuing with the care could lead to further disorganization and physiologic and behavioral stress.

Reference: Gardner SL, Goldson E. The neonate and the environment: impact on development. In: Gardner SL, Carter BS, Enzman-Hines M, Niermeyer S, eds. Merenstein & Gardner's Handbook of Neonatal Intensive Care: An Interprofessional Approach. 9th ed. St. Louis, MO: Elsevier; 2021:348-373.

13. **(B)** Bright light is detrimental to the developing brain due to overstimulation of the immature central nervous system and can lead to the development of physiologic and behavioral defense mechanisms, maladaptions, and poor outcomes. The premature infant has limited ability for visual attentiveness. Visual stimulation is tiring to the premature infant and a reduction in visual stimuli is desirable. Monitoring may be somewhat reassuring but does not explain the importance of a neurodevelopmentally supportive NICU environment. Day–night cycling of light is beneficial for promotion of diurnal rhythms and sleep patterns.

Reference: Gardner SL, Goldson E. The neonate and the environment: impact on development. In: Gardner SL, Carter BS, Enzman-Hines M, Niermeyer S, eds. Merenstein & Gardner's Handbook of Neonatal Intensive Care: An Interprofessional Approach. 9th ed. St. Louis, MO: Elsevier; 2021:343-344, 356-357.

14. **(D)** Skin-to-skin contact provides tactile stimulation, promotes physiologic stability, and improves maternal milk production. Vestibular, not olfactory, sensations occur with the rise and fall of the parent's chest. It is important to document the length of kangaroo care time as well as the infant and parent response to the activity. Standing transfer may decrease the stress of movement from incubator to parent chest.

References: Spruill CT. Developmental support. In: Verklan MT, Walden M, Forest S, eds. Core Curriculum for Neonatal Intensive Care Nursing. 6th ed. St. Louis, MO: Elsevier; 2021:186.

Gardner SL, Goldson E. The neonate and the environment: impact on development. In: Gardner SL, Carter BS, Enzman-Hines M, Niermeyer S, eds.

Merenstein & Gardner's Handbook of Neonatal Intensive Care: An Interprofessional Approach. 9th ed. St. Louis, MO: Elsevier; 2021:361-366.

15. **(C)** The early dominant sleep states of light/active (rapid eye movement [REM]) sleep and deep/quite (non-REM) influence the reaction of a newborn to stimuli and must be taken into account when providing developmentally supportive care. As the infant matures, more time is spent in the quiet alert state. Oxygen consumption is lowest during deep sleep. In the quiet alert state, the infant can maximally attend and respond to parents.

Reference: Gardner SL, Goldson E. The neonate and the environment: impact on development. In: Gardner SL, Carter BS, Enzman-Hines M, Niermeyer S, eds. Merenstein & Gardner's Handbook of Neonatal Intensive Care: An Interprofessional Approach. 9th ed. St. Louis, MO: Elsevier; 2021:340-342.

16. **(D)** External stimulation of the visual system should be modulated to promote circadian rhythm development in the NICU infant. Infants less than 35 weeks have an incompetent pupillary reflex and need their eyes protected from light. Music may be used for infants who are greater than 32 weeks' gestation and must be a specific type (lullabies) with appropriate monitoring for volume and time interval. Further study is also needed on this topic. Medications should not be mixed with feedings because they alter the taste and may cause rejection of the feeding. This can cause sensory confusion related to negative and pleasurable tastes. Infant massage may be too overstimulating for many preterm or ill infants. Skin-to-skin care is a better option for families to practice. Infant massage may be introduced later when the sensory integration process is more intact for the infant.

References: Gardner SL, Goldson E. The neonate and the environment: impact on development. In: Gardner SL, Carter BS, Enzman-Hines M, Niermeyer S, eds. Merenstein & Gardner's Handbook of Neonatal Intensive Care: An Interprofessional Approach. 9th ed. St. Louis, MO: Elsevier; 2021:343-344, 356-357.

Spruill CT. Developmental support. In: Verklan MT, Walden M, Forest S, eds. Core Curriculum for Neonatal Intensive Care Nursing. 6th ed. St. Louis, MO: Elsevier; 2021:178 [Table 11.2].

17. **(C)** The brain is a chain of communicating cells, and every touch, movement, and emotion affect its wiring and development. A very preterm infant (e.g., 24 weeks' gestation) has an immature brain structure with a smooth cortex, and few sulci will form during the first year of life. The brain triples in size during the first year of life and the quality of brain development is shaped by both genetic history and environmental factors.

References: Gardner SL, Goldson E. The neonate and the environment: impact on development. In: Gardner SL, Carter BS, Enzman-Hines M, Niermeyer S, eds. Merenstein & Gardner's Handbook of Neonatal Intensive Care: An Interprofessional Approach. 9th ed. St. Louis, MO: Elsevier; 2021:334-406.

Gardner SL, Goldson E. The neonate and the environment: impact on development. In: Gardner SL, Carter BS, Enzman-Hines M, Niermeyer S, eds. Merenstein & Gardner's Handbook of Neonatal Intensive Care: An Interprofessional Approach. 9th ed. St. Louis, MO: Elsevier; 2021:342.

Spruill CT. Developmental support. In: Verklan MT, Walden M, Forest S, eds. Core Curriculum for Neonatal Intensive Care Nursing. 6th ed. St. Louis, MO: Elsevier; 2021:185-186.

18. **(A)** Preterm infants do not have significant quiet sleep cycles until approximately 36 weeks' gestation; hence, a third sleep state called transitional sleep is identified in preterm infants. Transitional sleep is not a sleep state between REM and non-REM, but rather an additional type of sleep state because preterms do not have organized REM and non-REM sleep states. Transitional sleep is characterized by quiet sleep with a period of closed eyes, regular or periodic breathing, no body movements, and no REM. Transitional sleep does not decrease sleep time.

References: Gardner SL, Goldson E. The neonate and the environment: impact on development. In: Gardner SL, Carter BS, Enzman-Hines M,

Niermeyer S, eds. Merenstein & Gardner's Handbook of Neonatal Intensive Care: An Interprofessional Approach. 9th ed. St. Louis, MO: Elsevier; 2021:342.

Spruill CT. Developmental support. In: Verklan MT, Walden M, Forest S, eds. Core Curriculum for Neonatal Intensive Care Nursing. 6th ed. St. Louis, MO: Elsevier; 2021:185-186.

19. **(C)** Consider is deciding on the best response using the knowledge the nurse has gathered from the cues and clues. Cues are behaviors that the nurse observes the infant having and if they are stress or stability cues. Clues are items that the nurse may observe in the environment or the situation that lead to the infant's reaction. Connect is the nurse using cues and clues to see if there is a pattern of behavior/event related to stressors and the best response process.

Reference: Spruill CT. Developmental support. In: Verklan MT, Walden M, Forest S, eds. Core Curriculum for Neonatal Intensive Care Nursing. 6th ed. St. Louis, MO: Elsevier; 2021:179.

20. **(C)** Infant massage has been demonstrated to have many positive effects in stable preterm infants. Current research has shown that infant massage is best utilized for medically stable preterm infants at a variety of gestational ages. At this time their son may be too overstimulated by massage when he is dealing with respiratory and blood pressure problems. The nurse can guide the family to more situationally appropriate types of touch such as facilitated tuck. Massage can be done by parents, health care personnel, and a massage therapist.

References: Spurill CT. Developmental support. In: Verklan MT, Walden M, Forest S, eds. Core Curriculum for Neonatal Intensive Care Nursing. 6th ed. St. Louis, MO: Elsevier; 2021:186-187.

Gardner SL, Goldson E. The neonate and the environment: impact on development. In: Gardner SL, Carter BS, Enzman-Hines M, Niermeyer S, eds. Merenstein & Gardner's Handbook of Neonatal Intensive Care: An Interprofessional Approach. 9th ed. St. Louis, MO: Elsevier; 2021:359-361.

21. **(B)** Safe Sleep "dressing" may include a sleep sac or blanket up to the nipple line. Infants should always have access to their hands for self-consoling behaviors. Safe Sleep protocols need to be initiated in the NICU well before discharge, giving the infant enough time to adjust to the supine sleeping and to pattern the behavior for families. The infant's needs are assessed and individualized. For example, infants may be excluded based on airway obstructions or birth defects. Once Safe Sleep protocols are started, an infant is placed supine after feeds. Infants who are "Safe Sleep" should not be completely swaddled. Appropriately identified NICU infants should be in a sleeper and/or wrapped only to the nipple level. Patterning behavior for the family with the Safe Sleep program includes minimizing the amount of blankets and bedding in the bed.

Reference: Gardner SL, Goldson E. The neonate and the environment: impact on development. In: Gardner SL, Carter BS, Enzman-Hines M, Niermeyer S, eds. Merenstein & Gardner's Handbook of Neonatal Intensive Care: An Interprofessional Approach. 9th ed. St. Louis, MO: Elsevier; 2021:373-374.

Goldstein MH, Stewart DL, Keels EL, Moon RY, Committee on Fetus and Newborn, Task Force on Sudden Infant Death Syndrome. Transition to a safe home sleep environment for the NICU patient. *Pediatrics.* 2021;148(1):e2021052046. doi:10.1542/peds.2021-052046.

22. **(D)** To have the parent/family be a partner in the care, it is important to help them learn about their infant and how their infant reacts. Identifying cues and clues that they can use to care for their infant helps them gain competency and comfort with their care. Parents can experience and learn alongside the nurse when feedings are done. Parents should be doing all the "firsts" so that common care practices such as bathing are items that they are comfortable doing with minimal assistance. Infant-driven feeding rather than specific feeding times is more conducive to the infant and the family.

References: Spruill CT. Developmental support. In: Verklan MT, Walden M, Forest S, eds. Core Curriculum for Neonatal Intensive Care Nursing. 6th ed. St. Louis, MO: Elsevier; 2021:187-188.

Gardner SL, Goldson E. The neonate and the environment: impact on development. In: Gardner SL, Carter BS, Enzman-Hines M, Niermeyer S, eds. Merenstein & Gardner's Handbook of Neonatal Intensive Care: An Interprofessional Approach. 9th ed. St. Louis, MO: Elsevier; 2021:346.

23. **(D)** Skin assessment falls under the core measure of developmentally supportive activities of daily living, specifically under the attribute of skin care. Other attributes under this core measure include positioning and feeding. Caregiving activity modification falls under the protected sleep core measure, under the attribute of care strategies that are individualized for each infant and documented. Physical and auditory privacy falls under the healing environment core measure, under the attribute of a quiet, dimly lit, private environment that promotes safety and sleep. Resource availability for developmental care implementation falls under the healing environment core measure. The attribute is evidence-based policies, procedures, and resources are available to sustain the healing environment over time.

Reference: Spruill CT. Developmental support. In: Verklan MT, Walden M, Forest S, eds. Core Curriculum for Neonatal Intensive Care Nursing. 6th ed. St. Louis, MO: Elsevier; 2021:180 [Table 11.3].

24. **(B)** Alerting the infant to changes has two goals: one is to allow the infant to have a smoother state transition and the other allows the caretaker to observe for subtle signs of discomfort or engagement. Bathing should be a relaxing, soothing experience for the infant. He or she should be in a tucked position for an immersion bath, using a blanket, towel, or hands to keep the infant calm and comfortable. Infants should be comforted as quickly as possible. This decreases the negative effects that physiologic changes may have and helps to establish trust versus mistrust with the caregivers. Longer periods of crying usually take longer to console. Caregiving should be based on the infant and family schedule. This is often the major challenge NICUs have in coordinating the needs of the unit with the needs of the family.

Reference: Gardner SL, Goldson E. The neonate and the environment: impact on development. In: Gardner SL, Carter BS, Enzman-Hines M, Niermeyer S, eds. Merenstein & Gardner's Handbook of Neonatal Intensive Care: An Interprofessional Approach. 9th ed. St. Louis, MO: Elsevier; 2021:348-358.

25. **(A)** Cycled lighting will improve the circadian entrainment based on retinal exposure to light and dark. Infants who do not receive cycled lighting take up to 3 weeks after discharge to develop a circadian rhythm. Cycled lighting has been shown to improve weight gain and feeding efficiency and to also improve the progression to oral feeding (less time). While the rates of retinopathy of prematurity have not been shown to decrease with decreased light levels studies have shown that there is a decrease in negative biochemical and physical effects related to lighting levels.

Reference: Gardner SL, Goldson E. The neonate and the environment: impact on development. In: Gardner SL, Carter BS, Enzman-Hines M, Niermeyer S, eds. Merenstein & Gardner's Handbook of Neonatal Intensive Care: An Interprofessional Approach. 9th ed. St. Louis, MO: Elsevier; 2021:339, 343-344, 381-383.

26. **(C)** All environmental structures, furnishings, and even care items like adhesives need to be assessed for risk and replaced when appropriate with nontoxic items, avoiding such things as volatile organic compounds and di(2-ethylhexyl)phthalate (DEHP), which is a plastic softener and found in items from food packaging to intravenous bags and tubings. The Environmental Working Group has reported that at least 287 chemicals, including neurotoxins, have been found in neonatal cord blood and are transmitted to the developing fetus by maternal exposure. Not all facilities are LEED certified. LEED is a benchmark organization and a resource for designs that are environmentally responsible and human healthy.

Cleaning of surfaces and furniture does not require toxic chemicals; in fact, they can be cleaned using soap and water.

Reference: Spruill CT. Developmental support. In: Verklan MT, Walden M, Forest S, eds. Core Curriculum for Neonatal Intensive Care Nursing. 6th ed. St. Louis, MO: Elsevier; 2021:183.

27. **(C)** The interaction between genes and the environment is bidirectional, and early positive nurturing experiences provided during critical periods of development may reverse the effects of adverse early experiences. Developmental care interventions do support modifying epigenetic mechanisms, but positive parental nurturing and positive early life experiences create the best optimal outcomes. Early synaptic connections are affected during critical periods of brain development and have lasting effects. To protect against epigenetic factors, caregivers need to adapt the environment to the infant's needs, not have the infant adapt to the NICU environment. Beyond in utero, early life experiences and epigenetic impact have been shown to alter the hypothalamic–pituitary–adrenal axis function which regulates the stress and behavior responses.

References: Spruill CT. Developmental support. In: Verklan MT, Walden M, Forest S, eds. Core Curriculum for Neonatal Intensive Care Nursing. 6th ed. St. Louis, MO: Elsevier; 2021:172-173.

Gardner SL, Goldson E. The neonate and the environment: impact on development. In: Gardner SL, Carter BS, Enzman-Hines M, Niermeyer S, eds. Merenstein & Gardner's Handbook of Neonatal Intensive Care: An Interprofessional Approach. 9th ed. St. Louis, MO: Elsevier; 2021:348-356.

28. **(B)** The infant is in an awake, alert state demonstrating signs of self-regulation. This is an appropriate time to do some gestationally appropriate activities. And, by looking at the mother, the infant is signaling readiness to interact. Although the infant is showing signs of self-regulation, brief periods of eye contact would be the best option rather than continuous contact. The infant closing their eyes would be a sign of stress. Infant massage has demonstrated many positive benefits in healthy stable preterm infants, this infant needs to be assessed further for stability and as a candidate for massage.

References: Spruill CT. Developmental support. In: Verklan MT, Walden M, Forest S, eds. Core Curriculum for Neonatal Intensive Care Nursing. 6th ed. St. Louis, MO: Elsevier; 2021:178, 186-187.

Gardner SL, Goldson E. The neonate and the environment: impact on development. In: Gardner SL, Carter BS, Enzman-Hines M, Niermeyer S, eds. Merenstein & Gardner's Handbook of Neonatal Intensive Care: An Interprofessional Approach. 9th ed. St. Louis, MO: Elsevier; 2021:358-366.

Chapter 10

Radiographic Evaluation

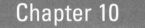

1. Which chest x-ray findings best represent primary surfactant deficiency?
   A. Hypoexpansion, air bronchograms, reticulogranular pattern
   B. Hyperexpansion, fluid in the fissure, air bronchograms
   C. Bilateral streakiness, hyper expansion, reticulogranular pattern
   D. Hypoexpansion, sail sign, fluid in the fissure

2. During a physical examination, an infant's point of maximal impulse is noted to be to the right of the mediastinum. The nurse should anticipate which of the following conditions?
   A. Left-sided pneumothorax
   B. Levocardia
   C. Right-sided pleural effusion
   D. Left-sided atelectasis

3. A 3-cm increase in abdominal girth, visible bowel loops, and increased apnea episodes are noted upon clinical examination. The nurse should anticipate an order for which type of x-ray?
   A. Anterior/posterior (A/P) chest
   B. A/P abdomen
   C. A/P abdomen and cross-table lateral
   D. Lateral decubitus and A/P chest

4. A newly born late preterm infant is admitted to neonatal intensive care unit (NICU) with grunting, flaring, retractions, and a maternal history of chorioamnionitis. An anteroposterior chest x-ray is immediately obtained and reveals generalized opacity. The nurse should anticipate that the infant is afflicted with which of the following conditions?

   A. Surfactant deficiency
   B. Congenital diaphragmatic hernia
   C. Pneumonia
   D. Bronchopulmonary dysplasia

5. An abdominal x-ray finding reveals a double bubble. The nurse should anticipate this finding to be indicative of which condition?
   A. Colonic obstruction
   B. Meconium ileus
   C. Pneumoperitoneum
   D. Duodenal atresia

6. An infant has an x-ray taken after intubation. The nurse should anticipate which of the following reflect the proper placement of the endotracheal tube?
   A. One centimeter below the carina
   B. Midway between the thoracic inlet and carina
   C. At the level of the clavicles
   D. The fifth thoracic vertebrae

7. An infant undergoes placement of an umbilical arterial catheter. The nurse should anticipate which of the following reflect proper placement for a high-lying catheter per chest/abdominal x-ray?
   A. Thoracic vertebrae 3–4
   B. Thoracic vertebrae 6–9
   C. Lumbar vertebrae 1–3
   D. Thoracic vertebrae 11–12

8. A premature infant has an umbilical venous catheter placed upon admission to the NICU until a percutaneously inserted central line can be inserted. The nurse should be aware that the proper radiologic placement is at which of the following locations?
   A. In close proximity to the foramen ovale
   B. Just below the junction of the inferior vena cava and right atrium
   C. At the junction of the superior vena cava and right atrium
   D. In the portion of the inferior vena cava located below the diaphragm

ANSWERS AND RATIONALES

1. **(A)** Hypoexpansion due to atelectasis, air bronchograms from atelectasis of the alveoli interspersed with open airways and a reticulogranular pattern, and open alveoli interspersed with atelectatic alveoli are the classic findings of surfactant deficiency. Hyperexpansion does not occur with surfactant deficiency. Fluid in the fissures is common in transient tachypnea of the newborn because there is a delay in the clearance of lung fluid after birth. Bilateral streakiness is found with pneumonia related to the infectious processes. The sail sign is a common finding with pneumomediastinum and reflects elevation of the thymus gland from the free air.

References: Trotter C. Radiologic evaluation. In: Verklan MT, Walden M and Forest S, eds. *Core Curriculum for Neonatal Intensive Care Nursing*. St. Louis, MO: Elsevier; 2021:223-225.

Weinert DM, Martinez-Rios C. Diagnostic imaging of the neonate. In: *Fanaroff & Martin's Neonatal-Perinatal Medicine Diseases of the Fetus and Infant*. 10th ed., vol. 1. Philadelphia, PA: Elsevier Saunders; 2015:537-539.

Weinman JP, Bronsert BM, Strain JD. Diagnostic imaging in the neonate. In: Gardner S, Carter B, Enzman-Hines M, Niermeyer S, eds. *Merenstein & Gardner's Handbook of Neonatal Intensive Care: An Interprofessional Approach*. 9th ed. St. Louis, MO: Elsevier; 2021:201-202 [essay].

2. **(A)** A tension pneumothorax on the left will shift the mediastinum to the right, moving the point of maximal impulse (PMI) to the right. Levocardia is the normal position of the heart, which places the PMI to the left of the sternum. A pleural effusion on the right would push the mediastinal structures to the left, pushing the PMI to the left. Atelectasis on the left would pull the mediastinal structures to the left; this would position the PMI further to the left.

References: Trotter C. Radiologic evaluation. In: Verklan MT, Walden M and Forest S, eds. *Core Curriculum for Neonatal Intensive Care Nursing*. St. Louis, MO: Elsevier; 2021:226.

Gardner S, Niermeyer S. Immediate newborn care after birth. In: Gardner S, Carter B, Enzman-Hines M, Niermeyer S, eds. *Merenstein & Gardner's Handbook of Neonatal Intensive Care: An Interprofessional Approach*. 9th ed. St. Louis, MO: Elsevier; 2021:117 [essay].

3. **(C)** Anterior–posterior (A/P) abdomen and cross-table lateral films will determine the presence of free air, given the concern for pneumoperitoneum per the clinical examination. Because free air rises, the cross-table lateral has the capability of showing free air positioned just under the abdominal wall. Although a lateral decubitus film will also reveal free air, it requires a high level of skill to position the infant properly. An A/P chest x-ray will reveal pathology of the lungs, not the abdomen. An A/P abdominal film is helpful but may not confirm the presence of free air due to the angle of penetration.

References: Trotter C. Radiologic evaluation. In: Verklan MT, Walden M and Forest S, eds. *Core Curriculum for Neonatal Intensive Care Nursing*. St. Louis, MO: Elsevier; 2021:220.

Weinman JP, Bronsert BM, Strain JD. Diagnostic imaging in the neonate. In: Gardner S, Carter B, Enzman-Hines M, Niermeyer S, eds. *Merenstein & Gardner's Handbook of Neonatal Intensive Care: An Interprofessional Approach*. 9th ed. St. Louis, MO: Elsevier; 2021:201-202 [essay].

4. **(C)** Given the history of maternal chorioamnionitis and the opacity of the film, pneumonia would be the most likely scenario. Surfactant deficiency would reflect a reticulogranular pattern with air bronchograms on the x-ray. The film for an infant with congenital diaphragmatic hernia would reveal bowel in the chest with a shifted mediastinum. In contrast, the film for an infant with bronchopulmonary dysplasia would show cystic changes of the lung.

References: Gardner S, Enzman-Hines M, Nyp M. Respiratory diseases. In: Gardner S, Carter B, Enzman-Hines M, Niermeyer S, eds. *Merenstein & Gardner's Handbook of Neonatal Intensive Care: An Interprofessional Approach*. 9th ed. St. Louis, MO: Elsevier; 2021:729-731 [essay].

Trotter C. Radiologic evaluation. In: Verklan MT, Walden M and Forest S, eds. *Core Curriculum for Neonatal Intensive Care Nursing*. St. Louis, MO: Elsevier; 2021:222-225.

5. **(D)** Duodenal atresia is classically seen radiologically as a double bubble as air in the stomach presents as the first bubble and the dilated duodenum filled with air is the second bubble. Colonic obstruction and meconium ileus reflect multiple dilated loops of bowel per abdominal x-ray. Pneumoperitoneum is a large, single, dark area of free air on abdominal x-ray.

References: Trotter C. Radiologic evaluation. In: Verklan MT, Walden M and Forest S, eds. *Core Curriculum for Neonatal Intensive Care Nursing*. St. Louis, MO: Elsevier; 2021:234-235.

Eklund MJ, Hill JG, Swift CC. In: Bissinger R, Eklund M. eds. *Neonatal Imaging*. 1st ed. The National Certification Corporation; Chicago; 2018:122-126.

6. **(B)** Proper placement on an endotracheal tube is midway between the thoracic inlet and the carina. Placement 1 cm below the carina or at the fifth thoracic vertebrae would result in a right mainstem bronchial placement. Placement at the level of the clavicles is too high and places the infant at risk for self-extubation.

References: Trotter C. Radiologic evaluation. In: Verklan MT, Walden M and Forest S, eds. *Core Curriculum for Neonatal Intensive Care Nursing*. St. Louis, MO: Elsevier; 2021:238.

Eklund MJ, Hill JG, Swift CC. In: Bissinger R, Eklund M. eds. *Neonatal Imaging*. 1st ed. The National Certification Corporation; 2018:21.

7. **(B)** Accurate high umbilical arterial catheter placement is between thoracic vertebrae 6 and 9. Low placement is between lumbar vertebrae 3 and 4. Placing the catheter at thoracic vertebrae 3–4, 11–12, and lumbar vertebrae 1–3 will avoid the areas of the celiac, mesenteric, and renal arteries.

References: Trotter C. Radiologic evaluation. In: Verklan MT, Walden M and Forest S, eds. *Core Curriculum for Neonatal Intensive Care Nursing*. St. Louis, MO: Elsevier; 2021:238.

Eklund MJ, Hill JG, Swift CC. In: Bissinger R, Eklund M. eds. *Neonatal Imaging*. 1st ed. The National Certification Corporation; 2018:100-106.

8. **(B)** An umbilical venous catheter should not be placed within the structure of the heart. The foramen ovale is located between the right and left atria, and this catheter location could lead to perforation and cardiac tamponade. A properly placed umbilical venous catheter is located just below the junction of the inferior vena cava and right atrium. An umbilical venous catheter should not be located in the superior vena cava. This location would reflect a catheter that was placed too deep and has the possibility of migrating into the right atrium. An umbilical venous catheter should not be located below the diaphragm for long-term placement. In an emergency situation, the Umbilical venous catheter (UVC) may be inserted a few centimeters until blood return is obtained but should not be left in that position for long-term administration of fluids or medications.

Reference: Trotter C. Radiologic evaluation. In: Verklan MT, Walden M and Forest S, eds *Core Curriculum for Neonatal Intensive Care Nursing*. St. Louis, MO: Elsevier; 2021:239.

Chapter 11

Pharmacology

1. An infant needs to rapidly achieve a therapeutic plasma drug concentration of a medication. Rather than wait for a plateau level (steady state) to be achieved, the care provider will order a:
   A. loading dose.
   B. maintenance dose.
   C. medication with no first-pass effect.
   D. medication with rapid cell entry properties.

2. The potassium-sparing diuretic spironolactone (Aldactone) is not useful in emergency situations such as florid pulmonary edema because:
   A. there is risk of an allergic reaction to the drug.
   B. the onset of action is approximately 48 hours.
   C. the intravenous form of the drug is highly caustic to veins.
   D. more than one dose results in hypokalemia and cardiac dysrhythmias.

3. An infant has liver disease and is receiving a drug that is highly metabolized by the liver. To achieve the desired pharmacodynamic response to the drug, the nurse would expect the drug's dose to be:
   A. higher than the standard dose.
   B. lower than the standard dose.
   C. the same as the standard dose.
   D. the same as the standard dose but given more frequently.

4. Which of the following determines dosing interval of a medication?
   A. Half-life
   B. Drug distribution
   C. Steady state
   D. Minimum effective concentration

5. An infant is receiving vancomycin for methicillin-resistant *Staphylococcus aureus (MRSA)*. The vancomycin trough level is 12 mcg/mL. What does this indicate to the nurse?
   A. The drug will cause no toxicities or adverse effects.
   B. The dose will not need to be changed for the duration of treatment.
   C. The dosing interval should be lengthened.
   D. The nurse will need to continue monitoring for desired, adverse, and toxic effects.

6. A provider orders a trough level of a medication. The nurse knows to draw the specimen:
   A. just before a dose.
   B. an hour after administering the drug dose.
   C. at any time after a dose.
   D. at the midpoint between two doses.

7. The lactation consultant is visiting the mother of a 35-week gestation infant. The mother states she is exclusively breastfeeding and has a urinary tract infection. The mother has questions about taking antibiotics while breastfeeding. The lactation consultant informs the mother some antimicrobial drugs are contraindicated for mothers when breastfeeding a premature neonate. A class of antimicrobial drugs contraindicated with breastfeeding a preterm infant is:
   A. aminoglycosides.
   B. cephalosporins.
   C. penicillins.
   D. sulfonamides.

8. Intravenous is the best route of administration in the neonatal population because:
   A. the ratio of body surface area in the neonate is higher than the body surface area of the adult.
   B. intravenously administered medications bypass many absorptive barriers.
   C. intramuscularly and subcutaneously administered medications are absorbed too rapidly.
   D. intravenously administered medications do not have to cross cell membranes to be absorbed.

9. An infant receiving a standard dose of caffeine for apnea of prematurity who continues to have apneic episodes is exhibiting which of the following responses to the medication?
   A. Desired effect
   B. Subtherapeutic effect
   C. Side effect
   D. Toxic effect

10. Drug distribution relies on many factors including which of the following?
    A. Half-life
    B. Drug interactions
    C. Plateau (steady-state) drug level
    D. Vascular perfusion of the tissue or organ

11. While precepting a new nurse in the neonatal intensive care unit (NICU), the preceptor includes which of the following statements when teaching about immunizations?
    A. Most immunizations are given starting at 1 month of age.
    B. The preferred site of administration is the deltoid area of the upper arm.
    C. Live virus vaccines are preferred over inactivated vaccines for infants being cared for in the NICU.
    D. Vaccines should be held when the neonate is on pressor agents.

ANSWERS AND RATIONALES

1. **(A)** A loading or priming dose rapidly establishes a therapeutic plasma drug level. It is calculated by multiplying the volume of distribution by the desired plasma drug concentration. The loading dose establishes a desired level. Maintenance dosing is

initiated after the loading dose to maintain the therapeutic level. The maintenance dose is smaller than the loading dose. With the first-pass effect, the medication enters hepatic metabolism before entering the circulation. The amount of drug available afterward may be significantly reduced. A medication without the first-pass effect will achieve a higher plasma concentration but will not reach a therapeutic level until multiple doses have been administered. The ability of a medication to enter the cell does not influence the therapeutic plasma concentration.

Reference: Ku L, Hornik C, Buschbach D. Pharmacology in neonatal care. In: Gardner SL, Carter BS, Enzman-Hines MI, Niermeyer S, eds. *Merenstein & Gardner's Handbook of Neonatal Intensive Care: An Interprofessional Approach.* 9th ed. St. Louis, MO: Elsevier; 2021:229-232.

2. **(B)** Spironolactone is an aldosterone antagonist and mild diuretic with a slow onset of action, taking up to 48 hours to take effect. This agent would be of limited value in acute pulmonary edema. Although allergic reactions can occur with any drug, the probability of an allergic reaction to spironolactone is small. Spironolactone is a steroid derivative and does not contain a sulfa ring as do loop and thiazide diuretics. Spironolactone is not available in intravenous form. Spironolactone prevents sodium reabsorption in the distal nephron and allows potassium reabsorption. Serum potassium levels therefore may rise with spironolactone use. Hence, the term *potassium sparing* is used when describing this drug's action.

Reference: Burchum JR, Rosenthal LD. *Lehne's Pharmacology for Nursing Care.* 11th ed. St. Louis, MO: Elsevier; 2022:460.

3. **(B)** Most drugs are metabolized into inactive metabolites. Until the drug is metabolized, the effects of the parent drug are ongoing. Drug metabolism, which occurs primarily in the liver, is impeded in the presence of hepatic disease. To prevent drug toxicity, a smaller than standard dose is expected. In the presence of liver disease, providing a standard dose, higher than standard dose, or more frequent dosing of a standard dose of a drug metabolized by the liver may result in toxic drug levels.

Reference: Domonoske CD. Pharmacology. In: Verklan MT, Walden M, Forest S, eds. *Core Curriculum for Neonatal Intensive Care Nursing.* 6th ed. St. Louis, MO: Elsevier; 2021:198, 201.

4. **(A)** Half-life is the time required for the amount of a drug to decline to half its original concentration. The half-life determines the dosing interval. Drugs with a short half-life must be given more frequently than drugs with a long half-life. Drug distribution refers to the movement of drugs through various body compartments after they are absorbed or injected. The volume of distribution is used to estimate a loading dose. Steady state refers to the state of equilibrium obtained when a drug is administered repeatedly at the same dose. Steady state is achieved after four to five half-lives. Minimum effective concentration (MEC) is defined as the minimum plasma drug level needed to achieve the desired therapeutic effects. Drugs must be present in concentrations greater than the MEC to be effective. Medications given as multiple doses over an extended period should be administered before the drug plasma level falls below the MEC; however, the MEC does not determine the dosing interval.

References: Adams MP, Urban CQ, Sutter RE. *Pharmacology: Connections to Nursing Practice.* 5th ed. Hoboken, NJ: Pearson; 2022:26-44.

Burchum JR, Rosenthal LD. *Lehne's Pharmacology for Nursing Care.* 11th ed. St. Louis, MO: Elsevier; 2022:24-43.

Domonoske CD. Pharmacology. In: Verklan MT, Walden M, Forest S, eds. Core Curriculum for Neonatal Intensive Care Nursing. 6th ed. St. Louis, MO: Elsevier; 2021:191-196.

Ku L, Hornik C, Buschbach D. Pharmacology in neonatal care. In: Gardner SL, Carter BS, Enzman-Hines MI, Niermeyer S, eds. *Merenstein & Gardner's Handbook of Neonatal Intensive Care: An Interprofessional Approach.* 9th ed. St. Louis, MO: Elsevier; 2021:230.

5. **(D)** The therapeutic range of a drug indicates that the drug is above the MEC but below the toxic level. A trough level represents the lowest concentration of a drug in the bloodstream and is obtained at the end of a dosing interval, that is, just before a dose. The goal vancomycin trough level is 10–15 mcg/mL. Individual patient response to drugs can be highly variable. Side effects, toxicities, or even no effect may occur at levels within therapeutic range. For this reason, and although the trough level is in the goal range, the nurse should continue to monitor for desired, adverse, and toxic effects. The dose may need to be adjusted during treatment. Lengthening the dosing interval could result in the trough level dropping below the minimum therapeutic range.

References: Adams MP, Urban CQ, Sutter RE. *Pharmacology: Connections to Nursing Practice.* 5th ed. Hoboken, NJ: Pearson; 2022:39-43.

Burchum JR, Rosenthal LD. *Lehne's Pharmacology for Nursing Care.* 11th ed. St. Louis, MO: Elsevier; 2022:39-41.

Gomella TL, Eyal FG, Bany-Mohammed F. *Gomella's Neonatology: Management, Procedures, On-Call Problems, Disease, and Drugs.* 8th ed. New York: McGraw-Hill Education; 2020:1311-1312.

6. **(A)** When a drug is given repeatedly, its concentration in blood fluctuates between doses. The interval between drug administration and serum sampling is determined by the pharmacokinetics and pharmacodynamics of the drug. A trough level represents the lowest concentration of a drug in the bloodstream and is obtained at the end of a dosing interval, that is, just before a dose. A peak level represents the highest concentration of a drug in the bloodstream and is obtained after a dose has been given. A random level is drawn at any time after a dose is given. A random level could be drawn at a midpoint between two doses, but this level reflects neither the highest (peak) nor lowest (trough) concentration of a drug in the bloodstream.

Reference: Domonoske CD. Pharmacology. In: Verklan MT, Walden M, Forest S, eds. *Core Curriculum for Neonatal Intensive Care Nursing.* 6th ed. St. Louis, MO: Elsevier; 2021:192.

7. **(D)** In general, drugs administered to a breastfeeding woman enter breast milk by passive diffusion. Most antimicrobials are safe for nursing infants. However, sulfonamides are contraindicated in breastfeeding mothers especially with preterm, ill, or stressed infants or infants with glucose-6-phosphate dehydrogenase deficiency. Sulfonamides compete with bilirubin for binding to serum albumin, allowing for free bilirubin levels to rise. Aminoglycosides, cephalosporins, and penicillins are all used in the neonatal population and are safe for the breastfeeding infant.

Reference: McClary JD. Principles of drug use during lactation. In: Martin RJ, Fanaroff AA, Walsh MC, eds. *Fanaroff and Martin's Neonatal-Perinatal Medicine: Diseases of the Fetus and Infant.* 11th ed. Philadelphia, PA: Elsevier; 2019:717.

8. **(B)** Intravenously administered medications bypass many absorptive barriers, such as the skin, gastrointestinal tract, lungs, muscle, and subcutaneous tissue. It is the most effective method of medication administration because the drug is delivered directly into the bloodstream. The ratio of body surface area in the neonate is greater than that of the adult, which provides a greater absorption rate for medications administered topically and percutaneously. Minimal subcutaneous tissue and muscle mass in the neonate significantly limit absorption of medications, especially in the low-birth-weight neonate. Regardless of the route of medication administration for the neonate, most all medications must cross the cell membrane to be absorbed.

Reference: Domonoske CD. Pharmacology. In: Verklan MT, Walden M, Forest S, eds. *Core Curriculum for Neonatal Intensive Care Nursing.* 6th ed. St. Louis, MO: Elsevier; 2021:196.

9. **(B)** A subtherapeutic effect occurs when the effects of a medication are less than the desired outcome of the medication. The desired effect of caffeine therapy is reduced apneic episodes, which has not been achieved in this scenario. A desired effect occurs when the

desired outcome of the medication is achieved. Side effects are in addition to the desired effects. Side effects of caffeine include tachycardia, increased wakefulness, gastrointestinal distension, gastrointestinal bleeding, and diuresis. Toxic effects result from a medication overdose or unexpected high serum levels of the medication. Toxic effects of caffeine include cardiac dysrhythmias and seizures.

References: Adams MP, Urban CQ, Sutter RE. *Pharmacology: Connections to Nursing Practice.* 5th ed. Hoboken, NJ: Pearson; 2022:383.

Churchman L. Apnea. In: Verklan MT, Walden M, Forest S, eds. *Core Curriculum for Neonatal Intensive Care Nursing.* 6th ed. St. Louis, MO: Elsevier; 2021:422.

Domonoske CD. Pharmacology. In: Verklan MT, Walden M, Forest S, eds. *Core Curriculum for Neonatal Intensive Care Nursing.* 6th ed. St. Louis, MO: Elsevier; 2021:192.

10. **(D)** Drug distribution refers to the movement of drugs through various body compartments after they are absorbed or injected. Drug distribution is determined by blood flow to tissues, the ability of a drug to exit the vascular system, and the ability of the drug to enter cells. Organ size, amount of drug transporters, and drug permeability also all play a role in drug distribution. Half-life refers to the time required for the level of a drug in the body to decrease by 50%. Half-life is a percentage, not a specific amount. Half-life determines the dosing interval of a drug. Drug interactions can affect the amount of a medication in circulation and may reduce the amount of medication available for distribution. A plateau or steady state refers to the state of equilibrium obtained when a drug is administered repeatedly at the same dose. Steady state is achieved after four to five half-lives.

References: Adams MP, Urban CQ, Sutter RE. *Pharmacology: Connections to Nursing Practice.* 5th ed. Hoboken, NJ: Pearson; 2022:34.

Burchum JR, Rosenthal LD. *Lehne's Pharmacology for Nursing Care.* 11th ed. St. Louis, MO: Elsevier; 2022:33, 40.

Ku L, Hornik C, Buschbach D. Pharmacology in neonatal care. In: Gardner SL, Carter BS, Enzman-Hines MI, Niermeyer S, eds. *Merenstein & Gardner's Handbook of Neonatal Intensive Care: An Interprofessional Approach.* 9th ed. St. Louis, MO: Elsevier; 2021:230.

11. **(D)** Because vasopressors may reduce blood flow to muscle and subcutaneous tissues, vaccines should be held when the neonate is on pressure agents. Most immunizations are given starting at 2 months of age. An exception is the first-dose hepatitis B vaccine which is recommended to be given at birth depending on birth weight and maternal hepatitis B surface antigen status. The preferred site of administration is the anterolateral aspect of the upper thigh. The deltoid is used in children over 1 year of age. Live virus vaccines should not be administered in the neonatal intensive care unit due to concerns of virus transmission.

References: American Academy of Pediatrics (AAP), The American College of Obstetricians and Gynecologists (ACOG). Perinatal infections. In: Kilpatrick SJ, Papile L, eds. *Guidelines for Perinatal Care.* 8th ed. Elk Grove Village, IL: AAP; 2017:380.

Domonoske CD. Pharmacology. In: Verklan MT, Walden M, Forest S, eds. *Core Curriculum for Neonatal Intensive Care Nursing.* 6th ed. St. Louis, MO: Elsevier; 2021:205.

Chapter 12

Care of the Extremely Low-Birth-Weight Infant

1. The nurse is expecting the delivery of an infant at 24 weeks postconceptional age, with an estimated fetal weight of 800 g. Which of the following elements of the delivery room setup is most specifically geared toward the extremely low-birth-weight infant?
   A. Prewarmed radiant warmer
   B. Polyethylene bag/wrap
   C. Prewarmed blankets
   D. Stockinet hat

2. The nurse is expecting the delivery of a 24-week postconceptional age infant with an estimated fetal weight of 800 g. At delivery, the infant is noted to be apneic. The attending physician intubates and orders the nurse to deliver positive pressure ventilation with a fraction of inspired oxygen (FiO_2) of 0.30 while the respiratory care practitioner applies the oxygen saturation monitor. Based on the patient-specific data, which of the following is the most accurate interpretation of this order?
   A. This is an inappropriate order because blended oxygen is not available in the delivery room.
   B. This is an appropriate order because even brief hyperoxia can result in negative sequelae in the extremely low-birth-weight infant.
   C. This is an inappropriate order because apneic infants all require resuscitation with 100% oxygen until their condition is stabilized.
   D. This is an inappropriate order because apneic infants must be resuscitated with 100% oxygen until pulse oximetry indicates that their oxygen saturation is greater than 98%.

3. The registered nurse (RN) is using a hybrid warmer to manage the thermal needs of a 750-g infant born yesterday at 24 weeks postconceptional age. When considering optimal thermal support for this infant, the RN understands that this is best accomplished by:
   A. using a humidity setting of greater than 70% while maintaining the device in the radiant warmer mode.
   B. using a humidity setting of greater than 50% while maintaining the device in the radiant warmer mode.
   C. using a humidity setting of greater than 70% while maintaining the device in the incubator mode.
   D. using a humidity setting of greater than 50% while maintaining the device in the incubator mode.

4. The RN is caring for a stable 2-day-old infant born at 27 weeks postconceptional age with a birthweight of 900 g. The nurse identifies which of the following as the best approach to initiating feedings for most patients with this clinical profile?
   A. Starting feedings as soon as possible with small volumes of probiotic supplements.
   B. Starting feedings as soon as possible with small volumes of colostrum or human milk.
   C. Maintaining nothing-by-mouth status for the first week of life.
   D. Starting feedings as soon as possible with full-strength premature formula.

5. The RN is caring for a stable 2-day-old infant born at 27 weeks postconceptional age. The infant is receiving nasal continuous positive airway pressure and trophic feedings. The RN

understands that which of the following represents appropriate, routine care for this infant?

A. Use of an orogastric Replogle tube set to low, continuous suction

B. Use of a vented indwelling orogastric feeding tube, capped between feedings

C. Use of a vented indwelling orogastric feeding tube

D. Use of an in-and-out orogastric feeding tube for feedings (no indwelling orogastric tube is maintained)

6. The RN is caring for an infant born the previous shift at 25 weeks' gestation. Although the infant has spontaneous respiratory effort, the RN understands this infant is extremely high risk for the diagnosis of apnea of prematurity, and that appropriate routine care would be to:

A. recognize the treatment of apnea of prematurity at this stage requires intubation and mechanical ventilation.

B. recognize aminophylline should be ordered in the first 3 days of life.

C. recognize caffeine citrate should be ordered in the first 3 days of life.

D. recognize apnea and, once symptoms manifest, notify the provider.

ANSWERS AND RATIONALES

1. **(B)** Polyethylene bags or wraps are specifically indicated for the extremely low–birth-weight (ELBW) infant at delivery because of the potential for extreme evaporative thermal losses due to transdermal water loss. Evaporative heat loss is the most common form of heat loss for the ELBW neonate. Use of a prewarmed warmer and prewarmed blankets is recommended for all newborns after delivery. Stockinet hats have not been found to be sufficiently efficacious in maintaining thermal stability. A plastic or wool cap has been shown to provide superior benefits.

References: Abiramalatha T, Ramaswamy VV, Bandyopadhyay T, et al. Delivery room interventions for hypothermia in preterm neonates: a systematic review and network meta-analysis. *JAMA Pediatr.* 2021;175(9):e210775. doi:10.1001/jamapediatrics.2021.0775.

Aziz K, Lee HC, Escobedo MB, et al. Part 5: neonatal resuscitation: 2020 American Heart Association guidelines for cardiopulmonary resuscitation and emergency cardiovascular care. *Circulation.* 2020;142(suppl 2): S524-S550.

Bissenger R, Annibale D, Fanning BA. *Golden Hours: Care of the Very Low Birth Weight Neonate.* 2nd ed. Chicago, IL: National Certification Corporation; 2019.

Forest S. Care of the extremely low birth weight infant. In: Verklan T, Walden M, Forest S, eds. *Core Curriculum for Neonatal Intensive Care Nursing.* 6th ed. St. Louis, MO: Elsevier; 2021:380.

Pappas BE, Robey DL. Neonatal delivery room resuscitation. In: Verklan T, Walden M, Forest S, eds. *Core Curriculum for Neonatal Intensive Care Nursing.* 6th ed. St. Louis, MO: Elsevier; 2021:69-85.

2. **(B)** Blended oxygen is recommended in the delivery room. It is expected that a newborn of this gestational age will need supplemental oxygen for resuscitation, but hyperoxia is to be avoided to avoid negative sequelae and oxygen should be titrated based upon pulse oximeter targets. The Neonatal Resuscitation Program recommends an initial oxygen concentration of 0.21-**0.3** for positive pressure ventilation in newborns less than 35 weeks gestation. A target SpO_2 of 98% is too high for a newborn of this gestational age who is receiving oxygen.

References: Aziz K, Lee HC, Escobedo MB, et al. Part 5: neonatal resuscitation: 2020 American Heart Association guidelines for cardiopulmonary

resuscitation and emergency cardiovascular care. *Circulation.* 2020;142(suppl 2): S524-S550.

Bissenger R, Annibale D, Fanning BA. *Golden Hours: Care of the Very Low Birth Weight Neonate.* 2nd ed. Chicago, IL: National Certification Corporation; 2019.

Madar J, Roehr CC, Ainsworth S, et al. European Resuscitation Council guidelines 2021: newborn resuscitation and support of transition of infants at birth. *Resuscitation.* 2021;161:291-326.

Weiner GM, Zaichkin J, eds. *Textbook of Neonatal Resuscitation.* 8th ed. Itasca, IL: American Academy of Pediatrics, American Heart Association; 2021.

Sweet DG, Carnierlli V, Greisen G, et al. European consensus guidelines on the management of respiratory distress syndrome – 2019 update. *Neonatology.* 2019;115(4):432-450.

Thakre R. Highlights of newborn resuscitation science, 2020. *J Neonatol.* 2021;35(1):24-28.

Welsford M, Nishiyama C, Shortt C, et al. Initial oxygen use for preterm newborn resuscitation: a systematic review with meta analysis. *Pediatrics.* 2019;143(1):e20181828. doi:10.1542/peds.2018-1828.

3. **(C)** Use of humidity greater than 70% is recommended for initial care of the ELBW infant. If the device is in the radiant warmer mode, humidity will be lost. Only with the device in the incubator mode can the set humidity be retained.

References: Bissenger R, Annibale D, Fanning BA. *Golden Hours: Care of the Very Low Birth Weight Neonate.* 2nd ed. Chicago, IL: National Certification Corporation; 2019.

Dixon KL, Carter B, Harriman T, Doles B, Sitton B, Thompson J. Neonatal thermoregulation: a golden hour protocol update. *Adv Neonatal Care.* 2021;21(4):280-288.

Glass L, Valdez A. Preterm infant incubator humidity levels: a systematic review. *Adv Neonatal Care.* 2021;21(4):297-307.

4. **(B)** Small-volume feedings (trophic feeds) of colostrum/human milk are recommended in the first 1–2 days of life to stimulate normal development of the bowel, facilitate growth, and support the neonatal gut microbiome. The safety and the efficacy of probiotic supplements are not yet fully established for this population and the American Academy of Pediatrics does not recommend for infants with a birth weight less than 1000 g. Delaying feedings in the stable patient may lead to bowel atrophy and prolong the need for total parental nutrition and central venous access.

References: Cerasani J, Ceroni F, De Cosmi V, et al. Human milk feeding and preterm infants' growth and body composition: a literature review. *Nutrients.* 2020;12(4):1155. doi:10.3390/nu12041155.

Committee on Nutrition, Section on Breastfeeding, Committee on Fetus and Newborn, Collaborators: Daniels S, Corkins M, de Ferranti S, et al. Donor human milk for the high-risk infant: preparation, safety, and usage options in the United States. *Pediatrics.* 2017;139(1):e20163440. doi:10.1542/peds.2016-3440.

Pannaraj PS, Li F, Cerini C, et al. Association between breast milk bacterial communities and establishment and development of the infant gut microbiome. *JAMA Pediatr.* 2017;171(7):647-654.

Poindexter B, AAP Committee on Fetus and Newborn. Use of probiotics in preterm infants. *Pediatrics.* 2021;147(6):e2021051485. doi:10.1542/peds.2021-051485.

Wight N, Kim J, Rhine W, et al. *Nutritional Support of the Very Low Birth Weight (VLBW) Infant: A Quality Improvement Toolkit.* Stanford, CA: California Perinatal Quality Care Collaborative; 2018.

5. **(C)** Although the use of a vented orogastric tube in the setting of providing feedings may be a challenge, it is crucial to provide venting of the air that enters the gastric space to prevent gastric distension from nasal continuous positive airway pressure. Capping the orogastric tube between feedings may lead to abdominal distention due to accumulation of air in the gastrointestinal tract. Use of suction is contraindicated in the setting of enteral feedings. Repeated placement of an in-and-out orogastric feeding tube is contraindicated due to noxious stimulation and pain which may compromise the infant's neurodevelopmental status.

References: Fernandes N, Chawla S. Mechanical ventilation for neonates. In: Sarnaik AP, Venkataraman ST, Kuch BA, eds. *Mechanical Ventilation in Neonates and Children.* Cham, Switzerland: Springer; 2022:129-155.

Leibel SL, Castro M, McBride T, et al. Comparison of continuous positive airway pressure versus high flow nasal cannula for oral feeding preterm infants (CHOmP): randomized pilot study. *J Matern Fetal Neonatal Med.* 2022;35(5):951-957.

6. **(C)** Nearly all ELBW infants are diagnosed with apnea of prematurity and the current recommendations for the infant with spontaneous respiratory effort are to support with continuous positive airway pressure (CPAP) as needed and initiate caffeine therapy before 3 days of life. Caffeine is preferred over aminophylline as it has a longer half-life so it can be dosed daily and does not require checking drug levels.

References: Eichenwald EC, Committee on Fetus and Newborn. Apnea of prematurity. *Pediatrics.* 2016;137(1). doi:10.1542/peds.2015-3757.

Jensen EA. Prevention of bronchopulmonary dysplasia: a summary of evidence-based strategies. *NeoReviews.* 2019;20(4):e189-e201.

Churchman L. Apnea. In: Verklan MT, Walden M, Forest S, eds. *Core Curriculum for Neonatal Intensive Care Nursing.* 6th ed. St. Louis, MO: Elsevier; 2021:417-424.

Shenk EE, Bondi DS, Pellerite MM, Sriram S. Evaluation of timing and dosing of caffeine citrate in preterm neonates for the prevention of bronchopulmonary dysplasia. *J Pediatr Pharmacol Ther.* 2018;23(2):139-145.

Chapter 13

Care of the Late Preterm Infant

1. Which of the following states contributes to hyperbilirubinemia in late preterm infants?
   A. Poor coordination of sucking and swallowing leading to dehydration
   B. Increase in hepatic update and conjugation
   C. Decrease in enterohepatic circulation
   D. Increased activity of hepatic uridine diphosphate glucuronyltransferase enzyme

2. A 35 2/7-week infant of a diabetic mother was delivered vaginally, weighing 3.5 kg. Rupture of membranes occurred 8 hours prior to delivery. Fluid was clear and nonodorous. Fetal monitoring strip revealed occasional variable decelerations with moderate variability. Immediately after birth, the infant demonstrated tachypnea, grunting, retractions, and cyanosis. Continuous positive airway pressure was provided in the delivery room. Upon admission into the neonatal intensive care unit (NICU), the initial arterial blood gas revealed a combined respiratory and metabolic acidosis with hypoxia. Initial chest x-ray revealed a reticulogranular pattern. Admission vital signs: heart rate 155 beats per minute; respiratory rate 68 breaths per minute; peripheral blood pressure 62/42 mm Hg; pre- and postductal oxygen saturations 88%. Which of the following differential diagnoses most likely reflects this presentation?
   A. Persistent pulmonary hypertension (PPHN) of the newborn
   B. Pneumonia
   C. Respiratory distress syndrome
   D. Transient tachypnea of the newborn

3. A 36-week-gestation infant has been stable and cared for on the mother/baby unit. Discharge criteria of a late preterm infant include which of the following?
   A. Weight loss not greater than 12%
   B. Twenty-four hours of successful oral feeding
   C. Follow-up appointments made for metabolic and hearing screening
   D. Older than 24 hours of age

4. What is the most common cause of rehospitalization of the late preterm infant between 6 and 12 months of life?
   A. Hyperbilirubinemia
   B. Early-onset sepsis
   C. Apnea
   D. Respiratory illnesses

5. A 35 3/7-week-gestational-age infant is placed on the mother's chest after a vaginal delivery and covered with a warm blanket. Apgars are 8 and 9 at 1 and 5 minutes of life, respectively. Axillary skin temperature at 1 hour of age is 35.1°C (95.2°F). What is the most likely cause of hypothermia in the late preterm infant during the transition period?
   A. Low metabolic rate
   B. Large temperature gradient between the environment and the neonate
   C. Decreased surface area
   D. Decreased brown fat utilization

6. What are the common contributing factors that predispose a late preterm infant to hypoglycemia?
   A. Increased glycogen stores and increased glucose utilization
   B. Decreased glycogen stores and decreased glucose utilization
   C. Decreased glycogen stores and increased glucose utilization
   D. Increased glycogen stores and decreased glucose utilization

7. Identify the potential long-term sequelae of a preterm infant delivered at 35 1/7 weeks gestation:
   A. Improved school performance at 6 years of age
   B. Increased risk for cerebral palsy
   C. Increased risk for seizures
   D. Decreased health care utilization during the first 5 years of life

8. A 35 3/7-week newborn exclusively breastfeeding in couplet care with a first-time mother has a bilirubin level of 5.4 at 24 hours of age, which is low/intermediate risk. Maternal and infant blood type is O+. Follow-up bilirubin levels remain below phototherapy requirements during initial hospitalization. Which of the following factors is most likely to prompt a readmission related to hyperbilirubinemia?
   A. Late preterm infant's often have more feeding difficulties predisposing them to dehydration leading to hyperbilirubinemia.
   B. Late preterm infants have the same success rate with oral feeding as term infants.

C. Early follow-up is not recommended for this population.

D. Late preterm infants are less likely to have hyperbilirubinemia secondary to accelerated maturation and increased concentration of uridine diphosphoglucuronate glucuronosyltransferase.

9. The NICU team attends the delivery of a late preterm infant born at 34 5/7 weeks. At 10 minutes of life, the team observed grunting, flaring, and subcostal retractions. The infant is treated with continuous positive airway pressure (CPAP) and transferred to the NICU for further care. Which of the following is most accurate about the effects of CPAP in this late preterm infant?
   A. Limits gas exchange
   B. Decreases lung compliance
   C. Increases total airway resistance
   D. Increases functional residual capacity

10. The nurse should understand that infants born between which weeks of pregnancy are considered to be late preterm?
   A. 33 0/7–36 6/7 weeks
   B. 34 0/7–36 6/7 weeks
   C. 35 0/7–37 6/7 weeks
   D. 33 6/7–37 6/7 weeks

11. During the first month of life late preterm newborns are more likely to be readmitted to the hospital for which reason?
   A. Hyperbilirubinemia
   B. Malrotation
   C. Congenital heart disease
   D. Inborn error of metabolism

12. A nurse is caring for a preterm newborn at 35 6/7 weeks gestation. When educating the mother on feeding, the nurse should emphasize which of the following regarding late preterm infants?
   A. They are at decreased risk for feeding difficulties secondary to increased oromotor tone.
   B. They are at risk for increased feeding difficulties secondary to decreased oromotor tone.
   C. They have less trouble orally feeding within the first few days of life.
   D. They expend less energy learning to eat than do term infants.

13. The nurse is caring for a 34 5/7-week newborn that is having episodes of apnea and bradycardia. When educating the family on apnea of prematurity, which of the following is the appropriate explanation?
   A. "A late preterm infant is more likely to have brief periods where they 'forget' to breathe (apnea) causing heart rate drops (bradycardia). This is caused by the physiologic immaturity of the preterm infant."
   B. "The administration of caffeine will result in cessation of the apnea events."
   C. "Your baby shouldn't be having apnea/bradycardia events at this gestation, and we will be doing more extensive testing to diagnose why these events are occurring."
   D. "Extremely preterm infants have apnea of prematurity secondary to immature brain development when born. Late preterm infants don't have these events."

14. When discharging an infant from the newborn nursery, what information is most important for the family to understand for the first few days post discharge to prevent rehospitalization given the infant is a late preterm?
   A. Signs and symptoms of illness, hyperbilirubinemia, and dehydration
   B. Car seat safety and sibling reactions
   C. Development care and needed immunizations
   D. Safe sleep and car seat safety

15. The late preterm newborn is more at risk to develop which condition within a few hours after birth?
   A. Hyponatremia
   B. Hypernatremia
   C. Hypoglycemia
   D. Hyperglycemia

16. The nurse is preparing a 36-week newborn for discharge home after spending 4 days in the NICU. The nurse provides teaching on newborn care placing an emphasis on warning signs that should warrant a call to the pediatrician. Which statement by the parents determine they understand what signs/symptoms to look for post discharge?
   A. "Our baby should have 6–8 wet diapers per day, so we know the baby is getting enough milk."
   B. "We should not worry about our baby becoming more yellow as each day passes."
   C. "Our baby will not wake up and cry when it's time to eat."
   D. "We should call the pediatrician not 911 if the baby becomes unresponsive."

17. A mother in labor and delivery gave birth to a 35 3/7-week newborn. The mother tells the nurse that she is excited that her baby was not born prematurely. What is the appropriate response the nurse should give the mother?
   A. "Your baby is premature and should to be monitored more closely in the NICU."
   B. "It's great that you were able to stay pregnant until you made it to term."
   C. "Your baby is considered a late preterm newborn, and we will need to closely monitor for problems that late preterm often encounter."
   D. "Any baby over 35 weeks is considered term."

18. The nurse frequently assesses the respiratory status of a 34 2/7-week newborn based on the understanding that late preterm newborns are at increased risk of respiratory distress syndrome because of which factor?
   A. Surfactant insufficiency
   B. Inability to clear fluid from the lungs
   C. Meconium aspirations syndrome
   D. PPHN

19. The nurse is providing newborn care to a 36 5/7-week gestation newborn. Based on the nurse's understanding of gestational age, which terminology best describes the newborn?
   A. Term
   B. Preterm
   C. Late preterm
   D. Post term

20. Which newborn at 36 hours of life is at the highest level of risk for hyperbilirubinemia?
    A. 39-week exclusively breastfeeding newborn, Asian ethnicity
    B. 35 5/7-week newborn formula feeding, Caucasian ethnicity
    C. 39-week newborn formula feeding, Hispanic ethnicity
    D. 36-week newborn exclusively breastfeeding, Asian ethnicity

21. The nurse is working with a mother and her late preterm newborn on feeding skills. Which of the following is the most appropriate statement when educating the mother on why her infant has not been successful at completing each feeding?
    A. Late preterm infants have immature brain development leading to low oral-motor tone with difficulty coordinating sucking and swallowing.
    B. The infant should be able to complete each feeding without difficulty because they have fully developed brains by 34 weeks gestation.
    C. The infant may have difficulty completing each feeding secondary to the immature intestinal development.
    D. Late preterm infants have feeding patterns similar to term infants.

22. A late preterm infant at 34 weeks' gestation, weighing 1250 g, was admitted to NICU for respiratory distress, which resolved within 48 hours of admission. NICU course was complicated by intrauterine growth restriction, hypoglycemia, hyperbilirubinemia, polycythemia, and metabolic acidosis. Infant began enterally feeding within the first 24 hours of life with a premature formula. At 5 days of age infant was noted to have abdominal distention, hematochezia, acidosis, and hypotension. This infant most likely suffers from which disease process?
    A. Herpes simplex virus infection
    B. Group B Strep infection
    C. Bowel obstruction
    D. Necrotizing enterocolitis

ANSWERS AND RATIONALES

1. **(A)** Late preterm infants have a decrease in oromotor tone, which leads to the inability to generate higher intraoral pressures during sucking and contributes to the incoordination of sucking and swallowing. Lack of such coordination can lead to poor feeding and dehydration, which in turn can lead to hyperbilirubinemia. The immaturity of the gastrointestinal system also decreases the ability of hepatic uptake and conjugation. Late preterm infants have an immature gastrointestinal maturity, resulting in decreased activity of hepatic uridine diphosphate glucuronyl transferase enzyme and increased enterohepatic circulation.

References: Boardman JP, Groves AM, Ramasethu J. The preterm infant. In: Boardman J, Groves A, Ramasethu J, eds. *Avery & McDonald's Neonatology: Pathophysiology and Management of the Newborn.* 8th ed. Wolters Kluwer, Netherlands; 2021:336-341.

Parsons K, Jain L. The late preterm infant. In: Martin R, Fanaroff A, Walsh M, eds. *Neonatal-Perinatal Medicine: Diseases of the Fetus and Infant.* 11th ed. Philadelphia, PA: Elsevier; 2020:654-669.

American Academy of Pediatrics. *Neonatal Care: A Compendium of AAP Clinical Practice Guidelines and Policies.* Itasca, IL: American Academy of Pediatrics; 2019.

2. **(C)** Persistent pulmonary hypertension (PPHN) is usually associated with hypotension and decreased saturation in the lower extremities dependent on the degree of right to left shunting. Although the presenting symptoms of pneumonia are similar to those described, additional characteristics that correlate with pneumonia include a fetal monitoring tracing showing decreased variability, prolonged rupture of membranes (longer than 24 hours), and purulent or foul-smelling amniotic fluid. Fetal hyperinsulinemia contributes to delayed maturation of the lungs, which inhibits the production of surfactant and increases the risk of surfactant deficiency related to respiratory distress syndrome. The reticulogranular pattern is suggestive of respiratory distress syndrome. Transient tachypnea of the newborn (TTN) is usually self-limiting and rarely requires supplemental oxygen at a level higher than 40%. These infants usually have mild cyanosis and may have blood gas values that reveal a mild respiratory alkalemia.

References: Boardman JP, Groves AM, Ramasethu J. The preterm infant. In: Boardman J, Groves A, Ramasethu J, eds. *Avery & McDonald's Neonatology: Pathophysiology and Management of the Newborn.* 8th ed. Wolters Kluwer, Netherlands; 2021:336-341.

Parsons K, Jain L. The late preterm infant. In: Martin R, Fanaroff A, Walsh M, eds. *Neonatal-Perinatal Medicine: Diseases of the Fetus and Infant.* 11th ed. Philadelphia, PA: Elsevier; 2020:654-669.

3. **(B)** Weight loss must not exceed more than 8%. Discharge of the late preterm infant must take into consideration the potential physiological immaturity; the infant must demonstrate the ability to successfully feed for at least 24 hours. Poor feeding and dehydration are common reasons for readmission. Metabolic and hearing screening must be completed before discharge, and follow-up appointments arranged 24–48 hours after discharge. The American Academy of Pediatrics recommends a length of stay of no less than 48 hours.

References: Boardman JP, Groves AM, Ramasethu J. The preterm infant. In: Boardman J, Groves A, Ramasethu J, eds *Avery & McDonald's Neonatology: Pathophysiology and Management of the Newborn.* 8th ed. Wolters Kluwer, Netherlands; 2021:336-341.

Parsons K, Jain L. The late preterm infant. In: Martin R, Fanaroff A, Walsh M, eds. *Neonatal-Perinatal Medicine: Diseases of the Fetus and Infant.* 11th ed. Philadelphia, PA: Elsevier; 2020:654-669.

4. **(D)** Bilirubin levels generally peak at 5–7 days. Late preterm infants are at an increased risk for sepsis. Early-onset sepsis is caused by maternal intrapartum transmission and presents at less than 72 hours and up to 7 days of life. Apnea of prematurity presents within the first week of life. The most common cause of rehospitalization between 6 and 12 months of age is respiratory illness.

References: Boardman JP, Groves AM, Ramasethu J. Care of the normal newborn. In: Boardman J, Groves A, Ramasethu J, eds. *Avery & McDonald's Neonatology: Pathophysiology and Management of the Newborn.* 8th ed. Wolters Kluwer, Netherlands; 2021:238-249.

Boardman JP, Groves AM, Ramasethu J. The preterm infant. In: Boardman J, Groves A, Ramasethu J, eds. *Avery & McDonald's Neonatology: Pathophysiology and Management of the Newborn.* 8th ed. Wolters Kluwer, Netherlands; 2021:336-341.

Parsons K, Jain L. The late preterm infant. In: Martin R, Fanaroff A, Walsh M, eds. *Neonatal-Perinatal Medicine: Diseases of the Fetus and Infant.* 11th ed. Philadelphia, PA: Elsevier; 2020:654-669.

American Academy of Pediatrics. *Neonatal Care: A Compendium of AAP Clinical Practice Guidelines and Policies.* Itasca, IL: American Academy of Pediatrics; 2019.

5. **(B)** The late preterm infant has an increased metabolic rate, thereby decreasing the ability to generate heat. The smaller size of late preterm infants leads to an increased ratio of surface area to body weight, causing the infant to lose heat easily to the environment. Late preterm infants are susceptible to the large temperature gradient between the infant and environment. The late preterm infant has decreased brown fat storage and rapidly depletes the brown fat storage.

References: Boardman JP, Groves AM, Ramasethu J. Care of the normal newborn. In: Boardman J, Groves A, Ramasethu J, eds. *Avery & McDonald's Neonatology: Pathophysiology and Management of the Newborn.* 8th ed. Wolters Kluwer, Netherlands; 2021:238-249.

Boardman JP, Groves AM, Ramasethu J. The preterm infant. In: Boardman J, Groves A, Ramasethu J, eds. *Avery & McDonald's Neonatology: Pathophysiology and Management of the Newborn*. 8th ed. Wolters Kluwer, Netherlands; 2021:336-341.

Parsons K, Jain L. The late preterm infant. In: Martin R, Fanaroff A, Walsh M, eds. *Neonatal-Perinatal Medicine: Diseases of the Fetus and Infant*. 11th ed. Philadelphia, PA: Elsevier; 2020:654-669.

6. **(C)** Glycogen is accumulated in the third trimester and stored in the brown fat and hepatic system; thus late preterm infants do not have as much glycogen as term infants. The high metabolic rate of the late preterm infant results in an increase in glucose utilization. Decreases in substrate availability to meet the metabolic demands place the late preterm infant at risk to develop hypoglycemia.

References: Boardman JP, Groves AM, Ramasethu J. The preterm infant. In: Boardman J, Groves A, Ramasethu J, eds. *Avery & McDonald's Neonatology: Pathophysiology and Management of the Newborn*. 8th ed. Wolters Kluwer, Netherlands; 2021:336-341.

Parsons K, Jain L. The late preterm infant. In: Martin R, Fanaroff A, Walsh M, eds. *Neonatal-Perinatal Medicine: Diseases of the Fetus and Infant*. 11th ed. Philadelphia, PA: Elsevier; 2020:654-669.

7. **(B)** Late preterm infants have demonstrated poor school performance, poorer cognitive performance, and developmental delays through 6 years of age. The brain of a late preterm infant remains immature and continues to grow until the age of 2. Late preterm infants are born before their nervous systems have fully developed potentially leading to cerebral palsy. Late preterm infants are not at risk for an increase in seizures. Studies have identified an increase in health care utilization during the first year of life.

References: Parsons K, Jain L. The late preterm infant. In: Martin R, Fanaroff A, Walsh M, eds. *Neonatal-Perinatal Medicine: Diseases of the Fetus and Infant*. 11th ed. Philadelphia, PA: Elsevier; 2020:654-669.

American Academy of Pediatrics. *Neonatal Care: A Compendium of AAP Clinical Practice Guidelines and Policies*. Itasca, IL: American Academy of Pediatrics; 2019.

8. **(A)** Late preterm newborns as opposed to term infants are more likely to have feeding difficulty secondary to low oromotor tone, function, and neural maturation which then predisposes them to dehydration and hyperbilirubinemia. Without adequate lactation support, adequate milk intake and early follow-up, studies have shown that late preterm newborns are at higher risk for rehospitalization for hyperbilirubinemia. Late preterm infants are at increased risk for hyperbilirubinemia secondary to delayed maturation and lower concentrations of uridine diphosphoglucuronate glucuronosyltransferase. The late preterm newborn is two times more likely to have significantly elevated bilirubin levels with higher concentrations 5–7 days after birth.

References: Boardman JP, Groves AM, Ramasethu J. The preterm infant. In: Boardman J, Groves A, Ramasethu J, eds. *Avery & McDonald's Neonatology: Pathophysiology and Management of the Newborn*. 8th ed. Wolters Kluwer, Netherlands; 2021:336-341.

Parsons K, Jain L. The late preterm infant. In: Martin R, Fanaroff A, Walsh M, eds. *Neonatal-Perinatal Medicine: Diseases of the Fetus and Infant*. 11th ed. Philadelphia, PA: Elsevier; 2020:654-669.

9. **(D)** Gas exchange is improved by preventing atelectasis during expiration. It increases lung compliance by stabilizing the chest wall functional residual capacity. There is a decrease in total airway resistance. Continuous positive pressure ventilation helps to maintain positive pressure in the airways during spontaneous breathing, helping to improve oxygenation of alveoli that are partially or completely open. Functional residual capacity increases when alveoli are prevented from closing by maintaining a continuous positive transpulmonary pressure throughout the respiratory cycle.

References: Parsons K, Jain L. The late preterm infant. In: Martin R, Fanaroff A, Walsh M, eds. *Neonatal-Perinatal Medicine: Diseases of the Fetus and Infant*. 11th ed. Philadelphia, PA: Elsevier; 2020:654-669.

Fanaraff A, Fanaraff J. Continuous positive airway pressure. In: Fanaroff A, Fanaroff J, *Klaus and Fanaroff Care of the High-Risk Neonate*. 7th ed. St. Louis, MO: Elsevier; 2020:211-226.

10. **(B)** Preterm birth is described as on or before the last day of the 37th week of gestation. In 2005, the National Institute of Child Health and Human development of the National Institute of Health recommended the terminology "late preterm" be used to identify infants born between 34 0/7 and 36 6/7 weeks gestation and have an increased risk for morbidity and mortality than term infants.

References: Boardman JP, Groves AM, Ramasethu J. The preterm infant. In: Boardman J, Groves A, Ramasethu J, eds. *Avery & McDonald's Neonatology: Pathophysiology and Management of the Newborn*. 8th ed. Wolters Kluwer, Netherlands; 2021:326-341.

Parsons K, Jain L. The late preterm infant. In: Martin R, Fanaroff A, Walsh M, eds. *Neonatal-Perinatal Medicine: Diseases of the Fetus and Infant*. 11th ed. Philadelphia, PA: Elsevier; 2020:654-669.

American Academy of Pediatrics. *Neonatal Care: A Compendium of AAP Clinical Practice Guidelines and Policies*. Itasca, IL: American Academy of Pediatrics; 2019.

11. **(A)** Hyperbilirubinemia is more prevalent, prolonged, and protracted in the late preterm newborn than in the term infant. Poor feeding contributes to dehydration which in turn exacerbates physiologic jaundice. Jaundice is the most common cause of rehospitalization specifically in the late preterm population. Malrotation is an intestinal rotation anomaly that is caused by the absent or incomplete bowel rotation during embryologic life. Congenital heart disease is one of the most common structural abnormalities in newborns. Inborn errors of metabolism are rare, and neonates may have otherwise normal prenatal and delivery histories. These infants present with food intolerance and increasing lethargy, and late onset of seizures could indicate an inborn error of metabolism.

References: Boardman JP, Groves AM, Ramasethu J. The preterm infant. In: Boardman J, Groves A, Ramasethu J, eds. *Avery & McDonald's Neonatology: Pathophysiology and Management of the Newborn*. 8th ed. Wolters Kluwer, Netherlands; 2021:336-341.

Boardman JP, Groves AM, Ramasethu J. Structural cardiac disease and cardiomyopathies. In: Boardman J, Groves A, Ramasethu J, eds. *Avery & McDonald's Neonatology: Pathophysiology and Management of the Newborn*. 8th ed. Wolters Kluwer, Netherlands; 2021:459-490.

Fanaraff A, Fanaraff J. Continuous positive airway pressure. In: Fanaroff A, Fanaroff J, *Klaus and Fanaroff Care of the High-Risk Neonate*. 7th ed. St. Louis, MO: Elsevier; 2020: 211-226.

Parsons K, Jain L. The late preterm infant. In: Martin R, Fanaroff A, Walsh M, eds. *Neonatal-Perinatal Medicine: Diseases of the Fetus and Infant*. 11th ed. Philadelphia, PA: Elsevier; 2020:654-669.

12. **(B)** Late preterm newborns have poor coordination of sucking and swallowing secondary to neurol immaturity and decreased oromotor tone producing decreased intraoral pressure during sucking. Late preterm newborns often have difficulty orally feeding within the first few days after birth due to suck–swallow incoordination and may need gavage feeding. Late preterm infants expend more energy when learning to bottle/breastfeed and are more likely to fatigue.

References: Boardman JP, Groves AM, Ramasethu J. The preterm infant. In: Boardman J, Groves A, Ramasethu J, eds. *Avery & McDonald's Neonatology: Pathophysiology and Management of the Newborn*. 8th ed. Wolters Kluwer, Netherlands; 2021:336-341.

Parsons K, Jain L. The late preterm infant. In: Martin R, Fanaroff A, Walsh M, eds. *Neonatal-Perinatal Medicine: Diseases of the Fetus and Infant*. 11th ed. Philadelphia, PA: Elsevier, Netherlands; 2020:654-669.

13. **(A)** The respiratory control system is immature in the preterm infant which results in respiratory breaks of variable duration. The reduced respiratory drive results in hypoventilation or cessation of respirations also known as apnea. By 34 weeks gestation the incidence of apnea of prematurity decreases to 20% and the incidence decreases even more at 35–36 weeks. In the late preterm

newborn, the prevalence of apnea is reported to be between 4% and 7%. Caffeine is a respiratory stimulant and can be used for the treatment of apnea of prematurity for infants less than 28 weeks gestation at birth. However, caffeine administration is generally stopped by 34 weeks gestation in preparation for discharge.

References: Boardman JP, Grove, Netherlands s AM, Ramasethu J. The preterm infant. In: Boardman J, Groves A, Ramasethu J, eds. *Avery & McDonald's Neonatology: Pathophysiology and Management of the Newborn.* 8th ed. Wolters Kluwer, Netherlands; 2021:336-341.

Parsons K, Jain L. The late preterm infant. In: Martin R, Fanaroff A, Walsh M, eds. *Neonatal-Perinatal Medicine: Diseases of the Fetus and Infant.* 11th ed. Philadelphia, PA: Elsevier; 2020:654-669.

American Academy of Pediatrics. *Neonatal Care: A Compendium of AAP Clinical Practice Guidelines and Policies.* Itasca, IL: American Academy of Pediatrics; 2019.

14. **(A)** Late preterm newborns are at increased risk for rehospitalization. The most common reasons for rehospitalization are suspected sepsis, hyperbilirubinemia, and feeding difficulty leading to dehydration. It has been documented that the late preterm newborns at higher risk are the ones born to first time mothers, breastfed infants, labor and delivery complications, in addition to recipients of public insurance and Asian/Pacific Islander decent. Early follow-up within 24–48 hours of discharge to check bilirubin levels, weight checks, and to ensure the infant is properly feeding. Although car seat safety is an important part of the discharge plan along with an appreciation of sibling reactions, safe sleep, developmental care, and an awareness of needed immunizations, these issues are not the most common reasons for rehospitalization.

References: Boardman JP, Groves AM, Ramasethu J. The preterm infant. In: Boardman J, Groves A, Ramasethu J, eds. *Avery & McDonald's Neonatology: Pathophysiology and Management of the Newborn.* 8th ed. Wolters Kluwer, Netherlands; 2021:336-341.

Parsons K, Jain L. The late preterm infant. In: Martin R, Fanaroff A, Walsh M, eds. *Neonatal-Perinatal Medicine: Diseases of the Fetus and Infant.* 11th ed. Philadelphia, PA: Elsevier; 2020:654-669.

15. **(C)** Hyponatremia does not typically occur in the healthy late preterm newborn. There are three common reasons for hyponatremia: inability to excrete a water load, excessive sodium losses, and inadequate sodium intake. Hypernatremia is not a common concern in the healthy late preterm newborn within the first couple days after birth. Hypernatremia is a greater concern when the late preterm newborn becomes dehydrated from poor feeding. Hypernatremia occurs as the result of increased insensible water losses, inadequate water intake, or excess sodium administration. Hypoglycemia is another component that can affect the late preterm infants transition after birth. Hypoglycemia is three times greater in preterm infants than term infants with two-thirds of those infants requiring intravenous dextrose containing fluids. Hyperglycemia is less frequently seen in newborn infants than hypoglycemia.

References: Boardman JP, Groves AM, Ramasethu J. The preterm infant. In: Boardman J, Groves A, Ramasethu J, eds. *Avery & McDonald's Neonatology: Pathophysiology and Management of the Newborn.* 8th ed. Wolters Kluwer, Netherlands; 2021:336-341.

Parsons K, Jain L. The late preterm infant. In: Martin R, Fanaroff A, Walsh M, eds. *Neonatal-Perinatal Medicine: Diseases of the Fetus and Infant.* 11th ed. Philadelphia, PA: Elsevier; 2020:654-669.

16. **(A)** Late preterm newborns are at risk for dehydration secondary to inadequate intake specifically breastfed infants. It is important to educate the caregivers on urine/stool frequency, bathing/skincare (umbilical cord care), common signs and symptoms of illness, instructions regarding jaundice, discuss sleeping patterns and positions, feeding readiness, thermometer use, and instructions on the appropriate responses to an emergency. Late preterm newborns are 2.4 times more likely to develop significant hyperbilirubinemia than term infants. Jaundice was the most common cause of rehospitalization in both term and late preterm infants. Early follow-up and

monitoring is imperative to properly screen for proper milk intake and reduce the risk of bilirubin encephalopathy.

References: Boardman JP, Groves AM, Ramasethu J. The preterm infant. In: Boardman J, Groves A, Ramasethu J, eds. *Avery & McDonald's Neonatology: Pathophysiology and Management of the Newborn.* 8th ed. Wolters Kluwer, Netherlands; 2021:336-341.

Parsons K, Jain L. The late preterm infant. In: Martin R, Fanaroff A, Walsh M, eds. *Neonatal-Perinatal Medicine: Diseases of the Fetus and Infant.* 11th ed. Philadelphia, PA: Elsevier; 2020:654-669.

17. **(C)** The late preterm infant is defined as an infant born between 34 0/7 and 36 6/7 weeks gestation; a term gestation is greater than 37 weeks. Late preterm newborns account for approximately 7% of births annually in the United States. Late preterm newborns look very similar to the term newborn and many times are cared for in the newborn nursery. These infants have immature physiology and metabolism resulting in magnified risks that should be addressed. Many newborn nurseries care for late preterm newborns ≥35 weeks gestation in addition to a weight requirement defined by the institution. These infants are more likely to be readmitted to the hospital for jaundice, concerns for infection, dehydration, and feeding difficulties.

References: Boardman JP, Groves AM, Ramasethu J. Care of the normal newborn. In: Boardman J, Groves A, Ramasethu J, eds. *Avery & McDonald's Neonatology: Pathophysiology and Management of the Newborn.* 8th ed. Wolters Kluwer, Netherlands; 2021:238-249.

Parsons K, Jain L. The late preterm infant. In: Martin R, Fanaroff A, Walsh M, eds. *Neonatal-Perinatal Medicine: Diseases of the Fetus and Infant.* 11th ed. Philadelphia, PA: Elsevier; 2020:654-669.

18. **(A)** Late preterm infants born with fetal lung structure and immature functional capacity are at increased risk for respiratory distress. The immature lung structure may be associated with intrapulmonary fluid absorption, surfactant insufficiency, and inefficient gas exchange. Respiratory distress syndrome results from primary absence of surfactant production and affects most premature infants. Surfactant is produced by type II pneumocytes. These are the prominent cells in the alveolus between 34 and 36 weeks of gestation. TTN is characterized by delayed clearance of lung fluid leading to transient pulmonary edema. TTN often follows an uneventful delivery of the late preterm or term newborn and the major symptom is persistent tachypnea. Meconium aspiration syndrome (MAS) is typically seen in term to postterm neonates. MAS is the cause of respiratory failure which can be multifactorial which can involve airway blockage, surfactant inactivation, inflammation, and pulmonary artery hypertension. PPHN is caused by acute respiratory distress with hypoxemia and acidemia secondary to decreased pulmonary blood flow caused by elevated pulmonary vascular resistance.

References: Blackburn S. Respiratory system. In: Blackburn S, ed. *Maternal, Fetal, & Neonatal Physiology: A Clinical Perspective.* 5th ed. St. Louis, MO: Elsevier; 2018:297-350.

Boardman JP, Groves AM, Ramasethu J. The preterm infant. In: Boardman J, Groves A, Ramasethu J, eds. *Avery & McDonald's Neonatology: Pathophysiology and Management of the Newborn.* 8th ed. Wolters Kluwer, Netherlands; 2021:336-341.

Parsons K, Jain L. The late preterm infant. In: Martin R, Fanaroff A, Walsh M, eds. *Neonatal-Perinatal Medicine: Diseases of the Fetus and Infant.* 11th ed. Philadelphia, PA: Elsevier; 2020:654-669.

19. **(C)** Infants born between 34 0/7 and 36 6/7 weeks gestation are classified as late preterm.

References: Boardman JP, Groves AM, Ramasethu J. The preterm infant. In: Boardman J, Groves A, Ramasethu J, eds. *Avery & McDonald's Neonatology: Pathophysiology and Management of the Newborn.* 8th ed. Wolters Kluwer, Netherlands; 2021:336-341.

Parsons K, Jain L. The late preterm infant. In: Martin R, Fanaroff A, Walsh M, eds. *Neonatal-Perinatal Medicine: Diseases of the Fetus and Infant.* 11th ed. Philadelphia, PA: Elsevier; 2020:654-669.

Parsons K, Jain L. Post-term pregnancy. In: Martin R, Fanaroff A, Walsh M, eds. *Neonatal-Perinatal Medicine: Diseases of the Fetus and Infant.* 11th ed. Philadelphia, PA: Elsevier; 2020:364-385.

20. (D) Hyperbilirubinemia is caused by decreased clearance of bilirubin. Significant hyperbilirubinemia within the first 36 hours is usually caused by hemolysis. Exclusively breastfed infants are at increased risk due to the potential for dehydration. However, term infants usually breastfeed adequately to stay hydrated. Late preterm newborns are at increased risk of developing significant hyperbilirubinemia which is more prevalent, pronounced, and lasts longer in this population. Late preterm newborns often have difficulty exclusively breastfeeding secondary to decreased oromotor tone, creating lower intraoral pressure during sucking which can lead to less volume intake and dehydration. Caucasian and Hispanic infants are not at any greater risk; Asian infants have increased risk.

References: Blackburn S. Bilirubin metabolism. In: Blackburn S, ed. *Maternal, Fetal, & Neonatal Physiology: A Clinical Perspective.* 5th ed. St. Louis, MO: Elsevier; 2018:589-608.

Boardman JP, Groves AM, Ramasethu J. The preterm infant. In: Boardman J, Groves A, Ramasethu J, eds. *Avery & McDonald's Neonatology: Pathophysiology and Management of the Newborn.* 8th ed. Wolters Kluwer, Netherlands; 2021:336-341.

Parsons K, Jain L. The late preterm infant. In: Martin R, Fanaroff A, Walsh M, eds. *Neonatal-Perinatal Medicine: Diseases of the Fetus and Infant.* 11th ed. Philadelphia, PA: Elsevier; 2020:654-669.

21. (A) The late preterm infant brain is immature at birth and will continue to grow until age 2. Neuronal immaturity and decreased oromotor tone cause the late preterm infant to have poor coordination and a weaker suck which can lead to poor caloric intake and dehydration in comparison to term infants. Most late preterm infants typically respond well to enteral feedings. It is known that the peristaltic functions, deglutition, and sphincter control of the late preterm infant are not as mature as the term counterparts.

References: Blackburn S. Bilirubin metabolism. In: Blackburn S, ed. *Maternal, Fetal, & Neonatal Physiology: A Clinical Perspective.* 5th ed. St. Louis, MO: Elsevier; 2018:589-608.

Boardman JP, Groves AM, Ramasethu J. The preterm infant. In: Boardman J, Groves A, Ramasethu J, eds. *Avery & McDonald's Neonatology: Pathophysiology and Management of the Newborn.* 8th ed. Wolters Kluwer, Netherlands; 2021:336-341.

Parsons K, Jain L. The late preterm infant. In: Martin R, Fanaroff A, Walsh M, eds. *Neonatal-Perinatal Medicine: Diseases of the Fetus and Infant.* 11th ed. Philadelphia, PA: Elsevier; 2020:654-669.

22. (D) Herpes simplex virus (HSV) is common in the neonatal population. It has been noted that half the infants born with HSV are premature between 30 and 37 weeks gestation with additional complications consistent with prematurity. These infants typically present in the first few days after birth. The infants born at term many times discharge home and return with symptoms by 1 week of life. Clinical presentation typically includes central nervous system involvement, skin lesions, and can have multisystem involvement. Group B *Streptococcus* (GBS) sepsis may include hypothermia or hyperthermia, lethargy, irritability, hypotonia, respiratory distress, feeding difficulties, bleeding problems, and abdominal distension. Early onset GBS sepsis is usually seen within the first 72 hours of life. There is a universal screening for antenatal GBS and antibiotic prophylaxis for mothers colonized. Late onset GBS sepsis occurs regardless of maternal antibiotic treatment. Necrotizing enterocolitis (NEC) is multifactorial predominantly seen in preterm infants. The incidence increases in infants that are growth restricted secondary to altered placental function. This is the most common gastrointestinal emergency in the neonatal intensive care unit. Most NEC cases are present between 28 and 32 weeks gestation; however, it can be seen in late preterm infants. Additional risk factors that place infants at higher risk for NEC are intrauterine growth restriction and packed red blood cell transfusion. Common presentation of infants with NEC are metabolic acidosis, bloody stools, abdominal distention, emesis, and abdominal discoloration. Bowel obstruction can present with vomiting, poor feeding, and/or abdominal distention. Infants with malrotation which is an emergency usually present with bilious emesis.

References: Boardman JP, Groves AM, Ramasethu J. The preterm infant. In: Boardman J, Groves A, Ramasethu J, eds. *Avery & McDonald's Neonatology: Pathophysiology and Management of the Newborn.* 8th ed. Wolters Kluwer, Netherlands; 2021:336-341.

Boardman JP, Groves AM, Ramasethu J. Disorders of the gastrointestinal tract. In: Boardman J, Groves A, Ramasethu J, eds. *Avery & McDonald's Neonatology: Pathophysiology and Management of the Newborn.* 8th ed. Wolters Kluwer, Netherlands; 2021:546-563.

Parsons K, Jain L. The late preterm infant. In: Martin R, Fanaroff A, Walsh M, eds. *Neonatal-Perinatal Medicine: Diseases of the Fetus and Infant.* 11th ed. Philadelphia, PA: Elsevier; 2020:654-669.

Parsons K, Jain L. Intrauterine growth restriction. In: Martin R, Fanaroff A, Walsh M, eds. *Neonatal-Perinatal Medicine: Diseases of the Fetus and Infant.* 11th ed. Philadelphia, PA: Elsevier; 2020:260-285.

Parsons K, Jain L. Viral infections in the neonate. In: Martin R, Fanaroff A, Walsh M, eds. *Neonatal-Perinatal Medicine: Diseases of the Fetus and Infant.* 11th ed. Philadelphia, PA: Elsevier; 2020:844-911.

PATHOPHYSIOLOGY

Chapter 14

Cardiovascular Disorders

1. A large ventricular septal defect (VSD) may not be immediately evident at birth due to:
   A. elevated pulmonary vascular resistance.
   B. patency of the ductus venosus.
   C. patent ductus arteriosus (PDA) that prevents flow through the VSD.
   D. decreased pulmonary vascular resistance.

2. In an infant with tetralogy of Fallot, the severity of symptoms will be most affected by which of the following?
   A. Degree of pulmonary edema
   B. Size of the VSD
   C. Degree of right ventricular (RV) outflow obstruction
   D. Size of the PDA

3. A 500-g infant with a PDA is being treated with indomethacin. When formulating a plan of care, the nurse should monitor which of the following parameters most closely, because of the treatment with indomethacin?
   A. Urinary output
   B. Blood pressure and pulses
   C. Liver enzymes and bilirubin levels
   D. Activity level and state of arousal

4. An infant presents with cyanosis at birth and is later diagnosed with transposition of the great vessels per echocardiography. The nurse recognizes that the degree of cyanosis depends on which of the following factors?
   A. Volume of cardiac output
   B. Amount of obstruction to the pulmonary circuit
   C. Quantity of pulmonary edema
   D. Volume of mixing between pulmonary and systemic circulations

5. A balloon septostomy is done for an infant with transposition of the great vessels to achieve which of the following?
   A. Increase pulmonary and systemic mixing at the atrial level
   B. Increase cardiac output by creating a VSD
   C. Decrease pulmonary and systemic mixing at the ventricular level
   D. Create a parallel circulation between the venous and arterial circuits

6. While performing a screening for critical congenital heart disease (CHD), by pulse oximetry, on an infant nearing discharge a nurse notes a difference of 2% between preductal and postductal readings. The nurse should do which of the following?

   A. Notify the neonatologist immediately.
   B. Consider this a negative screen.
   C. Retest in 1 hour.
   D. Instruct the family to schedule a repeat test after discharge.

7. Which of the following percentages should the nurse utilize to select the appropriately sized blood pressure bladder cuff size in relation to the infants' mid arm circumference?
   A. 25%
   B. 50%
   C. 85%
   D. 75%

8. An infant with a VSD presents with a loud, pansystolic murmur at birth but is otherwise asymptomatic. The nurse would anticipate the subsequent development of symptoms at 1–2 months of age due to which of the following?
   A. Pulmonary hypertension
   B. Closure of a PDA
   C. Development of congestive heart failure
   D. Increased cardiac load due to nutritional weight gain

9. A hyperoxia test is ordered for an infant presenting with tachypnea and mild cyanosis. An arterial blood gas is drawn from the right radial artery with a PaO_2 of 200 mm Hg. The nurse should anticipate that this result is indicative of:
   A. respiratory disease.
   B. persistent pulmonary hypertension.
   C. cyanotic heart disease.
   D. complex CHD.

10. An infant has a history of episodic supraventricular tachycardia that resolves spontaneously. An echocardiogram is performed, and there is slurred upstroke of the QRS and the presence of a delta wave. The nurse should suspect which of the following conditions?
    A. Coarctation of the aorta
    B. Wolff-Parkinson-White (WPW) syndrome
    C. DiGeorge syndrome
    D. Atrioventricular canal defect

11. An infant has bounding pulses in the brachial and femoral arteries per nursing assessment. The nurse should document these pulse palpations as:
    A. 1 plus (+).
    B. 2 plus (+).

C. 3 plus (+).

D. 4 plus (+).

12. An infant with profound acidosis has vasopressor-resistant hypotension. The nurse should understand which of the following as a contributing factor?
    A. The heart is being overburdened by vasopressor administration.
    B. The acidosis has no relation to the hypotension.
    C. The heart does not respond well to catecholamines in the presence of acidosis.
    D. Acidosis is a direct side effect of vasopressor administration.

13. An infant is receiving furosemide (Lasix) for management of congestive heart failure. The nurse should anticipate which of the following results from the arterial blood gas and electrolyte panel?
    A. Hypochloremic metabolic alkalosis
    B. Metabolic acidosis from hyperkalemia
    C. Respiratory acidosis from chronic heart failure
    D. Hyperchloremic metabolic alkalosis

14. A chest radiograph is ordered for an infant with a suspected PDA. The nurse should anticipate which of the following findings?
    A. Boot-shaped heart
    B. Decreased pulmonary vascular markings
    C. Increased pulmonary vasculature with cardiomegaly
    D. An egg-on-a-string appearing heart

15. A nurse is caring for an infant diagnosed with a small VSD that is isolated and not near the aortic valve. Which of the following is an accurate statement regarding the defect?
    A. Small defects will often close spontaneously.
    B. It is likely to require surgical intervention within first month of life.
    C. It requires prompt medical management soon after delivery.
    D. Repair can be done during a cardiac catheterization.

16. Adenosine is the drug of choice for which of the following cardiac arrhythmias?
    A. Premature atrial contractions
    B. Sinus tachycardia
    C. Premature ventricular contractions
    D. Supraventricular tachycardia

17. The nurse should recognize which of the following as characteristics of fetal circulation?
    A. The ventricles function in parallel in utero.
    B. There are two shunts.
    C. The atria pumps blood directly into the pulmonary circulation.
    D. The placenta is a high-resistance circuit.

18. An infant of a diabetic mother presents with pallor, poor feeding, tachypnea, a large heart on chest radiographs, and systolic ejection murmur. These factors are most likely related to which of the following?
    A. PDA
    B. Peripheral pulmonic stenosis
    C. Cardiomyopathy
    D. Coarctation of the aorta

19. A term infant has Apgar scores of 8 and 9 at 1 and 5 minutes, respectively. At 12 hours of life, a nurse auscultates a functional or innocent murmur. The nurse should:
    A. monitor for any increase in quality or intensity.
    B. notify the neonatologist of the finding.
    C. suspect a congenital heart lesion.
    D. anticipate an order for an electrocardiogram.

20. An infant is receiving digoxin. The nurse should be aware that the presence of concurrent hypokalemia may result in which of the following?
    A. Decrease the effectiveness of digoxin
    B. Precipitate digoxin toxicity at lower serum levels
    C. Lead to hypertensive episodes
    D. Precipitate bleeding events

21. A nurse is caring for an infant who has undergone surgical repair of a VSD. The nursing plan of care should include recognition of which of the following complications?
    A. Cardiac arrhythmias
    B. Pulmonary hypotension
    C. Pulmonary hypertension
    D. RV failure

22. A nurse is caring for an infant with WPW syndrome. The plan of care should include which of the following for the prevention of supraventricular tachycardia associated with WPW?
    A. Adenosine
    B. Hydralazine
    C. Digoxin
    D. Propranolol

23. An infant is 24 hours post procedure for the placement of a tunneled central catheter and suddenly exhibits a period of tachycardia followed by profound bradycardia. The nurse verifies endotracheal tube placement and determines heart sounds inaudible with no palpable pulses. There is display of an electrical rhythm on electrocardiogram. The nurse should anticipate:
    A. escalation of positive pressure ventilation.
    B. administration of antibiotics.
    C. pericardial tap.
    D. pharmacologic closure of the PDA.

24. A 26-week-gestation infant has a blood pressure of 33 mm Hg systolic, 18 mm Hg diastolic, and a mean arterial pressure of 23 mm Hg. The nurse should interpret this as:
    A. normotensive.
    B. hypovolemic.
    C. hypertensive.
    D. hypotensive.

25. An infant has an arterial blood gas drawn while receiving 80% FiO_2. The pH is 7.2, the $PaCO_2$ is 69 mm Hg, and the PaO_2 is 175 mm Hg. The nurse should interpret these results as originating from which body system or process?
    A. Pulmonary
    B. Cardiac
    C. Metabolic
    D. Infectious

26. An infant is born with known complex CHD. The nurse knows to take extra care with ongoing abdominal assessments. The parents ask why the nurse needs to be so vigilant about the infant's abdomen. The nurse bases her answers on which of the following?
    A. The cardiologist is required to answer that information.
    B. Infants with CHD are at risk for liver disease.
    C. The incidence of necrotizing enterocolitis is higher in babies with CHD.
    D. Infants with CHD frequently spit up.

27. An infant with hypotension is being treated with dopamine at a dosage of 15 mcg/kg/min through a peripheral intravenous (IV) catheter. Which of the following should be assessed hourly by the nurse?
    A. Femoral pulses
    B. Heart sounds
    C. Infusion site
    D. Urinary output

28. An infant is 24 hours postoperative from corrective CHD surgery requiring cardiopulmonary bypass with urinary output since surgery of less than 0.5 mL/kg/day. This finding is most likely to be indicative of:
    A. customary urinary output following cardiopulmonary bypass.
    B. failure of surgical repair.
    C. potential infection.
    D. chronic renal failure.

29. A hypotensive infant is diagnosed with a ductal-dependent lesion. The nurse should include which of the following treatments as the most crucial in the plan of care?
    A. Administration of antibiotics
    B. Initiation of supplemental oxygen
    C. Initiation of IV prostaglandin E1 infusion
    D. Administration of 5 mL/kg normal saline bolus

30. Which of the following cardiac lesions can be palliated with a transcatheter balloon valvuloplasty?
    A. PDA
    B. Hypoplastic left heart syndrome
    C. Peripheral pulmonary artery stenosis
    D. Aortic stenosis

31. An infant exhibits intermittent periods of cyanosis after birth. The nurse should anticipate that the infant may be afflicted with which of the following conditions?
    A. VSD
    B. PDA
    C. Truncus arteriosus
    D. Atrial septal defect (ASD)

32. When assessing an infant diagnosed with coarctation of the aorta, the nurse should expect which of the following symptoms?
    A. Lower extremities warm to touch
    B. Blood pressure gradient > 10 mm Hg between upper and lower extremities
    C. 4 plus (+) pulses in lower extremities
    D. Upper extremities cool to touch

33. An infant is receiving chlorothiazide (Diuril) with laboratory results as follows: sodium 137 mEq/L, potassium 2.2 mEq/L, and chloride 105 mEq/L. Which of the following medications should the nurse expect to be ordered to be given along with the chlorothiazide to prevent the side effect demonstrated by the lab values?
    A. Furosemide (Lasix)
    B. Sodium chloride (NaCl)
    C. Spironolactone (Aldactone)
    D. Digoxin

34. After cardiac surgery, the nurse should include which of the following interventions in the nursing plan of care to meet the developmental needs of the infant?
    A. Administer sedatives sparingly.
    B. Limit parental visits.
    C. Provide care every hour.
    D. Use positional devices and facilitate sucking.

35. An infant with congestive heart failure is receiving digoxin. The nurse should expect which of the following effects from the medication?
    A. Increased cardiac output
    B. Increased urine output
    C. Decreased blood pressure
    D. Increased heart rate

36. An infant with a VSD has been receiving furosemide (Lasix) for 2 weeks. The nurse should anticipate that the electrolyte panel may exhibit which of the following?
    A. Hyperchloremia
    B. Hyperkalemia
    C. Hyperglycemia
    D. Hypokalemia

37. An infant is maintained on prostaglandin E1 at 0.1 mcg/kg/min for a diagnosis of transposition of the great vessels. The nurse should consider which of the following side effects when formulating the plan of care?
    A. Hyperthermia
    B. Hypertension
    C. Hyperglycemia
    D. Hypercalcemia

38. A term infant requires intubation for respiratory distress at birth. The pulse oximeter probe reads: right hand 75% saturation and left foot 92% saturation. The nurse should anticipate which of the following conditions?
    A. Sepsis
    B. Respiratory distress syndrome
    C. Transposition of the great arteries
    D. Truncus arteriosus

39. Tetralogy of Fallot is a combination of which of the following cardiac defects?
    A. VSD, ASD, coarctation of the aorta, and PDA
    B. VSD, pulmonary valve stenosis, RV hypertrophy, and aortic stenosis
    C. VSD, obstruction of the RV outflow tract, RV hypertrophy, and overriding aorta
    D. ASD, PDA, coarctation of the aorta, and overriding aorta

40. An infant is diagnosed with hypoplastic left heart syndrome. The nurse should be aware that historically the treatment approach was:
    A. multistage surgical repair.
    B. heart transplant.
    C. single-stage surgical repair.
    D. palliative care.

41. Which of the following symptoms would be most important for the nurse to assess for an infant with suspected pulmonary edema?
    A. Tachycardia
    B. Tachypnea
    C. Hypothermia
    D. Hypotension

42. A 35.5 weeks' gestation infant has a maternal medication history of prenatal vitamins, occasional aspirin, and recent indomethacin use. The infant at birth exhibits a heart rate of 200, respiratory rate of 80, rales, central cyanosis, and poor perfusion. The nurse should recognize these symptoms as indicative of which of the following?
    A. Neonatal abstinence syndrome
    B. Ibuprofen withdrawal
    C. Premature closure of the ductus arteriosus
    D. PDA

43. An infant has a Blalock-Taussig shunt placed. Upon transfer from the operating room, the nurse notes a cerebral near-infrared spectroscopy attached to the forehead. The nurse should expect this device to provide data on which of the following?
    A. Central venous pressure
    B. Brain activity
    C. Seizure activity
    D. Cerebral oxygenation

44. The nurse is caring for an infant whose heart rate has increased to 260. The blood pressure remained within normal limits, and perfusion was 2 seconds for the first 30 minutes. After 30 minutes the capillary refill increased to 5 seconds. The nurse should anticipate which of the following actions as the highest priority?
    A. Transesophageal probe placement
    B. Defibrillation
    C. Cardioversion
    D. Initiation of chest compressions

45. An infant is ordered to receive adenosine. Which method of medication administration should the nurse utilize?
    A. Retrograde infusion
    B. Rapid IV push
    C. Slow IV push
    D. Intramuscular

46. The nurse initiates a milrinone infusion for an infant who recently underwent open heart surgery. Which vital sign should the nurse monitor closely related to this infusion?
    A. Respirations
    B. Degree of pain
    C. Temperature
    D. Blood pressure

47. A nurse is caring for an infant with pulmonary hypertension per echocardiogram. The plan of care should include avoidance of which of the following conditions in order to prevent the infant from worsening?
    A. Hypoxia and agitation
    B. Hyperoxia and alkalosis
    C. Hypoxia and alkalosis
    D. Hyperoxia and agitation

48. The nurse should monitor an infant who has experienced pulmonary and intracranial hemorrhage for which of the following types of shock?
    A. Cardiogenic
    B. Septic
    C. Neurologic
    D. Hypovolemic

49. What should the nursing plan of care for an infant who is exhibiting signs of septic shock include?
    A. Provide a neutral thermal environment.
    B. Defer parental notification until further information is available.
    C. Administer of 5 mL/kg normal saline boluses.
    D. Increase frequency of neuro assessments to every hour.

50. An infant who is postoperative from a PDA ligation develops hypotension. The infant is given fluid boluses followed by dopamine and dobutamine at infusion rates of 10 mcg/kg/min. The infant remains hypotensive. The nurse should anticipate which of the following medications as an adjunct therapy?
    A. Fentanyl
    B. Hydrocortisone
    C. Caffeine
    D. Midazolam

51. An infant is receiving dopamine (Intropin) at an infusion rate of 3 mcg/kg/min for which of the following purposes?
    A. Increase of blood pressure
    B. Constriction of pulmonary vasculature
    C. Vasodilatation of renal vascular bed
    D. Vasoconstriction of peripheral veins

52. A 600-g infant is exhibiting hypotension related to bacterial sepsis. The nurse should expect which of the following treatment protocols to optimally treat the hypotension?
    A. Normal saline fluid bolus over 20 minutes followed by a dopamine (Intropin) infusion
    B. Dobutamine (Dobutrex) infusion
    C. Volume expander by given rapid push
    D. Hydrocortisone

53. An infant with tetralogy of Fallot exhibits persistent crying, which evolves into a "Tet spell." The nurse should place the infant in which of the following positions?
    A. Supine, legs extended
    B. Knee-to-chest
    C. Prone
    D. Side-lying

54. An infant is receiving digoxin. The nurse should hold the dose if the heart rate is:

A. 50.
B. 150.
C. 200.
D. 220.

55. The nurse is admitting a term infant who has just undergone stage 1 Norwood repair with a larger than average blood loss intraoperatively. Vitals signs are heart rate 200, blood pressure mean 30 mm Hg with a systolic of 36 mm Hg, and temperature 37°C (98.6°F). The nurse should assess the infant for which of the following conditions?
A. Hypovolemia
B. Hypocalcemia
C. Acidosis
D. Hypoglycemia

56. A nurse should expect the primary action of dobutamine (Dobutrex) is to improve cardiac output by predominantly increasing:
A. contractility.
B. vascular resistance.
C. heart rate.
D. pulmonary vascular resistance.

57. An infant fails a congenital heart screen with oxygen saturations in the low 90s while on room air. An echocardiogram shows normal structure of heart with the inability to rule out coarctation of the aorta. Which vessel prevents coarctation of the aorta from being ruled out?
A. Overriding pulmonary artery
B. Pulmonary vein
C. PDA
D. Ductus venosus

58. A nurse is caring for a 4-kg infant who has undergone cardiac surgery and is now 72 hours postop. The plan of care includes monitoring for adequate urine output postoperatively. The nurse should expect how many mL/hour of urinary output?
A. 1 mL/h
B. 2 mL/h
C. 3 mL/h
D. 4 mL/h

59. An infant who has a VSD is ready for discharge and is ordered to receive furosemide (Lasix) at home. Which of the following statements by the nurse to the mother is appropriate for discharge teaching?
A. If the infant looks puffy, an extra dose may be needed.
B. Give the Lasix the same time each day as ordered.
C. Please weigh the diapers with every diaper change.
D. Take the infant's blood pressure twice a week.

60. An infant is diagnosed with persistent pulmonary hypertension. The nurse should give priority to which of the following treatment measures?
A. Achieve paralysis
B. Administer furosemide (Lasix)
C. Administer sildenafil
D. Provide oxygen supplementation

61. What nursing measure would be a priority for the long-term care plan for an infant with congestive heart failure?

A. Restriction of caloric intake
B. Diuretics or afterload reducers
C. Physical therapy
D. Sedation

62. The nurse should expect an infant to have which of the following heart lesions when a chest radiograph reveals a heart that encompasses the entire chest?
A. Pulmonary atresia
B. Tricuspid atresia
C. Hypoplastic left heart syndrome
D. Ebstein malformation

63. An infant is diagnosed with transposition of the great arteries. The nurse should expect chest radiograph findings to reveal which type of cardiac silhouette?
A. Egg on a string
B. Wall-to-wall heart
C. Boot-shaped
D. Narrow cardiac silhouette

64. CHD is most often associated with which of the following?
A. Tobacco use
B. Opiate use during pregnancy
C. Alcohol use in the third trimester
D. Combination of genetic, environmental, and multifactorial influences

65. A hyperoxia test is performed on an infant. When interpreting the results, the nurse must consider which of the following factors?
A. Ambient light might affect the pulse oximetry readings.
B. A hyperoxia test is not as reliable as an echocardiogram.
C. A chest x-ray must be performed in conjunction with a hyperoxia test.
D. An infant not intubated cannot have a hyperoxia test performed.

66. A nurse attending the delivery of an infant with a known congenital heart lesion places the pulse oximetry probe on the right wrist knowing which of the following is true?
A. The right wrist is considered "preductal."
B. This is the easiest limb from which to obtain saturations.
C. This location will aid in diagnosis of the type of defect.
D. The right wrist is considered "postductal."

ANSWERS AND RATIONALES

1. **(A)** Large ventricular septal defects are not symptomatic at birth because the pulmonary vascular resistance is normally elevated at this time. As the pulmonary vascular resistance decreases over the first 6–8 weeks of life, the amount of shunted blood increases, and symptoms may develop. The ductus venosus converts to a ligament (over time) with removal of the placental circuit at birth. A patent ductus arteriosus (PDA) is the connection between the pulmonary artery and the aorta in utero rather than the ventricles.

Reference: Marcdante K, Kliegman R, Schuh A. Acyanotic congenital heart disease. In: Marcdante K, Kliegman R, eds. *Nelson Essentials of Pediatrics.* 9th ed. Philadelphia, PA: Elsevier Saunders; 2021:564-568.

2. **(C)** The presence of an obstruction to right ventricular (RV) outflow with a large ventricular septal defect (VSD) causes a right-to-left shunt at the ventricular level with arterial desaturation. The greater the obstruction and the lower the systemic vascular resistance, the greater the right-to-left shunt. Thus the clinical findings vary with the degree of RV outflow obstruction. Patients with mild obstruction are minimally cyanotic or acyanotic. Those with severe obstruction are deeply cyanotic from birth. Few of these infants are asymptomatic. In those with significant RV outflow obstruction, many have cyanosis at birth, and nearly all have cyanosis by age 4 months. A patent ductus is the connection between the pulmonary artery and aorta in utero and does not involve the cardiac septum. Pulmonary edema is a common occurrence in infants with congestive heart failure.

Reference: Pei-Ni J. Cardiovascular diseases. In: Bunik M, Hay Jr WW, Levin MJ, Abzug MJ, eds. *Current Diagnosis & Treatment: Pediatrics.* 26th ed. New York: McGraw Hill; 2022:556-557.

3. **(A)** Indomethacin is an inhibitor of prostaglandin synthesis. Most notably, it decreases blood flow to the renal system, thus decreasing renal perfusion and urinary output. If oliguria occurs, electrolytes should be monitored and renally excreted drugs should be adjusted appropriately. Gastrointestinal perfusion may also be decreased, but generally not to the extent of renal function. Blood pressure (BP) and pulses are not affected by the administration of indomethacin. Indomethacin has no impact on activity level and state of arousal.

References: Gomella T, Eyal F, Bany-Mohammed F. *Gomella's Neonatology.* 8th ed. New York: McGraw-Hill; 2020:1272.

4. **(D)** In transposition of the great vessels, the degree of cyanosis depends on the amount of mixing between the pulmonary and systemic circulations. Oxygenated pulmonary venous blood is returned to the lungs, and desaturated systemic blood is returned to the body. Thus the two circulations exist in parallel. Some mixing between them must occur to allow oxygenated blood to reach systemic circulation and the desaturated blood to reach the lungs. Pulmonary edema, cardiac output, and obstruction to the pulmonary circuit do not affect the degree of cyanosis and/or mixing of the pulmonary and systemic circulations.

Reference: Hirsch-Romano JC, Ohye RG, Bove EL, Doherty GM. Congenital heart disease. In: Doherty GM, ed. *Current Diagnosis & Treatment: Surgery.* 15th ed. New York: McGraw Hill; 2020:428-430. Available at: https://accessmedicine.mhmedical.com/content.aspx?bookid=2859&sectionid=242156948.

5. **(A)** When an infant has a restrictive atrial septal defect (ASD), a balloon atrial septostomy, a technique developed by William Rashkind in 1966, may be performed. The procedure involves inserting a balloon-tipped catheter across the foramen ovale into the left atrium. The balloon is then inflated and forcibly withdrawn so that the catheter tears the septum primum and enlarges the ASD. Mixing should increase immediately, with a corresponding increase in arterial oxygen saturation. The VSD is a connection between the right and left ventricles and is not the site of balloon septostomy. Parallel circuits do not allow for the mixing of blood flow.

Reference: Hirsch-Romano JC, Ohye RG, Bove EL, Doherty GM. Congenital heart disease. In: Doherty GM, ed. *Current Diagnosis & Treatment: Surgery.* 15th ed. New York: McGraw Hill; 2020:428-430. Available at: https://accessmedicine.mhmedical.com/content.aspx?bookid=2859&sectionid=242156948.

6. **(B)** A failed screen result is defined as: any oxygen saturation less than 90%; oxygen saturation is less than 95% in right hand and foot on three measures, each separated by 1 hour or there is a greater than 3% absolute difference in oxygen saturation between the right hand and foot on three measures, each separated by

1 hour. Any screening that is >95% in either extremity with no more than a 3% absolute difference in oxygen saturation between the upper and lower extremity would be considered a "pass" result, or "negative" screen.

Reference: Smith D. The newborn infant. In: Bunik M, Hay Jr WW, Levin MJ, Abzug MJ, eds. *Current Diagnosis & Treatment: Pediatrics.* 26th ed. McGraw Hill; 2022:15.

7. **(A)** The cuff bladder width should be approximately 50% of the infant's mid arm circumference. The BP reading will be falsely elevated if the cuff is too narrow and falsely low if the cuff is too large.

Reference: Marcdante K, Kliegman R. Cardiovascular system assessment. In: Marcdante K, Kliegman R, eds. *Nelson Essentials of Pediatrics.* 9th ed. Philadelphia, PA: Elsevier Saunders; 2022:554-555.

8. **(C)** Infants with small isolated defects are often asymptomatic. The murmur of a small defect may be detected within the first 24–36 hours of life, because the very restrictive opening permits the normal rapid fall in pulmonary arterial resistance and pressures. In term infants born at sea level with a large VSD, clinical deterioration may occur at any time from approximately 3–12 weeks after birth. In premature infants, pulmonary vascular muscular hypertrophy regresses more rapidly, with failure frequently noted at 1–4 weeks. Infants may present with signs of heart failure as the pulmonary vascular resistance falls and left-to-right shunting increases. Symptoms may include tachypnea, grunting respirations, and fatigue, particularly with enteral feeding attempts. Weight gain is slow, and excessive sweating is common. The ductus arteriosus closes shortly after birth and would not be a clinical factor at 1–2 months of age.

Reference: Harikrishnan KN, Vettukattil JJ. Congenital heart diseases. In: Elmoselhi A, ed. *Cardiology: An Integrated Approach.* New York: McGraw Hill; 2018:437-440. Available at: https://accessmedicine-mhmedical-com.wake.idm.oclc.org/content.aspx?bookid=2224&sectionid=171661563.

9. **(A)** A hyperoxia test is performed by administering 100% oxygen for 5–10 minutes and then measuring the arterial preductal PaO_2 (right radial artery). A significant increase in PaO_2 levels, particularly a PaO_2 level >150 mm Hg, makes the likely cause respiratory distress rather than cardiac in origin. Levels below 50–60 mm Hg may be related to transposition of the great vessels or from defects in pulmonary outflow. Mixing lesions may have PaO_2 values from 75 to 150 mm Hg. Infants with persistent pulmonary hypertension commonly present with hypoxia and hypoxemia.

Reference: Sadowski S, Verklan MT. Cardiovascular disorders. In: Verklan M, Walden M, Forrest S, eds. *Core Curriculum for Neonatal Intensive Care Nursing.* 6th ed. St. Louis: Elsevier Health Sciences; 2021:461.

Smith D. Cardiac problems in the newborn. In: Bunik M, Hay Jr WW, Levin MJ, Abzug MJ, eds. *Current Diagnosis & Treatment: Pediatrics.* 26th ed. McGraw Hill; 2022:41.

10. **(B)** Wolff-Parkinson-White (WPW) syndrome is a type of supraventricular tachycardia (SVT) that features reentrant tachycardia in which, during sinus rhythm, the impulse travels antegrade (from atria to ventricles) down the accessory connection, bypassing the atrioventricular (AV) node and creating ventricular preexcitation. The electrocardiogram commonly reveals early eccentric activation of the ventricle with a short PR interval and slurred upstroke of the QRS and the presence of a delta wave. Coarctation of the aorta, DiGeorge syndrome, and AV canal do not present with SVT.

Reference: Jone PN, Kim JS, Burkett D, Jacobsen R, Von Alvensleben J. Cardiovascular diseases. In: Bunik M, Hay WW, Levin MJ, Abzug MJ, eds. *Current Diagnosis & Treatment: Pediatrics.* 26th ed. New York: McGraw-Hill; 2022:596-599.

11. **(D)** Pulse volume is graded from 0 to 4: Absent: 0, Faint: 1+, Normal to average: 2+, Increased pulse: 3+, Strong, bounding: 4+.

Reference: Swartz MA. The peripheral vascular system. In: Swartz MH, ed. *Textbook of Physical Diagnosis: History and Examination*. 8th ed. Elsevier; 2021:327-340 [chapter 15].

12. **(C)** Acidosis can impair the myocardial response to catecholamines, thus further reducing contractility. Vasopressor administration is not a cause of acidosis. Acidosis is the result of anaerobic metabolism and is reflected by a decrease in blood pH. Hypotension may exist in the presence of acidosis, but hypotension is treated with fluid resuscitation followed by vasopressor administration.

Reference: Fuhrman BP, Zimmerman JJ, Clark RSB, et al. Shock states. In: Zimmerman JJ, Rotta AT, eds. *Fuhrman & Zimmerman's Pediatric Critical Care*. 6th ed. Elsevier; 2022:352-362 [chapter 34].

13. **(A)** Furosemide (Lasix) is a loop diuretic commonly used to treat or prevent congestive heart failure. It removes large amounts of potassium and chloride from the body, thus possibly causing hypochloremic metabolic alkalosis when used chronically. Electrolytes and fluid balance should be monitored during long-term therapy. Lasix is not associated with the occurrence of metabolic or respiratory acidosis.

Reference: Jone PN, Kim JS, Burkett D, Jacobsen R, Von Alvensleben J. Cardiovascular diseases. In: Bunik M, Hay WW, Levin MJ, Abzug MJ, eds. *Current Diagnosis & Treatment: Pediatrics*. 26th ed. New York: McGraw-Hill; 2022:554.

14. **(C)** Common clinical manifestations of a PDA include increased pulmonary vasculature and cardiomegaly on chest radiograph, bounding peripheral pulses, and an active precordium. A widening pulse pressure with a low diastolic BP may be present. Unexplained acidosis may be present. A boot-shaped heart is common in tetralogy of Fallot. An egg on a string-appearing heart is common with transposition of the great vessels.

Reference: Swanson T, Erickson L. Cardiovascular diseases and surgical interventions. In: Gardner S, Carter B, Enzman-Hines M, Niermeyer S, eds. *Merenstein & Gardner's Handbook of Neonatal Intensive Care: An Interprofessional Approach*. 9th ed. St. Louis, MO: Elsevier; 2021:851-853 [chapter 24].

15. **(A)** Fifty percent to seventy-five percent of all small VSDs will close spontaneously without treatment. About 20% of large defects will become smaller spontaneously. Surgery may be needed if the infant develops failure to thrive or congestive heart failure from a VSD. VSDs are not repaired via cardiac catheterization.

Reference: Swanson T, Erickson L. Cardiovascular diseases and surgical interventions. In: Gardner S, Carter B, Enzman-Hines M, Niermeyer S, eds. *Merenstein & Gardner's Handbook of Neonatal Intensive Care: An Interprofessional Approach*. 9th ed. St. Louis, MO: Elsevier; 2021:855-857 [chapter 24].

16. **(D)** Adenosine is the drug of choice for prompt conversion of paroxysmal SVT to sinus rhythm because of its success rate and its very short duration of action. It acts by directly inhibiting the AV nodal conduction and increases the AV nodal refractory period but has lesser effects on the sinoatrial node. Sinus tachycardia may be reflective of infection, dehydration, or shock and is generally treated with fluid resuscitation and antimicrobials. Premature atrial retractions or premature ventricular contractions do not require treatment with adenosine.

Reference: Pei-Ni J. Cardiovascular diseases. In: Bunik M, Hay Jr WW, Levin MJ, Abzug MJ, eds. *Current Diagnosis & Treatment: Pediatrics*. 26th ed. New York: McGraw Hill; 2022:599.

17. **(A)** The ventricles of the fetal heart work in parallel, not in series, as in postnatal circulation after transition. This parallel circulation results in well-oxygenated blood entering the left ventricle, which supplies the heart and brain, and less oxygenated blood entering the right ventricle, which supplies the rest of the body. These two separate circulations are maintained by the right atrium structure, which effectively directs entering blood to either the left atrium or the right ventricle, depending on its oxygen content. The placenta is a low-resistance circuit in utero, and fetal circulation occurs in the presence of three shunts: ductus venosus, ductus arteriosus, and foramen ovale.

Reference: Niermeyer S, Clarke S. Care at Birth. In: Gardner S, Carter B, Enzman-Hines M, Niermeyer S, eds. *Merenstein & Gardner's Handbook of Neonatal Intensive Care: An Interprofessional Approach*. 9th ed. St. Louis, MO: Elsevier; 2021:68-69 [chapter 4].

18. **(C)** Infants born to mothers with uncontrolled diabetes are at risk for transposition of the great vessels, VSDs, cardiomyopathy, and complex congenital heart disease. Coarctation of the aorta and peripheral pulmonic stenosis are not common findings in the infant of a diabetic mother. A patent ductus is unlikely to cause the specific constellation of clinical symptoms described.

Reference: Smith D. The newborn infant. In: Bunik M, Hay WW, Levin MJ, Abzug MJ, eds. *Current Diagnosis & Treatment: Pediatrics*. 26th ed. New York: McGraw-Hill; 2022:11 [chapter 2].

19. **(A)** Fifty percent of infants may have functional or innocent murmurs within the first 48 hours of delivery. These murmurs can be related to the incomplete transition to postnatal circulation reflecting left-to-right flow through a PDA, increased flow over the pulmonary valve associated with a fall in pulmonary vascular resistance, or mild bilateral peripheral pulmonary artery stenosis related to the size and pressure differential between the main pulmonary trunk and the pulmonary branches. Physician notification is not necessary given this is integral to normal transitional process. It would be appropriate to monitor for any increase in quality or intensity. The presence of a congenital heart lesion would likely be accompanied by other clinical symptoms.

Reference: Marcdante K, Kliegman R. Cardiovascular system assessment. In: Marcdante K, Kliegman R, eds. *Nelson Essentials of Pediatrics*. 9th ed. Philadelphia, PA: Elsevier Saunders; 2022:558.

20. **(B)** In infants with hypokalemia, toxicity may occur despite serum digoxin concentrations below 2.0 ng/mL, because potassium depletion sensitizes the myocardium to digoxin.

Reference: Bohannon K, Ho PM, Nolt V. Neonatal pharmacology; medications used in the neonatal intensive care unit. In: Gomella T, Eyal F, Bany-Mohammed F, eds. *Gomella's Neonatology: Management, Procedures, On-Call Problems, Diseases and Drugs*. 8th ed. New York: McGraw Hill; 2020:1252-1253.

21. **(A)** VSD closure complications may include right bundle branch block, third-degree heart block, aortic insufficiency, tricuspid insufficiency, and other common surgical complications such as infection or bleeding. Pulmonary hypotension or hypertension and RV failure are not common complications.

Reference: Swanson T, Erickson L. Cardiovascular diseases and surgical interventions. In: Gardner SL, Carter BS, Hines ME, Niermeyer S, eds. *Merenstein & Gardner's Handbook of Neonatal Intensive Care: An Interprofessional Approach*. 9th ed. St. Louis, MO: Elsevier; 2021:855-857 [chapter 24].

22. **(D)** Propranolol is the medication of choice for the prevention of SVT in infants with SVT caused by WPW syndrome. Hydralazine is an antihypertensive; adenosine is used for treatment of SVT for infants not diagnosed with WPW. Digoxin is not an effective agent for the treatment of SVT.

Reference: Chun T, Arya B. Perinatal arrhythmias. In: Sawyer T, Gleason C, eds. *Avery's Diseases of the Newborn*. 11th ed. Philadelphia, PA: Elsevier; 2024:828-843 [chapter 49].

23. **(C)** Pericardial tamponade has multiple known causes, but a new onset after a central line procedure may indicate an iatrogenic perforation of the vessel near the pericardial space. The result is a filling of the pericardial sac with blood and possibly fluid, thus causing a decline in cardiac function. Symptoms may include a period of initial tachycardia followed by bradycardia, pulsus paradoxus, PR depression, ST elevation, electrical alternans, declining or absent pulses, and quiet or absent heart sounds. When infants

have a rapid decompensation and death is an immediate concern, rapid needle decompression of the pericardial space is necessary. The administration of antibiotics will not resolve the tamponade nor will pharmacologically closure of the PDA. An increase in positive pressure ventilation may be needed but must follow resolution of the tamponade.

Reference: Ferri FF. Cardiac tamponade. In: *Ferri's Clinical Advisor 2022: 5 Books in 1*. St. Louis, MO: Elsevier Health Sciences; 2022.

24. **(D)** Normal BP for the first week of life is considered to be a mean arterial BP at least equal to the gestational age of the infant. This infant is hypotensive given the gestational age of 26 weeks and the mean arterial pressure of 23 mm Hg.

Reference: Batton B. Neonatal blood pressure standards. *Clin Perinatol*. 2020;47(3):469-485. doi:10.1016/j.clp.2020.05.008.

25. **(A)** $PaCO_2$ is commonly elevated with pulmonary disease, especially in the face of a normal PaO_2. The $PaCO_2$ is uncommonly elevated in the presence of cardiac or metabolic disease, which tends to reflect alterations in pH, PaO_2, and bicarbonate levels. The presence of infection can result in acidosis and hypoxia.

Reference: Barry J, Deacon J, Hernandez C, Jones MD. Acid-base homeostasis and oxygenation. In: Gardner SL, Carter BS, Hines ME, Niermeyer S, eds. *Merenstein & Gardner's Handbook of Neonatal Intensive Care: An Interprofessional Approach*. 9th ed. St. Louis, MO: Elsevier; 2021:186-193 [chapter 8].

26. **(C)** Infants with congenital heart disease (CHD) are at an increased risk for necrotizing enterocolitis. The reason for this is multifactorial in nature and is thought to be related to factors such as prostaglandin therapy, decreased blood flow to the gut, certain invasive procedure (line placement), and infection.

Reference: Dumitrascu Biris I, Mintoft A, Harris C, et al. Mortality and morbidity in preterm infants with congenital heart disease. *Acta Paediatr*. 2021;111(1):151-156. doi:10.1111/apa.16155.

27. **(C)** Dopamine can cause blanching and severe skin ischemia/ necrosis with infiltration. Dopamine is titrated based on BP readings versus femoral pulses or heart sounds. Dopamine can increase urinary output, but it is not clinically necessary to record urinary output every hour if the infant can void spontaneously.

Reference: Bohannon K, Ho PM, Nolt V. Neonatal pharmacology; medications used in the neonatal intensive care unit. In: Gomella T, Eyal F, Bany-Mohammed F, eds. *Gomella's Neonatology: Management, Procedures, On-Call Problems, Diseases and Drugs*. 8th ed. New York: McGraw Hill; 2020:1252-1253.

28. **(A)** It is normal to have oliguria for up to 48 hours after cardiopulmonary bypass. It is not indicative of repair failure, chronic renal failure, or potential infection given this infant is only 24 hours postop.

Reference: Fuhrman BP, Zimmerman JJ, Clark RSB, et al. Critical care after surgery for congenital cardiac disease. In: Zimmerman JJ, Rotta AT, eds. *Fuhrman & Zimmerman's Pediatric Critical Care*. 6th ed. Elsevier; 2022:380-410 [chapter 36].

29. **(C)** The single most important intervention for a ductal-dependent lesion is the infusion of intravenous (IV) prostaglandin E1 (PGE1) to ensure ductal patency and improve left-to-right shunting and systemic blood flow. The initial dose of PGE1 is usually 0.1 mcg/kg/min. PGE1 should then be titrated to the lowest effective dose and can be administered through an umbilical venous catheter, central line, intraosseous (IO) line, or peripheral IV line with equal efficacy, although central access is preferred. The administration of supplemental oxygen will prompt closure of the duct, and if perfusion is adequate, a normal saline bolus of 5 mL/kg is not needed. Antibiotics would only serve to treat bacterial infection.

Reference: Yue EL, Meckler GD. Congenital and acquired pediatric heart disease. In: Tintinalli JE, Ma OJ, Yealy DM, et al., eds. *Tintinalli's Emergency Medicine: A Comprehensive Study Guide*. 9th ed. New York: McGraw Hill; 2020.

30. **(D)** A balloon valvuloplasty can be performed in the catheterization laboratory for aortic stenosis immediately after the infant

has been stabilized with medical and pharmacologic treatment, including PGE1. It is the procedure of choice for reduction of transvalvular gradients in symptomatic infants. This procedure is an ideal palliative treatment option because mortality from surgical valvuloplasty early after diagnosis can be high due to the critical illness severity. Balloon valvuloplasty thus provides relief of the valvular gradient and allows for future surgical intervention to be performed on an unscarred chest. Hypoplastic left heart repair requires a series of surgical procedures to correct due to an underdeveloped left ventricle. It is desirable to achieve closure of the patent ductus for successful transition from intrauterine to extrauterine life. A balloon procedure is contraindicated for a PDA.

Reference: Murthy R, Moe TG, Van Arsdell GS, Nigro JJ, Karamlou T. Congenital heart disease. In: Brunicardi FC, Andersen DK, Billiar TR, et al., eds. *Schwartz's Principles of Surgery*. 11th ed. New York: McGraw Hill; 2019. Available at: https://accessmedicine.mhmedical.com/content.aspx?bookid=2576&sectionid=216207926.

31. **(C)** The anatomy of truncus arteriosus involves a single great artery originating from both the left and right ventricles. The blood flow to the lungs is directly dependent on the pulmonary vascular resistance. As the pulmonary vascularity changes, the pulmonary blood flow will also change, causing changes in the amount of blood flowing into the lungs. Intermittent changes in the pulmonary circulation may manifest as changes in cyanosis. Isolated atrial and VSDs are not generally associated with cyanosis.

Reference: Swanson T, Erickson L. Cardiovascular diseases and surgical intervention. In: Gardner SL, Carter BS, Hines ME, Niermeyer S, eds. *Merenstein & Gardner's Handbook of Neonatal Intensive Care: An Interprofessional Approach*. 9th ed. St. Louis, MO: Elsevier; 2021:872-873 [chapter 24].

32. **(B)** The narrowing of the aorta at the transverse aortic arch causes the BP and perfusion to be lower in the legs than in the arms. The BP (>10 mm Hg) is the most consistent factor in critical coarctation of the aorta and is present in 97% of cases. The pulses are decreased 92% of the time in the lower extremities; the lower extremities are cool to touch. The upper extremities would be warm to touch given there is no compromised perfusion.

Reference: Swanson T, Erickson L. Cardiovascular diseases and surgical intervention. In: Gardner SL, Carter BS, Hines ME, Niermeyer S, eds. *Merenstein & Gardner's Handbook of Neonatal Intensive Care: An Interprofessional Approach*. 9th ed. St. Louis, MO: Elsevier; 2021:857-858 [chapter 24].

33. **(C)** Spironolactone (Aldactone) is a potassium-sparing diuretic. Furosemide (Lasix) is a potassium-wasting diuretic. The sodium and chloride are normal and would not need supplementation. Digoxin is an inotrope to achieve maximal cardiac output.

Reference: Nyp M, Brunkhorst J, Reavey D, Pallotto EK. Fluid and electrolyte management. In: Gardner SL, Carter BS, Hines ME, Niermeyer S, eds. *Merenstein & Gardner's Handbook of Neonatal Intensive Care: An Interprofessional Approach*. 9th ed. St. Louis, MO: Elsevier; 2021:426-427 [chapter 14].

34. **(D)** Developmentally appropriate care for this infant should include nonnutritive sucking, cluster care, providing sedatives and analgesics as needed per activity, and pain assessments. Positioning devices and the tucked position keep the infant comfortable and promote normal alignment of the body. The parents should be encouraged to visit, assist with care, and be taught appropriate touch techniques.

Reference: Gardner S, Goldson E. The neonate and the environment impact on development. In: Gardner SL, Carter BS, Hines ME, Niermeyer S, eds. *Merenstein & Gardner's Handbook of Neonatal Intensive Care: An Interprofessional Approach*. 9th ed. St. Louis, MO: Elsevier; 2021:348-394 [chapter 13].

35. **(A)** Digoxin is an inotrope and increases cardiac output and is used to lower the heart rate in infants with tachycardia. The urine output may increase as the blood flow improves with increased cardiac output, but this is not the primary treatment goal.

Reference: Sadowski S, Verklan MT. Cardiovascular disorders. In: Verklan M, Walden M, Forrest S, eds. *Core Curriculum for Neonatal Intensive Care Nursing.* 6th ed. St. Louis, MO: Elsevier; 2021:491-492.

36. **(D)** Furosemide (Lasix) is a loop diuretic and is used to eliminate excess water. Potassium and chloride are excreted with the water, causing hypokalemia and hypochloremia that can lead to metabolic alkalosis. The blood sugar is not affected.

Reference: Sadowski S, Verklan MT. Cardiovascular disorders. In: Verklan M, Walden M, Forrest S, eds. *Core Curriculum for Neonatal Intensive Care Nursing.* 6th ed. St. Louis, MO: Elsevier; 2021:492.

37. **(A)** Prostaglandin E1 is a potent vasodilator. Apnea, fever, and hypotension are known side effects. Blood glucose levels are not affected.

Reference: Swanson T, Erickson L. Cardiovascular diseases and surgical intervention. In: Gardner SL, Carter BS, Hines ME, Niermeyer S, eds. *Merenstein & Gardner's Handbook of Neonatal Intensive Care: An Interprofessional Approach.* 9th ed. St. Louis, MO: Elsevier; 2021:850-851 [chapter 24].

38. **(C)** The infant has reversed differential cyanosis. This can be seen with transposition of the great arteries when the preductal saturations are lower than the post ductal saturations. The transposition of the arteries leads to two separate circulations. The deoxygenated blood goes out the right atrium to the aorta to the body (right hand); the pulse oximeter reading is lower. Sepsis and respiratory distress syndrome may lead to pulmonary hypertension, but the right pulse oximeter reading would be higher. Truncus arteriosus causes low saturations in both upper and lower extremities.

Reference: Yue EL, Meckler GD. Congenital and acquired pediatric heart disease. In: Tintinalli JE, Ma OJ, Yealy DM, et al., eds. Tintinalli's Emergency Medicine: A Comprehensive Study Guide. 9th ed. New York: McGraw Hill; 2020. Available at: https://accessmedicine.mhmedical.com/content.aspx?bookid=2353&sectionid=220290085.

39. **(C)** The four defects of tetralogy of Fallot are VSD, obstruction of the RV outflow tract, RV hypertrophy, and overriding aorta.

Reference: Swanson T, Erickson L. Cardiovascular diseases and surgical intervention. In: Gardner SL, Carter BS, Hines ME, Niermeyer S, eds. *Merenstein & Gardner's Handbook of Neonatal Intensive Care: An Interprofessional Approach.* 9th ed. St. Louis, MO: Elsevier MO; 2021:866-867 [chapter 24].

40. **(D)** Survival of infants with hypoplastic left heart syndrome in the 20th century was not greater than 25%. Currently about 65%–70% of all newborns will survive all three staged procedures but longer term survival is not easily achieved. Transplant is an option but there is a scarcity, and many infants die while waiting for a donor. There is not a single-stage surgical approach. Very few families opt for comfort care, and in some institutions, this is rarely offered as an option.

Reference: Swanson T, Erickson L. Cardiovascular diseases and surgical intervention. In: Gardner SL, Carter BS, Hines ME, Niermeyer S, eds. *Merenstein & Gardner's Handbook of Neonatal Intensive Care: An Interprofessional Approach.* 9th ed. St. Louis, MO: Elsevier; 2021:874-875 [chapter 24].

41. **(B)** Respirations greater than 60 bpm at rest are the first sign noted in congestive heart failure and pulmonary edema. Tachycardia occurs later to help compensate for decreased cardiac output. The infant will increase both heart rate and respirations to compensate before the infant drops the BP. Hypothermia may occur later with shock.

Reference: Hansen TN, Richardson CP, Diblasi RM. Neonatal pulmonary physiology. In: Gleason CA, Juul SE, eds. *Avery's Diseases of the Newborn.* 10th ed. Philadelphia, PA: Elsevier; 2018:618-631 [chapter 39].

42. **(C)** Maternal use of aspirin and indomethacin along with other nonsteroidal antiinflammatory drugs (prostaglandin inhibitors) can cause the ductus to close prematurely in utero.

Symptoms of pulmonary hypertension may be evident soon after birth. Infants with neonatal abstinence syndrome have central nervous system symptoms and feeding problems. There are no known side effects in infants no longer receiving ibuprofen. Symptoms from a PDA do not present at birth but in the first week of life.

Reference: Bohannon K, Ho PM, Nolt V. Neonatal pharmacology; medications used in the neonatal intensive care unit. In: Gomella T, Eyal F, Bany-Mohammed F, eds. *Gomella's Neonatology: Management, Procedures, On-Call Problems, Diseases and Drugs.* 8th ed. New York: McGraw Hill; 2020:1272.

43. **(D)** The near-infrared spectroscopy monitor assesses trends in renal, abdominal, or cerebral (if on forehead) oxygenation. An electroencephalograph would provide brain or seizure activity. It does not monitor central venous pressure.

Reference: Sadowski S, Verklan MT. Cardiovascular disorders. In: Verklan M, Walden M, Forrest S, eds. *Core Curriculum for Neonatal Intensive Care Nursing.* 6th ed. St. Louis, MO: Elsevier Health Sciences; 2021:492.

44. **(C)** The first line of therapy is synchronized cardioversion in a hemodynamically unstable patient with SVT. The drug of choice has become adenosine for acute management. If available, esophageal pacing is effective, but not the first line of treatment. Chest compressions are only needed if the heart rate is less than 60 with effective ventilation.

Reference: Tsaban G, Kastantino Y. Supraventricular tachycardia. In: *Ferri F, ed. Ferri's Clinical Advisor 2020.* Elsevier; 2020:1442-1444.

45. **(B)** Adenosine transiently blocks the conduction of the AV node. It is given rapidly by IV push due to its short half-life of 10 seconds or less.

References: Bohannon K, Ho PM, Nolt V. Neonatal pharmacology; medications used in the neonatal intensive care unit. In: Gomella T, Eyal F, Bany-Mohammed F, eds. *Gomella's Neonatology: Management, Procedures, On-Call Problems, Diseases and Drugs.* 8th ed. New York: McGraw Hill; 2020:1227.

46. **(D)** Milrinone is phosphodiesterase inhibitor that increases heart rate and contractility and is a vasodilator. Some patients may need volume infusion after a load of milrinone. The other vital signs are not affected.

Reference: Swanson T, Erickson L. Cardiovascular diseases and surgical interventions. In: Gardner S, Carter B, Enzman-Hines M, Niermeyer S, eds. *Merenstein & Gardner's Handbook of Neonatal Intensive Care: An Interprofessional Approach.* 9th ed. St. Louis, MO: Elsevier; 2021:850-851 [chapter 24].

47. **(A)** Maintaining adequate oxygenation is the primary goal in treating pulmonary hypertension. Hypoxia increases the pulmonary vascular restriction, which leads to worsening of the clinical condition. Also, the infant should be kept calm because agitation can also hypoxia can worsen. Hyperoxia and alkalosis can occur as the infant improves rapidly and must also be assessed for in the weaning phase but it is not seen in a worsening state.

Reference: Gardner S, Enzman-Hines M, Nyp M. Respiratory diseases. In: Gardner S, Carter B, Enzman-Hines M, Niermeyer S, eds. *Merenstein & Gardner's Handbook of Neonatal Intensive Care: An Interprofessional Approach.* 9th ed. St. Louis, MO: Elsevier; 2021:804-805 [chapter 23].

48. **(D)** Hypovolemic shock is a state of inadequate blood volume and can be seen with any condition that causes blood or fluid losses such as intraventricular hemorrhage, pulmonary hemorrhage, vomiting and diarrhea, severe third spacing, or large fluid loss from defects such a gastroschisis. Septic shock is caused from an infection. Cardiogenic shock results from cardiogenic dysfunction.

References: Sadowski S, Verklan, MT. Cardiovascular disorders. In: Verklan M, Walden M, Forrest S, eds. *Core Curriculum for Neonatal Intensive Care Nursing.* 6th ed. St. Louis, MO: Elsevier; 2021:496-498 [chapter 28].

49. **(A)** An infant with sepsis may have either hypothermia or hyperthermia. Infants in servocontrolled incubators may have these masked by the servocontrolled environment. The nurse should be aware to a sudden decrease in need for the incubator to supply a heat support for the infant. A neutral thermal environment also decreases oxygen consumption. The parents have the right to be included in any care discussions or changes in patient condition. A normal saline bolus of 5 mL/kg is insufficient to provide adequate volume resuscitation. Although neurologic assessments should be included in routine care, they do not need to be completed on an hourly basis.

Reference: Gardner S, Cammack B. Heat balance. In: Gardner S, Carter B, Enzman-Hines M, Niermeyer S, eds. *Merenstein & Gardner's Handbook of Neonatal Intensive Care: An Interprofessional Approach.* 9th ed. St. Louis, MO: Elsevier; 2021:137-147 [chapter 6].

50. **(B)** Hydrocortisone is a corticosteroid that is effective in the treatment of hypotension that is refractory to vasopressors and fluid boluses. A side effect of fentanyl and midazolam is hypotension. Caffeine is not used in hypotension treatment.

Reference: Bohannon K, Ho PM, Nolt V. Neonatal pharmacology; medications used in the neonatal intensive care unit. In: Gomella T, Eyal F, Bany-Mohammed F, eds. *Gomella's Neonatology: Management, Procedures, On-Call Problems, Diseases and Drugs.* 8th ed. New York: McGraw Hill; 2020:1269.

51. **(C)** Dopamine (Intropin) at a low dose is selective to the renal, mesenteric, cerebral, and coronary vasculature and will promote urinary output. Dopamine (Intropin) at 3 mcg/kg/min has little effect on the heart rate, BP, pulmonary or peripheral vasculature.

Reference: Bohannon K, Ho PM, Nolt V. Neonatal pharmacology; medications used in the neonatal intensive care unit. In: Gomella T, Eyal F, Bany-Mohammed F, eds. *Gomella's Neonatology: Management, Procedures, On-Call Problems, Diseases and Drugs.* 8th ed. New York: McGraw Hill; 2020:1253-1254.

52. **(A)** Babies with septic shock have a loss of vascular tone and also may have a "leaky" capillary bed. This may lead to a relative hypovolemic state. A normal saline bolus would be a prudent first step. Post bolus, Dopamine (Intropin) is considered the first line because it serves to be inotropic and vasoconstrictive serving to increase cardiac output and increasing the BP by decreasing the diameter of the blood vessels. A volume expander should not be given rapid push to a premature baby because of the risk of intraventricular hemorrhage. Hydrocortisone is usually reserved for hypotension refractory to first line treatments. Dobutamine (Dobutrex) is considered a secondary use vasopressor following fluid bolus and Dopamine administration.

Reference: Davis AL, Carcillo JA, Aneja RK, et al. American College of Critical Care medicine clinical practice parameters for hemodynamic support of pediatric and neonatal septic shock. *Crit Care Med.* 2017;45(6):1061-1093. doi:10.1097/CCM.0000000000002425.

53. **(B)** Infants who have tetralogy of Fallot and are feeding, crying, or doing any activity that requires more oxygen may exhibit trouble breathing with severe cyanosis. The knee-to-chest or squatting position is the best position to increase blood flow to the lungs. Supine with legs extended, prone, or side lying would not increase blood flow to the lungs.

Reference: Kliegman RM, St Geme JW, Blum NJ, Shah SS, Tasker RC, Wilson KM. Cyanotic congenital heart disease: lesions associated with decreased pulmonary blood flow. In: Kliegman RM, St Geme JW, Blum NJ, Shah SS, Tasker RC, Wilson KM, eds. *Nelson Textbook of Pediatrics.* 21st ed. Philadelphia, PA: Elsevier Inc.; 2020:2396-2407 [chapter 457].

54. **(A)** Digoxin can have toxic side effects of PR prolongation, sinus bradycardia, or sinoatrial block. A heart rate of 50 would be considered a toxic side effect. Toxicity usually first manifests as vomiting, dysrhythmia, or bradycardia. Bradycardia, not tachycardia, is a side effect of digoxin. A heart rate of 220 would be suspect for SVT whereas a heart rate of 150 is within the normal range for a neonate.

References: Bohannon K, Ho PM, Nolt V. Neonatal pharmacology; medications used in the neonatal intensive care unit. In: Gomella T, Eyal F, Bany-Mohammed F, eds. *Gomella's Neonatology: Management, Procedures, On-Call Problems, Diseases and Drugs.* 8th ed. New York: McGraw Hill; 2020:1252-1253.

Swanson T, Erickson L. Cardiovascular disorders and surgical interventions. In: Gardner S, Carter B, Enzman-Hines M, Niermeyer S, eds. *Merenstein & Gardner's Handbook of Neonatal Intensive Care: An Interprofessional Approach.* 9th ed. St. Louis, MO: Elsevier; 2021:848-849 [chapter 24].

55. **(A)** Blood, fluid loss, and third spacing can cause hypovolemia after surgery. Hypovolemia is a common cause of tachycardia. The infant could exhibit hypocalcemia, acidosis, and hypoglycemia after surgery, but these symptoms do not directly correlate with tachycardia and low BP.

Reference: Bohannon K, Ho PM, Nolt V. Neonatal pharmacology; medications used in the neonatal intensive care unit. In: Gomella T, Eyal F, Bany-Mohammed F, eds. Gomella's Neonatology: Management, Procedures, On-Call Problems, Diseases and Drugs. 8th ed. New York: McGraw Hill; 2020:617-625.

56. **(A)** Dobutamine (Dobutrex) is an inotropic vasopressor and increases myocardial contractility. It decreases systemic and pulmonary vascular resistance. It only slightly increases heart rate.

References: Jone PN, Kim JS, Burkett D, Jacobsen R, Von Alvensleben J. Cardiovascular diseases. In: Bunik M, Hay WW, Levin MJ, Abzug MJ, eds. *Current Diagnosis & Treatment: Pediatrics.* 26th ed. New York: McGraw-Hill; 2022:552.

Bohannon K, Ho PM, Nolt V. Neonatal pharmacology; medications used in the neonatal intensive care unit. In: Gomella T, Eyal F, Bany-Mohammed F, eds. *Gomella's Neonatology: Management, Procedures, On-Call Problems, Diseases and Drugs.* 8th ed. New York: McGraw Hill; 2020:1253.

57. **(C)** In the presence of a PDA the future closure of a PDA, the aorta can become constricted and a coarctation can develop. The ductus venosus is functionally eliminated at birth with the removal of the placental circuit. An overriding pulmonary artery or pulmonary vein does not anatomically influence the aorta as no vessel connection exists.

Reference: Jone PN, Kim JS, Burkett D, Jacobsen R, Von Alvensleben J. Cardiovascular diseases. In: Bunik M, Hay WW, Levin MJ, Abzug MJ, eds. *Current Diagnosis & Treatment: Pediatrics.* 26th ed. New York: McGraw-Hill; 2022:563.

58. **(D)** This infant should have 4–8 mL/h or 1–2 mL/kg/h urinary output postoperatively to ensure adequate renal perfusion 48 hours postsurgery. Any amount less than 4–8 mL/h would be inadequate.

Reference: Cyr AR, Alarcon LH. Physiologic monitoring of the surgical patient. In: Brunicardi FC, Andersen DK, Billiar TR, et al., eds. *Schwartz's Principles of Surgery.* 11th ed. McGraw Hill; 2019. Available at: https://accessmedicine.mhmedical.com/content.aspx?bookid=2576&sectionid=216205807.

59. **(B)** Furosemide (Lasix) is a potent diuretic and should be given as prescribed. The correct dose is established for each patient. Infants who have cardiac defects may develop congestive heart failure if they do not receive the diuretic as scheduled every day. If given in excess, it can cause dehydration and electrolyte disturbances. Weighing of diapers or BP checks are usually not required to be done in the home environment by the parent or caretaker.

Reference: Neofax. *IBM Micromedex.* 2022. Available at: https://www.micromedexsolutions.com/home/dispatch/.

60. **(D)** Oxygen is a proven pulmonary vasodilator and the first line of treatment in pulmonary hypertension. Paralysis is often used but is not a proven therapy. Furosemide (Lasix) is a diuretic and may decrease BP. A lower BP may exacerbate persistent pulmonary hypertension of the newborn. Sildenafil may be used in acquired or chronic pulmonary hypertension but is not considered a first-line therapy.

Reference: Carter N, Clark BS. Neonatology. In: Kleinman K, McDaniel L, Molloy M, eds. *The Harriet Lane Handbook: A Manual for Pediatric House Officers.* Philadelphia, PA: Elsevier; 2021:456-457 [chapter 18].

61. **(B)** Medications such as diuretics and afterload reducers are commonly prescribed for congestive heart failure. Diuretics help

maintain a normal circulating volume and help relieve pulmonary and hepatic congestion related to the back-pressure caused by the failing heart muscle. Afterload reducers reduce systemic vascular resistance to relieve the pressure the heart needs to pump against. Adequate calorie intake will ensure that the infant stays appropriate on the growth curve. Sedation is not used for congestive heart failure (CHF). Physical therapy may be a part of the treatment plan but does not supersede the importance of providing medications for the CHF and appropriate calories for adequate growth.

Reference: Swanson T, Erickson L. Cardiovascular diseases and surgical interventions. In: Gardner S, Carter B, Enzman-Hines M, Niermeyer S, eds. *Merenstein & Gardner's Handbook of Neonatal Intensive Care: An Interprofessional Approach.* 9th ed. St. Louis, MO: Elsevier; 2021:844-851 [chapter 24].

62. **(D)** Ebstein malformation on x-ray reveals extreme cardiomegaly with severity depending on the degree of tricuspid valve insufficiency and size of the atrial shunt. Hypoplastic left heart syndrome may have cardiomegaly, but not as severe as in Ebstein malformation. Tricuspid atresia has variable heart size, but size is nondiagnostic. Pulmonary atresia shows increased heart size with right atrial hypertrophy but not to the extent of Ebstein malformation.

Reference: Scholz T, Reinking BE. Congenital heart disease. In: Sawyer T, Gleason C, eds. *Avery's Diseases of the Newborn.* 11th ed. Philadelphia, PA: Elsevier; 2024:801-827 [chapter 50].

63. **(A)** The aorta is anterior to the main pulmonary artery in transposition of the great arteries, producing a narrow mediastinum or the appearance of an "egg on a string." Wall-to-wall heart is associated with Ebstein malformation. A boot-shaped heart is common with tetralogy of Fallot. A narrow cardiac silhouette can be associated with dehydration.

Reference: Scholz T, Reinking BE. Congenital heart disease. In: Sawyer T, Gleason C, eds. *Avery's Diseases of the Newborn.* 11th ed. Philadelphia, PA: Elsevier; 2024:801-827 [chapter 50].

64. **(D)** CHD has been found to be caused by genetic or environmental causes in up to 30% of cases and the remainder are thought to be multifactorial in nature. Tobacco, opiate, and alcohol are all known to be teratogens but do not directly correlate with the occurrence of congenital heart disease.

Reference: Libby P. Congenital heart disease in adolescents and adults. In: Bonow R, Mann D, Tomaselli G, Bhatt D, Solomon S, Braunwald E, eds. *Braunwald's Heart Disease: A Textbook of Cardiovascular Medicine.* 12th ed. Philadelphia, PA: Elsevier; 2022:1541-1586 [chapter 82].

65. **(B)** Ambient lighting has no effect on pulse oximetry readings during a hyperoxia test. A hyperoxia test is an important screening tool but it does not replace an echocardiogram for confirmation of a congenital heart defect. A chest x-ray is not related to a hyperoxia test.

An infant does not need to be intubated to have a hyperoxia test performed. A nasal cannula or oxygen hood device may be used to deliver oxygen to the infant.

Reference: Rohit M, Rajan P. Approach to cyanotic congenital heart disease in children. *Indian J Pediatr.* 2020;87:372-380. doi:10.1007/s12098-020-03274-3.

66. **(A)** The right wrist is considered "preductal" and gives readings on blood coming from the heart prior to where mixing occurs at the ductus arteriosus. The "preductal" blood has a similar oxygen saturation as the blood perfusing the heart and brain, which allows for a more accurate assessment of the success of a resuscitation in the delivery room. Oxygen saturation levels can be obtained from any extremity but will vary based on if it is a preductal or postductal reading. Both pre- and postductal readings are necessary as part of the diagnostic workup for congenital heart disease.

Reference: Weiner GM. Lesson 3. Initial steps of newborn care. In: *Textbook of Neonatal Resuscitation.* 8th ed. Itasca, IL: American Academy of Pediatrics; 2021:33-63.

Chapter 15

Pulmonary Disorders

1. Which one of the following statements about continuous positive airway pressure (CPAP) is true?
   A. CPAP and positive end expiratory pressure (PEEP) are synonymous.
   B. Nasal CPAP can be delivered using either a continuous or a variable-flow device to maintain constant airway pressure.
   C. The specified amount of pressure is delivered continuously only during the inspiratory phase of respiration.
   D. The specified amount of pressure is delivered continuously only during the expiratory phase of respiration.

2. Advantages of bubble CPAP include which of the following?
   A. It is not necessary to heat the gas.
   B. Pressure is generated by changing the flow rate of gases during inspiration and expiration to maintain a constant airway pressure in the alveoli if the nasal prongs remain in place.
   C. The system is inexpensive, simple, and readily available.
   D. The system delivers continuous positive pressure at two separate CPAP levels.

3. CPAP is most likely to be used with which of the following conditions?
   A. Congenital diaphragmatic hernia (CDH)
   B. Central apnea
   C. Pneumothorax
   D. Obstructive apnea

4. When choosing the appropriate size of nasal prongs for administering CPAP, the nurse knows that:
   A. prongs should loosely fit in the nares to avoid injury to the nasal septum.
   B. using moderate force, prongs should fill the nostrils completely.
   C. part of the prongs should remain outside the nose.
   D. the larger the prongs, the higher the airway resistance.

5. Which of the following factors interferes with transillumination of a pneumothorax?
   A. Dark room lighting
   B. Bright light from the transilluminator

C. Large-for-gestation infant

D. Darkly pigmented skin

6. A characteristic radiographic finding of a pneumomediastinum is:
   A. the "sail sign."
   B. a mediastinal shift toward the unaffected side.
   C. decreased heart size.
   D. the liver is clearly defined from the anterior abdominal wall on a right lateral view.

7. Subglottic stenosis may result from:
   A. multiple doses of surfactant.
   B. prolonged intubation.
   C. endotracheal tube (ETT) placed in the right mainstem bronchus.
   D. traumatic intubation.

8. Necrotizing tracheobronchitis is characterized by which of the following?
   A. Stridor
   B. Softening of the cartilaginous airway rings and a failure to support the round shape of the trachea
   C. Dilation of the trachea and bronchi
   D. Inflammation and granulation of the distal trachea

9. Which of the following statements about ventilation–perfusion matching (Va/Qc) is true?
   A. Alveolar underventilation results in a high Va/Qc ratio.
   B. A Va/Qc ratio of 1 indicates a shunt.
   C. The ideal ventilation–perfusion ratio is zero.
   D. Ventilation–perfusion mismatching is the most common reason for hypoxia.

10. The American Academy of Pediatrics recommendations for prevention of sudden infant death syndrome (SIDS) in healthy infants include:
    A. home cardiorespiratory monitoring.
    B. proper sleep position.
    C. limiting bedding to no more than two loose blankets in the crib.
    D. using bumper pads on crib slats.

11. Which of the following is considered a precursor or risk factor for SIDS?
    A. Prenatal and postnatal exposure to cigarette smoke
    B. Apnea
    C. Low environmental temperature
    D. Short QT interval

12. The obstetric provider requests that the high-risk neonatal team attend the emergency cesarean section delivery of a term infant with nonreassuring fetal status. Which of the following factors does the team consider to be the best indication for the need to resuscitate?
    A. Maternal general anesthesia
    B. A 1-minute Apgar score of 4
    C. The infant's clinical presentation and response
    D. Maternal administration of magnesium sulfate

13. Which of the following is considered a contraindication for chest physiotherapy?

A. Atelectasis

B. Neuromuscular compromise

C. Chest tube or gastrostomy tube in place

D. Pulmonary hemorrhage

14. An experienced nurse is orienting a new neonatal intensive care unit (NICU) nurse whose assignment includes a 40-day-old, former 25-week-gestation infant diagnosed with bronchopulmonary dysplasia (BPD). The experienced nurse provides which of the following explanations about BPD?
    A. BPD is characterized by altered lung development with decreased numbers of alveoli and abnormal blood vessel development.
    B. The primary cause of BPD is oxygen toxicity.
    C. BPD occurs exclusively in preterm infants with severe respiratory distress syndrome (RDS).
    D. BPD results from lung damage caused only by mechanical ventilation.

15. Pulmonary interstitial emphysema (PIE) results from extraneous air in the:
    A. subcutaneous tissue.
    B. pleural space.
    C. connective tissue of the peribronchovascular sheaths.
    D. alveoli trabeculae-visceral pleura.

16. A chest x-ray was obtained after oxygen requirements increased from 25% to 35% for an infant on nasal cannula at 1 L/min. The physical examination is unchanged from baseline. The x-ray shows a small pneumothorax on the left side. Which of the following actions is considered inappropriate?
    A. Monitoring the infant for additional changes in respiratory status
    B. Positioning the infant with the affected side down
    C. Ensuring that supplies needed for needle thoracentesis are at the bedside
    D. Placing the infant on nasal CPAP

17. Which pathophysiology is associated with meconium aspiration syndrome (MAS)?
    A. Atelectasis-prone lungs susceptible to volutrauma
    B. Hemodynamic impairment and restricted chest and/or diaphragmatic movement
    C. Gas interstitium compressing alveoli, airways, and pulmonary venules
    D. Uneven aeration, gas trapping, and surfactant inactivation

18. Which of the following statements about high-frequency ventilation (HFV) is true?
    A. HFV does not cause gas trapping.
    B. Gas exchange occurs even when tidal volume is less than anatomic dead space.
    C. The mean airway pressure used to support lung volume using HFV is lower than that required with conventional mechanical ventilation.
    D. HFV is not as effective as conventional mechanical ventilation for eliminating carbon dioxide.

19. During the assessment of an infant on HFV, the nurse notices increased chest wall motion. This finding suggests:
    A. improved compliance.
    B. inadequate amplitude.

C. gas trapping.

D. a large pneumothorax.

20. Which of the following factors is thought to decrease the severity of RDS in the at-risk population?

   A. Chronic intrauterine stress

   B. Second-born twin

   C. Male sex

   D. Cesarean section without labor

21. Upon auscultation of a recently extubated infant, the nurse hears continuous low-pitched breath sounds during inspiration and expiration. What adventitious breath sound is described here?

   A. Crackles

   B. Wheezes

   C. Rhonchi

   D. Stridor

22. A disadvantage of pulse oximetry is:

   A. a slow response to changes in oxygen saturation.

   B. a low correlation of SpO_2 and PaO_2 at lower saturations.

   C. there is no way to verify the reliability of the sensor.

   D. phototherapy can interfere with SpO_2 accuracy.

23. A radiology report corresponding to a chest x-ray states that lung fields are overaerated and clear. These findings are consistent with:

   A. pulmonary air leak.

   B. congenital lobar emphysema (CLE).

   C. hyperinflation.

   D. hydrothorax.

24. Which of the following is a possible cause of respiratory acidosis?

   A. Acetazolamide administration

   B. Maternal heroin addiction

   C. Diuretic therapy

   D. Apnea

25. An arterial blood gas (ABG) obtained on a full-term infant at 1 hour of age shows the following: pH 7.24, PCO_2 51, PO_2 40, and HCO_3 17. The best interpretation of these results is:

   A. compensated metabolic acidosis and hypoxemia.

   B. mixed respiratory and metabolic acidosis and hypoxemia.

   C. partially compensated metabolic acidosis and hypoxemia.

   D. respiratory acidosis and hypoxemia.

26. When obtaining a blood sample for capillary blood gas analysis, the nurse knows to:

   A. avoid the posterolateral aspect of the heel.

   B. hold the puncture site above the rest of the extremity to facilitate collection.

   C. avoid the calcaneus.

   D. squeeze the extremity to increase blood flow.

27. Which of the following statements about ETT-CPAP is true?

   A. Clean technique can be used when suctioning.

   B. There is a decreased risk for air leaks compared with nasal CPAP.

   C. There is increased work of breathing with prolonged use of ET-CPAP.

   D. This method is the preferred method for delivering noninvasive ventilation.

28. Mechanical ventilation is indicated for which of the following conditions?

   A. A large CDH

   B. PCO_2 of 50 mm Hg on blood gas

   C. Mild-to-moderate respiratory distress

   D. Mild pulmonary edema

29. Which of the following modes of mechanical ventilation describes the delivery of a synchronized breath, with each spontaneous breath meeting the threshold criteria, or the delivery of mechanical breaths at a preset regular rate if there is no spontaneous respiratory effort?

   A. Assist/control

   B. Pressure support ventilation

   C. Neurally adjusted ventilatory assist

   D. Synchronized intermittent mandatory ventilation

30. During suctioning of patients on mechanical ventilation, the nurse considers what additional action to maintain PEEP?

   A. Uses a closed suction system.

   B. Oxygenates with 100% oxygen prior to suctioning.

   C. Avoids suctioning to prevent interruption of PEEP.

   D. Routinely suctions every 2 hours to prevent atelectasis.

31. When caring for an infant requiring cardiorespiratory support and continuous monitoring, including pulse oximetry, the nurse realizes:

   A. the accuracy of pulse oximetry may be affected by vasoconstricting drugs such as epinephrine and dopamine.

   B. pulse oximetry eliminates the need for blood gas analysis.

   C. pulse oximetry is not accurate when a large alveolar–arterial gradient is present.

   D. pulse oximetry has a slow response time for determining oxygen saturation, and therefore readings may not accurately reflect the patient's current status.

32. While caring for a preterm infant on ventilator support and end-tidal CO_2 monitoring, the nurse is aware that:

   A. end-tidal CO_2 monitoring can be used with spontaneous, conventional, and HFV.

   B. end-tidal CO_2 monitoring is unreliable in infants with severe lung disease.

   C. end-tidal CO_2 monitoring has a better correlation with $PaCO_2$ than transcutaneous CO_2 monitoring.

   D. end-tidal CO_2 monitoring is slow to respond to changes in partial pressure of carbon dioxide in alveolar gas (P_ACO_2).

33. Which of the following ventilator parameters is favorable for extubation?

   A. Intermittent mandatory ventilation of 22–30/minute

   B. Peak inspiratory pressure of 20–24 cm H_2O

   C. Tidal volume of 6–8.5 mL/kg

   D. FiO_2 of 0.26

34. Which of the following factors is predictive of a low risk for RDS?

   A. A lecithin–sphingomyelin (L/S) ratio of 3:2

   B. The presence of phosphatidylglycerol (PG) in the presence of blood-contaminated amniotic fluid

   C. An L/S ratio of greater than 2:1 in the presence of blood-contaminated amniotic fluid

   D. The absence of PG in amniotic fluid

35. While caring for a 2-day-old 28-week-gestation intubated infant, the nurse recognizes that the infant requires endotracheal suctioning. Which of the following actions is appropriate?
    A. Use sterile normal saline before suctioning to mobilize and thin secretions.
    B. Turn the infant's head from side to side with suction passes to advance the catheter down the contralateral bronchus.
    C. Insert and remove the catheter several times to ensure removal of secretions.
    D. Provide nonnutritive sucking and/or body containment during suction procedure to minimize the infant's stress response to suctioning.

36. Compared with dexamethasone, low-dose hydrocortisone is associated with:
    A. an equivalent safety profile.
    B. an increase in adverse neurodevelopmental outcomes.
    C. a lower incidence of BPD/chronic lung disease.
    D. a lower risk of reduced brain growth.

37. The formation of respiratory bronchioles during the canalicular stage of fetal lung development is significant because it heralds:
    A. formation of the lung bud and initial branching of the airways.
    B. alveolar proliferation and development.
    C. rapid proliferation of pulmonary vasculature.
    D. primitive development of the gas exchange section of the lung.

38. A newborn infant with respiratory difficulty is diagnosed with a congenital chylothorax. A thoracentesis followed by placement of a tube thoracotomy for continuous drainage is performed. The nurse must monitor this patient closely for:
    A. apnea.
    B. air leak.
    C. infection.
    D. subcutaneous emphysema.

39. Lung development is completed by what age?
    A. 38–40 weeks of gestation
    B. 12–15 months of age
    C. 3–5 years of age
    D. 16–20 years of age

40. Surfactant improves lung function by:
    A. increasing opening pressure.
    B. inhibiting alveolar fluid clearance.
    C. promoting structural maturation of the lung.
    D. reducing surface tension at the air–liquid interface in the alveolus.

41. Which of the following populations of infants at 36 weeks of gestation is at increased risk for developing RDS?
    A. Infants of mothers abusing heroin
    B. Fetal exposure to chorioamnionitis
    C. Infants of class A, B, and C diabetic mothers
    D. Infants born to mothers receiving corticosteroids

42. Surfactant is produced in the lungs by:
    A. acini.
    B. type I pneumocytes.
    C. type II pneumocytes.
    D. surfactant protein A.

43. Early signs of respiratory disease in a neonate include:
    A. retractions.
    B. hypotension.
    C. acrocyanosis.
    D. respiratory rate of 30–40 breaths per minute.

44. Mechanically ventilated infants must be monitored for acid–base status. Prolonged, severe hypocapnia resulting in respiratory alkalosis places the infant at risk for:
    A. apnea.
    B. intraventricular hemorrhage.
    C. periventricular leukomalacia.
    D. gastroesophageal reflux disease.

45. In the delivery room a 1200-g infant at 30 weeks' gestation shows grunting, nasal flaring, and chest wall retractions. Which of the following pulmonary pathophysiologic conditions is most likely occurring?
    A. Pulmonary air leak syndrome
    B. RDS
    C. MAS
    D. Transient tachypnea of the newborn

46. Expiratory grunting represents the infant's attempt to:
    A. conserve energy.
    B. decrease upper airway resistance.
    C. overcome large airway obstruction.
    D. maintain a normal functional residual capacity.

47. To rule out group B streptococcal infection as an underlying cause of respiratory distress, which of the following studies would be most appropriate?
    A. Eye culture
    B. Blood cultures
    C. Cultures of nasopharyngeal secretions
    D. Cultures of axillary and rectal specimens

48. A radiographic picture of grainy lungs and prominent air bronchograms is characteristic of which of the following conditions?
    A. Pneumonia
    B. Pulmonary edema
    C. Pulmonary air leaks
    D. RDS

49. Results of an infant's ABG analysis are: pH 7.25, $PaCO_2$ 70, HCO_3 22, base deficit -4, PaO_2 50, and oxygen saturation 88%. These blood gas results are indicative of which acid–base condition?
    A. Metabolic acidosis
    B. Metabolic alkalosis
    C. Respiratory acidosis
    D. Respiratory alkalosis

50. An infant is being mechanically ventilated because of respiratory failure secondary to RDS. ABG results indicate a rising

PaCO$_2$. Breath sounds are coarse bilaterally, with bubbling of secretions observed in the ETT. The infant is extremely restless, with "seesaw" respirations. The ventilator is consistently sounding an alarm for high inspiratory pressure. The nurse's first action is to:
A. reposition the infant.
B. administer an analgesic.
C. silence the ventilator alarm.
D. suction the infant.

51. By 72 hours of life a small preterm infant who has been treated with surfactant for RDS develops a grade II–VI continuous murmur at the left upper sternal border. Bilateral rales are heard on auscultation. Bounding peripheral pulses with a widened pulse pressure are present. Urine output is less than 2 mL/kg/h. Blood gas analyses reveal increasing hypoxemia, hypercarbia, and metabolic acidosis with subsequent need for increased ventilatory support. These findings are most consistent with which condition?
A. Sepsis
B. Air leak
C. Pneumonia
D. Patent ductus arteriosus (PDA)

52. Which of the following is indicated for the management of an infant with RDS complicated by PDA?
A. Volume expansion
B. Indomethacin (Indocin)
C. Furosemide (Lasix)
D. Prostaglandin E1 (Alprostadil)

53. Which of the following is a complication associated with PDA?
A. Metabolic alkalosis
B. Pulmonary air leak
C. Pulmonary hypoplasia
D. Pulmonary hemorrhage

54. Nursing management of an acutely ill preterm infant with RDS is directed toward:
A. liberalizing administration of fluids.
B. handling frequently to provide developmental stimulation.
C. maintaining the infant in a neutral thermal environment.
D. decreasing inspired oxygen fraction (FiO$_2$) for oxygen saturation values of less than 88%.

55. When assessing a 3-day-old infant with RDS, the nurse calculates the infant's urine output to be more than 5 mL/kg/h for an 8-hour period. The nurse suspects that the increase in urine output is indicative of which of the following conditions?
A. Renal failure
B. Worsening pulmonary status
C. Development of chronic lung disease
D. Recovery phase of RDS

56. A maternal history of chorioamnionitis, fever, premature rupture of membranes longer than 24 hours, prolonged labor with intact membranes, and excessive obstetric manipulations predisposes the infant to which of the following conditions?
A. Congenital pneumonia
B. RDS
C. MAS
D. Transient tachypnea of the newborn

57. A 39-week, large-for-gestational-age infant was delivered by cesarean section. The Apgar scores were 8 and 9 at 1 and 5 minutes, respectively, and initial vital signs were stable. At 2 hours of age, the infant exhibits increased work of breathing and a pulse oximetry reading of 88% on room air. Blow-by oxygen raises the oxygen saturation to 96%. An ABG analysis reveals the following: pH 7.36, PaCO$_2$ 37, HCO$_3$ 24, and PaO$_2$ 65. Appropriate management for this infant would include which of the following interventions?
A. Administration of surfactant
B. Administration of inhaled nitric oxide (iNO)
C. Intubation and mechanical ventilation
D. Provision of supplemental oxygen to maintain PaO$_2$ at 70–80

58. The initial chest radiograph for a large-for-gestational-age term infant delivered by cesarean section reveals diffuse haziness with prominent perihilar streaking bilaterally and fluid in the fissures. This radiographic picture is consistent with which diagnosis?
A. RDS
B. MAS
C. PIE
D. Transient tachypnea of the newborn

59. Severe asphyxia of the full-term infant in the early neonatal period may result in which of the following conditions?
A. Pneumonia
B. Transient tachypnea of the newborn
C. Left-to-right shunting through the foramen ovale
D. Persistent pulmonary hypertension of the newborn

60. Central apnea is defined as:
A. absence of airflow and spontaneous respiratory effort.
B. absence of airflow with continued respiratory effort.
C. a condition with both neurologic and obstructive components.
D. a cyclical pattern of apnea for 5–10 seconds followed by breathing for 10–15 seconds.

61. The neonate's unique response to hypoxemia and carbon dioxide retention is characterized by:
A. an initial decrease in respiratory effort.
B. prolonged sustained increase in alveolar ventilation.
C. a brief period of increased respiration followed by respiratory depression.
D. an increase in minute ventilation above baseline until blood levels of oxygen and carbon dioxide normalize.

62. Which of the following nursing interventions may exacerbate apnea in preterm infants?
A. Limiting loud noises
B. Weighing on a cold scale
C. Controlling environmental temperature
D. Positioning with small rolls under the neck and shoulder

63. As the nurse prepares to administer a dose of caffeine to a preterm infant, the nurse determines that the infant is tachycardic, with a heart rate of 190 beats per minute. The infant is resting quietly in the incubator. The nurse's action is to:
A. administer the dose of caffeine.
B. wait 5 minutes before administering the dose.

C. withhold the dose and notify the physician or neonatal nurse practitioner (NNP).

D. remeasure the heart rate and administer the dose if heart rate is less than 180 beats per minute.

64. An infant requires frequent ABG monitoring, but obtaining ABG specimens is difficult in the infant. A transcutaneous oxygen and carbon dioxide monitor is ordered for this infant. The nurse knows that:
    A. no more ABG specimens will be needed.
    B. the umbilical arterial catheter can now be removed.
    C. use of this monitor will reduce the number of ABG specimens needed.
    D. there is a direct correlation between the transcutaneous oxygen and carbon dioxide values and the ABG values.

65. Aspiration pneumonitis acquired at delivery manifests within the first hours to days of life. Which of the following pathogens is most commonly associated with aspiration pneumonitis?
    A. *Chlamydia trachomatis*
    B. Respiratory syncytial virus
    C. Group β-hemolytic streptococci
    D. Fungi, especially *Candida* species

66. A 3.5-kg, postterm infant was born via cesarean section because of prolonged fetal bradycardia and thick meconium-stained fluid. At delivery the infant was limp, apneic, cyanotic, and bradycardic and required intubation. Suctioning of the trachea produced thick green material. On admission, the admitting nurse recognizes that this infant is at high risk for which of the following conditions?
    A. Pulmonary edema
    B. Nonspecific respiratory distress
    C. MAS
    D. Transient tachypnea of the newborn

67. A newborn term infant with MAS is intubated and conventional ventilation is started. When the infant is 3 hours of age, the cardiorespiratory monitor alarms for bradycardia and hypotension. The infant is extremely restless and cyanotic, with diminished breath sounds on the left side, poor peripheral pulses, asymmetric chest rise, and a mediastinal shift toward the right. The nurse suspects the development of which of the following conditions?
    A. Pleural effusion
    B. Tension pneumothorax
    C. Pulmonary hemorrhage
    D. PIE

68. A term infant is delivered vaginally after an uncomplicated labor and delivery. Immediately after birth, the infant becomes cyanotic with severe grunting, retracting, and nasal flaring. The infant is intubated, and positive pressure ventilation is started. On physical examination, breath sounds are diminished on the left side with displacement of cardiac sounds toward the right. The abdomen is scaphoid in appearance. A chest radiograph reveals dilated loops of bowel in the thoracic space with right mediastinal shift. The nurse prepares to assist with management of which of the following conditions?
    A. Tension pneumothorax
    B. Pneumomediastinum

C. CDH

D. Congenital pulmonary airway malformation (CPAM)

69. Factors that predispose an infant to BPD include which of the following?
    A. Hypovolemia
    B. Full-term birth
    C. Oxygen administration and mechanical ventilation
    D. Transient tachypnea of the newborn

70. Radiographic findings characteristic of severe BPD include which of the following?
    A. Pleural effusion
    B. Alveolar infiltrates
    C. Dark areas without parenchymal markings
    D. Cystic lung fields with hyperinflation and atelectasis

71. Which of the following is the appropriate management for ventilator-induced respiratory alkalosis?
    A. Increase the ventilator rate.
    B. Decrease minute ventilation.
    C. Increase peak inspiratory pressure.
    D. Decrease PEEP.

72. Which of the following statements about pulmonary physiology is accurate?
    A. Tidal volume is defined as the volume of air maximally inspired and maximally expired in one breath.
    B. Vital capacity is defined as the amount of air that moves into or out of the lungs with each normal respiration.
    C. Functional residual capacity is defined as the volume of gas that remains in the lungs after normal expiration.
    D. Physiologic dead space is defined as the volume of gas within the area of the pulmonary conducting airways that cannot engage in gas exchange.

73. Which of the following statements about the care of an infant with a chest tube is accurate?
    A. Repositioning of the patient should be minimized.
    B. Milking and stripping of the chest tube are routine interventions to ensure tube patency.
    C. Continuous bubbling in the water seal chamber is an indication that the chest tube is functioning effectively.
    D. Tube patency, fluctuation, and bubbling in the drainage system should be monitored and documented hourly.

74. A preterm infant being treated with mechanical ventilation for severe RDS suddenly has hypotension, muffled heart sounds, and bradycardia. The chest radiograph reveals a "halo" surrounding the heart. The nurse prepares to assist with management of which of the following conditions?
    A. Pneumothorax
    B. Pneumopericardium
    C. Pneumomediastinum
    D. PIE

75. Why is iNO useful in the treatment of persistent pulmonary hypertension?
    A. iNO supports cardiac function.
    B. iNO promotes bronchodilation.
    C. iNO decreases systemic arterial pressure.
    D. iNO is a potent selective pulmonary vasodilator.

76. The nurse anticipates that an infant will be scheduled for surgical reduction of a CDH:
    A. immediately after delivery.
    B. after surfactant therapy.
    C. after a trial period of treatment with iNO.
    D. once pulmonary stabilization has been achieved.

77. Which of the following is a long-term complication associated with CDH repair?
    A. Chylothorax
    B. Potter syndrome
    C. Gastroesophageal reflux
    D. Necrotizing enterocolitis

78. Initial blood gas analysis for an infant with RDS reveals the following: pH 7.28, $PaCO_2$ 65, PaO_2 85, and HCO_3 22. The most appropriate management for this infant, who is being mechanically ventilated, is to:
    A. decrease the ventilator rate.
    B. decrease the inspiratory time.
    C. increase the peak inspiratory pressure.
    D. increase the PEEP.

79. While being mechanically ventilated, an infant becomes agitated and cyanotic. The infant's respirations are vigorous but asynchronous from those of the ventilator. The best initial response is to:
    A. obtain a chest radiograph.
    B. suction the ETT.
    C. administer vecuronium.
    D. change the mode of ventilation from synchronized intermittent mandatory ventilation to assist-control ventilation.

80. Which of the following shifts the oxygen–hemoglobin dissociation curve to the left?
    A. Increase in pH
    B. Increase in $PaCO_2$
    C. Increase in temperature
    D. Increase in diphosphoglycerate level

81. A full-term infant has apnea at 10 hours of life. The most likely cause is:
    A. sepsis.
    B. placement on the back to sleep.
    C. hyperglycemia.
    D. apnea of prematurity.

82. Which of the following is a pathologic condition characterized by right ventricular hypertrophy and right-axis deviation on electrocardiogram, respiratory wheezing, hepatomegaly, and radiographic findings of cystic lesions with lung hyperinflation?
    A. Severe BPD
    B. RDS
    C. MAS
    D. PIE

83. An infant is admitted to the NICU from the delivery room exhibiting tachypnea, nasal flaring, cyanosis, and increased anteroposterior diameter of the chest. The amniotic fluid was characterized as thick "pea-stained" fluid. An initial ABG analysis determines that endotracheal intubation is warranted. Which of the following is most appropriate as an initial setting for this infant when synchronized intermittent mandatory ventilation is started?
    A. Low rate
    B. Low inspiratory time
    C. Low peak inspiratory pressure
    D. High PEEP

84. Hyponatremia associated with RDS in a preterm infant with no documented weight loss within the first few days of life is indicative of:
    A. total body sodium depletion.
    B. excessive evaporative loss.
    C. excessive total body water.
    D. high-volume urinary output.

85. Which of the following will optimize patient outcomes in the intubated extremely preterm infant with RDS who is 4 days old?
    A. Multiple laboratory specimen draws via heel stick
    B. Restriction of intravenous fluids at 100 mL/kg/day
    C. Frequent and scheduled endotracheal suctioning
    D. Administration of surfactant

86. Which of the following statements is true regarding inhaled nitrogen oxide (iNO)?
    A. iNO is inactivated after it combines with hemoglobin.
    B. iNO is an effective pulmonary vasodilator with a half-life of 3–5 minutes.
    C. iNO is initiated and maintained at 20 ppm until pulmonary vascular relaxation has occurred.
    D. Once pulmonary vascular relaxation has been accomplished, it is safe to halt administration of iNO because the half-life is so short.

87. The administration of surfactant at the time of delivery is termed:
    A. rescue therapy.
    B. assisted ventilation.
    C. prophylactic therapy.
    D. chemical resuscitation.

88. The care provider has ordered indomethacin (Indocin) for an infant diagnosed with a PDA. Which of the following would indicate to the nurse that it is safe to administer the medication?
    A. Serum creatinine level of 2.0 mg/dL
    B. Urine output of 0.5 mL/kg/h
    C. Platelet count of 110,000/mm^3
    D. Radiographic evidence of necrotizing enterocolitis

89. The most common cause of stridor in the infant is:
    A. choanal atresia.
    B. laryngomalacia.
    C. vocal cord paralysis.
    D. congenital subglottic stenosis.

90. A 38-week-gestation infant has apnea, hypotonia, cyanosis, and a heart rate of less than 100 beats per minute at delivery. When tactile stimulation and blow-by oxygen fail to induce spontaneous respiration, the nurse initiates positive pressure bag-and-mask ventilation, suspecting that the infant has which of the following conditions?

A. Idiopathic apnea
B. Obstructive apnea
C. Primary apnea associated with asphyxia
D. Secondary apnea associated with asphyxia

91. When an apnea monitor sounds an alarm 20 seconds after the cessation of breathing, the most appropriate immediate response is to:
A. assess breath sounds.
B. provide blow-by oxygen.
C. administer positive pressure ventilation with bag and mask.
D. provide gentle tactile stimulation of the chest and/or extremities.

92. Which of the following medications is used to treat apnea that is refractory to methylxanthine therapy?
A. Caffeine (Cafcit)
B. Doxapram (Dopram)
C. Theophylline (Theo-Dur, Slo-Bid)
D. Aminophylline (Phyllocontin, Truphylline)

93. A nursing intervention that helps alleviate apnea in preterm infants is:
A. performing endotracheal suction.
B. weighing on a cold scale.
C. controlling environmental temperature.
D. tapping on the outside of the incubator.

94. Which of the following is an advantage of caffeine (Cafcit) over theophylline (Theo-Dur, Slo-Bid) in the management of apnea of prematurity?
A. Caffeine is given only by mouth.
B. Caffeine requires twice-a-day dosing.
C. Caffeine is excreted more rapidly by the kidneys.
D. Caffeine has a longer half-life.

95. CPAP ventilation is indicated for an infant with which of following diagnoses?
A. Cleft palate
B. Choanal atresia
C. Laryngomalacia
D. Tracheoesophageal fistula

96. When the nurse is planning the care of the infant receiving CPAP ventilation at 8 cm H_2O, which of the following interventions should receive the least consideration?
A. Monitoring $PaCO_2$
B. Monitoring and documenting urine output
C. Monitoring vital signs and oxygen saturation via pulse oximetry
D. Maintaining a nasogastric tube to gravity drainage

97. Inclusion criteria for the use of extracorporeal membrane oxygenation (ECMO) include:
A. severe lung hypoplasia.
B. gestational age of 32 weeks.
C. bilateral grade IV intracranial hemorrhage.
D. left CDH without liver herniation in a full-term infant.

98. Which of the following is considered inclusion criteria for ECMO?

A. An oxygenation index of greater than 40 for 4 hours
B. A PaO_2 of 100 that is responsive to iNO
C. A pH of 7.35 that is responsive to pharmacologic and ventilator management
D. A pCO_2 less than 30 for 2 hours

99. Factors that predispose an infant to BPD include which of the following?
A. Full-term birth
B. Fluid restriction
C. Mechanical ventilation
D. Inspired oxygen concentration of 0.21

100. Diuretic therapy with furosemide (Lasix) has been shown to improve lung compliance in infants with BPD. Complications associated with its use include:
A. ototoxicity.
B. hyperkalemia.
C. hyperchloremia.
D. metabolic acidosis.

101. What are the caloric requirements for an infant with severe BPD?
A. 80–100 kcal/kg/day
B. 100–120 kcal/kg/day
C. 120–140 kcal/kg/day
D. 150–180 kcal/kg/day

102. High-dose dexamethasone administration for the treatment of BPD has been associated with an increased incidence of which of the following?
A. Pulmonary air leak
B. Pulmonary hypertension
C. Neurodevelopmental dysfunction
D. Severe retinopathy of prematurity

103. An infant born at an estimated 25 weeks' gestation who is now 56 weeks corrected postconceptual age remains mechanically ventilated on synchronized intermittent mechanical ventilation mode. The chest radiograph is consistent with severe BPD. The ventilator settings most appropriate for this infant would include a(n):
A. inspiratory time of 0.3–0.5 seconds.
B. respiratory rate of 50 breaths per minute.
C. inspired oxygen fraction (FiO_2) of 0.21 with a corresponding PaO_2 of 30.
D. PEEP of 8 cm H_2O.

104. An ABG analysis was obtained with the following results: pH 7.32, $PaCO_2$ 67, PaO_2 46, HCO_3 28, and base excess +4. What is the best interpretation of these results?
A. Uncompensated respiratory acidosis
B. Hypoxemia and respiratory alkalosis
C. Partially compensated metabolic acidosis
D. Partially compensated respiratory acidosis and hypoxemia

105. Dexamethasone has been ordered for an infant born at 25 weeks' gestation who is now 56 weeks corrected postconceptual age. The nurse expects which of the following as a result of dexamethasone administration?
A. Increased blood pressure
B. Increased ventilator support

C. Hypoglycemia

D. Biventricular atrophy on echocardiography

106. On physical examination of an infant with chronic BPD, the nurse notes inspiratory and expiratory wheezing, intercostal retractions, and an oxygen saturation of 68%. These signs alert the nurse to the possibility of bronchospasm. The most appropriate intervention would be administration of which of the following medications?

A. Caffeine (Cafcit)

B. Furosemide (Lasix)

C. Albuterol (Ventolin and Proventil)

D. Theophylline (Theo-Dur and Slo-Bid)

107. An intubated infant's pulse oximeter sounds an alarm because oxygen saturation is 75%. The nurse suctions the infant's airway, and pink-tinged secretions are obtained. The most appropriate action is to:

A. perform aggressive endotracheal suctioning.

B. transfuse platelets to reach a platelet count of 200,000/mm³.

C. transfuse red blood cells to reach a hemoglobin level of 15 mg/dL.

D. increase PEEP from 4 to 6 cm H_2O.

108. ECMO is indicated for which of the following conditions?

A. Bilateral pulmonary hypoplasia

B. BPD

C. Transient tachypnea of the newborn

D. Persistent pulmonary hypertension of the newborn

109. The most common congenital cystic malformation of the lung resulting in obstructive air trapping is:

A. bronchopulmonary sequestration (BPS).

B. CLE.

C. CDH.

D. CPAM.

110. An infant has a prenatal history of polyhydramnios. On physical examination, the infant appears normal. At first feeding, he becomes dusky with signs of respiratory distress, and suctioning of the nasopharynx/oropharynx is required. Further attempts to nipple-feed are met with the same results. The nurse suspects the cause of this infant's respiratory distress to be:

A. choanal atresia.

B. pulmonary hypoplasia.

C. congenital heart disease.

D. esophageal atresia with tracheoesophageal fistula.

111. Which of the following statements about the oxygen–hemoglobin dissociation curve is accurate?

A. The absence of cyanosis indicates a well-oxygenated infant.

B. A right-shifted curve indicates increased affinity of hemoglobin for oxygen.

C. The oxygen–hemoglobin dissociation curve reflects the affinity of hemoglobin for oxygen.

D. Hemoglobin's affinity for oxygen is primarily influenced by serum glucose and electrolyte values.

112. Which of the following can cause a pulse oximeter to display inaccurate oxygen saturation values?

A. Prematurity

B. Use of vasodilating drugs

C. Cyanotic heart disease

D. Decreased peripheral perfusion

113. A newborn infant requires supplemental oxygen, and oxygen administration is initiated via oxygen hood. An appropriate nursing intervention is to:

A. switch the infant to a nasal cannula.

B. do nothing, because no intervention is required.

C. ensure sufficient gas flow to prevent carbon dioxide retention.

D. obtain an order and change the patient to nasal CPAP ventilation.

114. Heliox, a mixture of helium and oxygen at a 4:1 ratio, has been demonstrated to have beneficial ventilatory effects in infants with:

A. pneumothorax.

B. intracranial hemorrhage.

C. necrotizing enterocolitis.

D. obstructive pulmonary disease.

115. Infants with micrognathia and glossoptosis require careful monitoring by the nurse for which of the following complications?

A. Cor pulmonale

B. Obstructive apnea

C. Subglottic stenosis

D. Reactive airway disease

116. A mother walked into labor and delivery with a history of rupture of membrane for more than 24 hours. Fetal monitoring showed a nonreassuring fetal heart rate pattern, and a stat cesarean section was done. A 24-week preterm infant was born with Apgar scores 3 and 6 at 1 and 5 minutes, respectively. The infant was intubated in the delivery room and transferred to the NICU. The infant remains on mechanical ventilation with stable vital signs. On day 2 of life, when the nurse suctions the ETT, she finds fresh blood coming out of the ETT. The nurse understands the possible cause for pulmonary hemorrhage after surfactant administration is:

A. a rapid decrease in intrapulmonary pressure.

B. a rapid increase in intrapulmonary pressure.

C. a rapid decrease in intrathoracic pressure.

D. a rapid decrease in intracardiac pressure.

117. Which of the following is included in the management of unilateral PIE?

A. Increase PEEP to open the alveoli.

B. Increase tidal volume.

C. Keep the involved area of the lung up.

D. Keep the involved area of the lung down.

118. Which pathophysiology is associated with transient tachypnea of newborn?

A. Ball-valve obstruction of the small airways

B. Reduced number of lung cells, airways, blood vessels, and alveoli

C. Failure of reabsorption of fetal lung fluid

D. Air within the lung parenchyma

119. A 40-year-old multigravida mother walked into the labor and delivery unit with no prenatal care. On assessment, contractions were occurring every 5 minutes, and vaginal exam showed station 0. Within 1 hour, an infant was born via spontaneous vaginal delivery. The Apgar scores were 8 and 8 at 1 and 5 minutes, respectively. The infant remained with the mother after delivery under the supervision of a mother baby nurse. At 48 hours of life, the infant was noted to have a respiratory rate in the 70s. The NNP ordered a chest x-ray, which showed a large stomach bubble and bowel gas in the left side of the chest. The NNP immediately asked the nurse to place an orogastric tube to empty the stomach and transferred the infant to the NICU for further management. This radiographic picture is consistent with which diagnosis?
    A. MAS
    B. CPAM
    C. CDH
    D. Pulmonary sequestration

120. Infants with persistent pulmonary hypertension have predominantly:
    A. a left-to-right shunt via the PDA and/or the patent foramen ovale.
    B. a right-to-left shunt via the PDA and/or the patent foramen ovale.
    C. a right-to-left shunt via the patent ductus venosus and/ or the patent foramen ovale.
    D. a left-to-right shunt via the patent ductus venosus and/ or the patent foramen ovale.

121. Infants with prenatally diagnosed CDH should all undergo early:
    A. chest x-ray to assess the degree of pulmonary hypertension.
    B. cardiac catheterization to evaluate the function of the left and right ventricles.
    C. echocardiography to ascertain the presence of associated heart defect, degree of pulmonary hypertension, and function of left and right ventricles.
    D. fluorescent in situ hybridization to rule out 22q11.2 deletion syndrome (DiGeorge syndrome).

122. A proposed cause of pulmonary hypoplasia in a fetus is:
    A. inadequate amniotic fluid volume.
    B. an excess of amniotic fluid volume.
    C. presence of congenital heart defect.
    D. presence of a tracheoesophageal fistula with an esophageal atresia.

123. The nurse is asked to start transcutaneous CO_2 monitoring on an infant. The nurse applies the electrode over the:
    A. abdomen or thigh.
    B. head or scalp.
    C. thorax or hand.
    D. wrist or hand.

124. A mother asks a registered nurse (RN) working in the NICU how the risk for RDS can be reduced. Which of the following is the most accurate information for the RN to convey to the mother?
    A. Giving antenatal corticosteroid therapy to the mother between 23 and 34 weeks' gestation
    B. Giving antenatal corticosteroid therapy to the mother just before delivery

C. Giving antenatal corticosteroid therapy to the mother at 18 weeks' gestation
    D. Giving antenatal corticosteroid therapy to the mother as soon as possible after unprotected sex

125. The most common bronchodilator used in the treatment of BPD is:
    A. albuterol.
    B. corticosteroids (Decadron).
    C. furosemide (Lasix).
    D. thiazide (Diuril).

126. Right-sided vocal cord paralysis is a complication of:
    A. ECMO.
    B. ligation of the PDA.
    C. BPD.
    D. pulmonary hypertension.

127. Bilateral vocal cord paralysis is a complication in which of the following conditions?
    A. Tracheoesophageal fistula
    B. ECMO
    C. Hypoxic ischemic encephalopathy
    D. PDA

128. An infant with unilateral vocal cord paralysis has notable stridor. What is the best position for this infant to decrease stridor?
    A. Side lying, on the contralateral side of the paralysis
    B. Side lying, on the ipsilateral side of the paralysis
    C. Supine
    D. Prone

129. Tracheal compression by a vascular ring is diagnosed most accurately by:
    A. chest x-ray.
    B. barium swallow.
    C. bronchoscopy.
    D. magnetic resonance imaging.

130. What is the most common congenital lung lesion in neonates?
    A. BPS
    B. CLE
    C. CPAM
    D. Pneumatocele

131. Which of the following is the treatment of choice for eventration of the diaphragm?
    A. ECMO
    B. Nitric oxide
    C. Lobectomy
    D. Plication of the diaphragm

132. A term infant admitted with CDH has severe pulmonary hypertension. The mother is asking the nurse why her baby is having pulmonary hypertension. The response by the nurse is based on which of the following etiologies?
    A. Structural remodeling of the pulmonary vessels
    B. Lack of surfactant in the lungs
    C. Failure to transition from fetal to neonatal circulation
    D. Accumulation of fluid in the lungs

ANSWERS AND RATIONALES

1. **(B)** Positive end expiratory pressure (PEEP) is defined as the amount of airway pressure in the lung at the end of expiration. Continuous positive airway pressure (CPAP) is a noninvasive mode of ventilation that provides continuous distending pressure to patients with a sustainable respiratory drive. Nasal CPAP delivers humidified gas via short nasal prongs or a nasal mask at varying pressures, which is measured in cm of H_2O pressure. Devices that provide nasal CPAP include the neonatal ventilator, a standalone nasal CPAP device, or via a bubble CPAP system. Ventilators provide gas while limiting the outflow of gases based on the pressure setting. With bubble CPAP, the expiratory tubing is submerged in a chamber of water, and the level of water to which the tubing is submerged determines the amount of pressure generated. The flow of gases is continuous with both the ventilator and the bubble mode of delivering CPAP. Standalone nasal CPAP devices use a specialized flow generator to deliver variable flow during inspiration and expiration to maintain a constant airway pressure. CPAP delivers a specified pressure during both inspiration and expiration.

References: Donn SM, Attar MA. Assisted ventilation of the neonate and its complications. In: Martin RJ, Fanaroff AA, Walsh MC, eds. *Fanaroff & Martin's Neonatal-Perinatal Medicine: Diseases of the Fetus and Infant.* 11th ed. Philadelphia, PA: Elsevier; 2020:1174-1177.

Gardner SL, Enzman-Hines M, Nyp M. Respiratory diseases. In: Gardner SL, Carter BS, Niermeyer S, eds. *Merenstein & Gardner's Handbook of Neonatal Intensive Care: An Interprofessional Approach.* 9th ed. St. Louis, MO: Elsevier; 2021:744-746.

Manley BJ, Davis PG, Yoder BA, Owen LS. Non-invasive respiratory support. In: Keszler M, Gautham KS, eds. *Goldsmith's Assisted Ventilation of the Neonate: An Evidence-Based Approach to Newborn Respiratory Care.* 7th ed. Philadelphia, PA: Elsevier; 2022:202-205.

Wilson J, Snapp B, Walters M. The pulmonary system. In: Koehn A, ed. *Neonatal Nurse Practitioner Certification Intensive Review: Fast Facts and Practice Questions.* New York: Springer Publishing Company, LLC; 2020:235-260.

2. **(C)** As long as heaters and a gas source are available, the bubble CPAP system can be inexpensive, readily available, and easily maintained. The system utilizes a one-liter bottle of sterile water and CPAP tubing. The depth of the expiratory end of the CPAP tube submerged in the water correlates with the amount of pressure generated. Commercially available devices are widely available. As with other methods of delivering CPAP, the gas must be heated. In bubble CPAP pressure is delivered continuously during inspiration and expiration. In variable-flow CPAP, bilevel pressure is used during inspiration and expiration. Special devices are used to deliver bilevel positive airway pressure.

References: Gardner SL, Enzman-Hines M, Nyp M. Respiratory diseases. In: Gardner SL, Carter BS, Niermeyer S, eds. *Merenstein & Gardner's Handbook of Neonatal Intensive Care: An Interprofessional Approach.* 9th ed. St. Louis, MO: Elsevier; 2021:744-746.

Manley BJ, Davis PG, Yoder BA, Owen LS. Non-invasive respiratory support. In: Keszler M, Gautham KS, eds. *Goldsmith's Assisted Ventilation of the Neonate: An Evidence-Based Approach to Newborn Respiratory Care.* 7th ed. Philadelphia, PA: Elsevier; 2022:203-205.

Sessions KL, Mvalo T, Kondowe D, Hosseinipour MC. Bubble CPAP and oxygen for child pneumonia care in Malawi: a CPAP Impact time motion study. *BMC Health Serv Res.* 2019;19:533. doi:10.1186/s12913-019-4364-y.

3. **(D)** CPAP is effective with obstructive apnea because it stabilizes the compliant chest wall and splints the upper airways and diaphragm. Studies demonstrate that CPAP is not effective in treating central apnea. Respiratory efforts cease during central apnea, and there is no evidence of obstruction or breathing motions. Because CPAP may cause gastric and intestinal distension, further compressing the lung(s), it is contraindicated in congenital diaphragmatic hernia (CDH). Swallowed air from CPAP further compresses the lung by the herniated portions of the gastrointestinal system. A pneumothorax may worsen with CPAP due to increased end expiratory pressure. If transpulmonary pressures remain high, air may continue to dissect into the visceral pleura.

References: Donn SM, Attar MA. Assisted ventilation of the neonate and its complications. In: Martin RJ, Fanaroff AA, Walsh MC, eds. *Fanaroff & Martin's Neonatal-Perinatal Medicine: Diseases of the Fetus and Infant.* 11th ed. Philadelphia, PA: Elsevier; 2020:1174-1177.

Gardner SL, Enzman-Hines M, Nyp M. Respiratory diseases. In: Gardner SL, Carter BS, Niermeyer S, eds. *Merenstein & Gardner's Handbook of Neonatal Intensive Care: An Interprofessional Approach.* 9th ed. St. Louis, MO: Elsevier; 2021:744-746.

Manley BJ, Davis PG, Yoder BA, Owen LS. Non-invasive respiratory support. In: Keszler M, Gautham, KS, eds. *Goldsmith's Assisted Ventilation of the Neonate: An Evidence-Based Approach to Newborn Respiratory Care.* 7th ed. Philadelphia, PA: Elsevier; 2022:203.

Wilson J, Snapp B, Walters M. The pulmonary system. In: Koehn A, ed. *Neonatal Nurse Practitioner Certification Intensive Review: Fast Facts and Practice Questions.* New York: Springer Publishing Company, LLC; 2020:235-260.

4. **(C)** Part of the prongs should remain outside the nose to keep the prong bridge from pressing into the septum. Prongs that are too small allow pressure to escape and increase the risk of frictional damage caused when they slip in and out of the nose. Prongs should be large enough to fill the nares completely without force. Prong size and airway pressure are inversely proportional, thus the larger the prong size, the lower the resistance.

References: Gardner SL, Enzman-Hines M, Nyp M. Respiratory diseases. In: Gardner SL, Carter BS, Niermeyer S, eds. *Merenstein & Gardner's Handbook of Neonatal Intensive Care: An Interprofessional Approach.* 9th ed. St. Louis, MO: Elsevier; 2021:744-746.

Manley BJ, Davis PG, Yoder BA, Owen LS. Non-invasive respiratory support. In: Keszler M, Gautham KS, eds. *Goldsmith's Assisted Ventilation of the Neonate: An Evidence-Based Approach to Newborn Respiratory Care.* 7th ed. Philadelphia, PA: Elsevier; 2022:205-208.

5. **(D)** Preliminary diagnosis of a pneumothorax by transillumination may be difficult in infants with darkly pigmented skin. Bright room lighting and inadequate light from the transilluminator can interfere with preliminary diagnosis. Transillumination is effective for preliminary diagnosis of a pneumothorax in large-for-gestation infants.

Reference: Crowley MA. Neonatal respiratory disorders. In: Martin RJ, Fanaroff AA, Walsh MC, eds. *Fanaroff & Martin's Neonatal-Perinatal Medicine: Diseases of the Fetus and Infant.* 11th ed. Philadelphia, PA: Elsevier; 2020:1221-1223.

6. **(A)** The classic radiographic sign of a pneumomediastinum is the "sail sign," which results from free air lifting the thymus. A mediastinal shift, decreased heart size, and free air above the liver on a right lateral x-ray are signs of a pneumothorax.

Reference: Crowley MA. Neonatal respiratory disorders. In: Martin RJ, Fanaroff AA, Walsh MC, eds. *Fanaroff & Martin's Neonatal-Perinatal Medicine: Diseases of the Fetus and Infant.* 11th ed. Philadelphia, PA: Elsevier; 2020:1221-1223.

7. **(B)** Narrowing of the subglottic diameter is usually associated with prolonged intubation. Pulmonary hemorrhage is a complication of surfactant administration. The risk of pneumothorax increases when the endotracheal tube (ETT) is in the right mainstem. Tracheal perforation may result from traumatic intubation using improper technique.

Reference: Crowley MA. Neonatal respiratory disorders. In: Martin RJ, Fanaroff AA, Walsh MC, eds. *Fanaroff & Martin's Neonatal-Perinatal Medicine: Diseases of the Fetus and Infant.* 11th ed. Philadelphia, PA: Elsevier; 2020:1221-1223.

8. **(D)** Necrotizing tracheobronchitis is a necrotic inflammatory process that involves the distal trachea and mainstem bronchi.

With this complication, normal tracheal mucosa is replaced with acute inflammatory cells, leading to mucosal sloughing and occlusion of the distal trachea, granulation, atelectasis, and impaired gas exchange. Stridor may be noted with subglottic stenosis, tracheomalacia, and bronchomalacia. Tracheomalacia and bronchomalacia develop due to softening of the cartilaginous airway rings and result in a failure to support the round shape of the trachea. Dilation of the trachea and bronchi caused by barotrauma can lead to tracheomegaly, tracheomalacia, and bronchomalacia.

Reference: Crowley MA. Neonatal respiratory disorders. In: Martin RJ, Fanaroff AA, Walsh MC, eds. *Fanaroff & Martin's Neonatal-Perinatal Medicine: Diseases of the Fetus and Infant.* 11th ed. Philadelphia, PA: Elsevier; 2020: 1221-1223.

9. **(D)** The V_a/Q_c ratio expresses the interaction between pulmonary ventilation and perfusion. Matching ventilation and perfusion is required for efficient gas exchange. Mismatching is the most common cause of hypoxia. Alveolar underventilation results in a low ventilation–perfusion ratio (lower value for numerator of the ratio). A ventilation–perfusion ratio of zero indicates a shunt; no ventilation takes place as blood passes through the lungs. The ideal ratio is 1:1, in which ventilation is perfectly matched to perfusion.

Reference: Gardner SL, Enzman-Hines M, Nyp M. Respiratory diseases. In: Gardner SL, Carter BS, Niermeyer S, eds. *Merenstein & Gardner's Handbook of Neonatal Intensive Care: An Interprofessional Approach.* 9th ed. St. Louis, MO: Elsevier; 2021:785-796.

10. **(B)** The American Academy of Pediatrics (AAP) recommends placing infants on their back during sleep time to decrease the risk of sudden infant death syndrome (SIDS). The prone position has been associated with fewer spontaneous arousals from sleep in term infants, a longer first quiet sleep period following feedings, fewer awakenings, and a decrease in heart rate variability. These characteristics lead to a higher arousal threshold and increased vulnerability to SIDS. Although home cardiorespiratory monitoring may be justified for infants at risk for recurrent apnea, bradycardia, and hypoxemia posthospital discharge, the AAP does not recommend its use for the prevention of SIDS in healthy infants. The AAP recommends keeping soft objects such as pillows, pillow-like toys, quilts, comforters, mattress toppers, sheepskins, and loose bedding away from the infant's sleep area. Bumper pads and similar products that attach to crib slats are not recommended by AAP. Such devices have been implicated in deaths due to suffocation, entrapment, and strangulation.

References: Gardner SL, Goldson E. The neonate and the environment impact on development. In: Gardner SL, Carter BS, Niermeyer S, eds. *Merenstein & Gardner's Handbook of Neonatal Intensive Care: An Interprofessional Approach.* 9th ed. St. Louis, MO: Elsevier; 2021:371-401.

Moon RY, Carlin RF, Hand I, The Task Force on Sudden Infant Death Syndrome and The Committee on Fetus and Newborn. Sleep-related infant deaths: updated 2022 recommendations for reducing infant deaths in the sleep environment. *Pediatrics.* 2022;150(1):e2022057990. doi:10.1542/peds. 2022-057990.

11. **(A)** Prenatal and postnatal cigarette smoke exposure is a major risk factor for SIDS. Evidence-based research does not support the theory that apnea is the pathophysiologic precursor to SIDS. A high environmental temperature and prolonged QT interval are associated with SIDS.

References: Gardner SL, Goldson E. The neonate and the environment impact on development. In: Gardner SL, Carter BS, Niermeyer S, eds. *Merenstein & Gardner's Handbook of Neonatal Intensive Care: An Interprofessional Approach.* 9th ed. St. Louis, MO: Elsevier; 2021:371-401.

Moon RY, Carlin RF, Hand I, The Task Force on Sudden Infant Death Syndrome and The Committee on Fetus and Newborn. Sleep-related infant deaths: updated 2022 recommendations for reducing infant deaths in the sleep environment. *Pediatrics.* 2022;150(1):e2022057990. doi:10.1542/peds.2022-057990.

12. **(C)** Although the need for resuscitation is based in part on anticipation of likely problems, the best indication for resuscitation need is the infant's clinical presentation and response. Apgar scores quantify the infant's initial clinical presentation in the first several minutes of life but do not determine whether resuscitation is needed. The initial steps of resuscitation are taken before 1 minute of life. Although maternal administration of general anesthesia or magnesium sulfate is antepartum and intrapartum factors related to neonatal depression at delivery, most of these infants do not require resuscitation.

Reference: Niermeyer S, Clarke SB. Care at birth. In: Gardner SL, Carter BS, Enzman-Hines M, Niermeyer S, eds. *Merenstein & Gardner's Handbook of Neonatal Intensive Care: An Interprofessional Approach.* 9th ed. St. Louis, MO: Elsevier; 2021:67-74.

13. **(D)** Pulmonary hemorrhage is an absolute contraindication for chest physiotherapy (CPT) due to the risk of exacerbation of bleeding. CPT is useful for the treatment of atelectasis and may be useful to facilitate removal of secretions in neonates with neuromuscular compromise because these neonates may have limited ability to cough and clear secretions. CPT is not contraindicated for infants with a chest tube or gastrostomy tube, although modified positioning is required.

Reference: Gardner SL, Enzman-Hines M, Nyp M. Respiratory diseases. In: Gardner SL, Carter BS, Niermeyer S, eds. *Merenstein & Gardner's Handbook of Neonatal Intensive Care: An Interprofessional Approach.* 9th ed. St. Louis, MO: Elsevier; 2021:729-746.

14. **(A)** Bronchopulmonary dysplasia (BPD) is characterized by altered lung development with decreased numbers of alveoli and abnormal blood vessel development as opposed to lung damage. Although oxygen toxicity has been attributed to the development of BPD, the causes are multifactorial and include prematurity, oxidant injury, inflammation and lung injury related to mechanical ventilation, arrested lung development, and abnormal repair processes of the lung. BPD may occur in smaller infants who do not necessarily have severe respiratory distress syndrome (RDS).

References: Fraser D. Respiratory distress. In: Verklan T, Walden M, Forest S, eds. *Core Curriculum for Neonatal Intensive Care Nursing.* 6th ed. St. Louis, MO: Elsevier; 2021:406-408.

Gardner SL, Enzman-Hines M, Nyp M. Respiratory diseases. In: Gardner SL, Carter BS, Niermeyer S, eds. *Merenstein & Gardner's Handbook of Neonatal Intensive Care: An Interprofessional Approach.* 9th ed. St. Louis, MO: Elsevier; 2021:772-784.

15. **(C)** Pulmonary interstitial emphysema (PIE) occurs when gases collect in the connective tissue of the peribronchovascular sheaths and is a complication of mechanical ventilation. Subcutaneous emphysema is a collection of extraneous air in the subcutaneous tissue. A pneumothorax is a collection of extraneous air in the pleural space. Pseudocysts occur when extraneous air collects in the alveoli trabeculae–visceral pleura.

Reference: Gardner SL, Enzman-Hines M, Nyp M. Respiratory diseases. In: Gardner SL, Carter BS, Niermeyer S, eds. *Merenstein & Gardner's Handbook of Neonatal Intensive Care: An Interprofessional Approach.* 9th ed. St. Louis, MO: Elsevier; 2021:768-784.

16. **(D)** Nasal CPAP may increase end expiratory pressure and worsen a pneumothorax and therefore should be avoided. Only supportive care is required for a mild pneumothorax without evidence of significant respiratory failure. Monitoring for additional changes in respiratory status is indicated because a mild pneumothorax has the potential of progressing and developing into a tension pneumothorax. Positioning the affected side down can minimize worsening of a pneumothorax. If a tension pneumothorax develops immediate emergency evacuation of free air by needle aspiration is required. Treatment delay can be avoided by having supplies readily available at the bedside.

References: Gardner SL, Enzman-Hines M, Nyp M. Respiratory diseases. In: Gardner SL, Carter BS, Niermeyer S, eds. *Merenstein & Gardner's Handbook of Neonatal Intensive Care: An Interprofessional Approach*. 9th ed. St. Louis, MO: Elsevier; 2021:768-784.

Wilson J, Snapp B, Walters M. The pulmonary system. In: Koehn A, ed. *Neonatal Nurse Practitioner Certification Intensive Review: Fast Facts and Practice Questions*. New York: Springer Publishing Company, LLC; 2020:235-260.

17. **(D)** Meconium aspiration syndrome (MAS) occurs when the term or postterm fetus aspirates meconium-stained amniotic fluid into the lungs due to stress occurring before, during, or immediately after delivery. MAS is radiographically characterized by uneven aeration with areas of atelectasis and gas trapping. Meconium can inactive both endogenous and exogenous surfactants and inhibit surfactant production. Atelectasis-prone lungs susceptible to volutrauma describes the pathophysiology associated with severe uniform lung disease, such as RDS. Hemodynamic impairment and restricted chest and/or diaphragmatic movement may be seen in severe necrotizing enterocolitis (NEC) or repaired gastroschisis with compartment syndrome. The pathophysiology of air leak syndromes involves gas that escapes into the pulmonary intersitium, compressing alveoli, airways, and pulmonary venules leading to ventilation perfusion mismatch.

References: Crowley MA. Neonatal respiratory disorders. In: Martin RJ, Fanaroff AA, Walsh MC, eds. *Fanaroff & Martin's Neonatal-Perinatal Medicine: Diseases of the Fetus and Infant*. 11th ed. Philadelphia, PA: Elsevier; 2020:1214-1215.

Wilson J, Snapp B, Walters M. The pulmonary system. In: Koehn A, ed. *Neonatal Nurse Practitioner Certification Intensive Review: Fast Facts and Practice Questions*. New York: Springer Publishing Company, LLC; 2020:235-260.

18. **(B)** The properties of convection and molecular diffusion are used during high-frequency ventilation (HFV) to deliver tidal volumes that are less than anatomic dead space. Gas exchange occurs during HFV due to the increased turbulence of gas molecules. HFV can cause gas trapping if used inappropriately. Sufficient exhalation time is required for optimal HFV management to prevent inadvertent PEEP and unwarranted lung overinflation. Depending on the type of HFV device and where the pressure is measured, the mean airway pressure used to support lung volume may be higher or lower than that used with conventional mechanical ventilation. HFV is as effective as conventional mechanical ventilation for eliminating for carbon dioxide.

References: Gardner SL, Enzman-Hines M, Nyp M. Respiratory diseases. In: Gardner SL, Carter BS, Niermeyer S, eds. *Merenstein & Gardner's Handbook of Neonatal Intensive Care: An Interprofessional Approach*. 9th ed. St. Louis, MO: Elsevier; 2021:759-784.

Wilson J, Snapp B, Walters M. The pulmonary system. In: Koehn A, ed. *Neonatal Nurse Practitioner Certification Intensive Review: Fast Facts and Practice Questions*. New York: Springer Publishing Company, LLC; 2020:235-260.

19. **(A)** Improved lung compliance, excessive peak inspiratory pressure (PIP) or amplitude, and machine failure may result in increased chest wall motion. Inadequate amplitude, gas trapping, or a massive pneumothorax may result in a lack of or decreased chest wall motion.

Reference: Gardner SL, Enzman-Hines M, Nyp M. Respiratory diseases. In: Gardner SL, Carter BS, Niermeyer S, eds. *Merenstein & Gardner's Handbook of Neonatal Intensive Care: An Interprofessional Approach*. 9th ed. St. Louis, MO: Elsevier; 2021:759-784.

20. **(A)** Chronic fetal stress increases endogenous corticosteroids, resulting in accelerated lung maturity and a decrease in the severity of RDS. Second-born twin, male sex, and cesarean section without labor are factors that predispose infants to developing RDS.

Reference: Gardner SL, Enzman-Hines M, Nyp M. Respiratory diseases. In: Gardner SL, Carter BS, Niermeyer S, eds. *Merenstein & Gardner's Handbook of Neonatal Intensive Care: An Interprofessional Approach*. 9th ed. St. Louis, MO: Elsevier; 2021:784-788.

21. **(C)** Rhonchi are characterized by continuous, low-pitched breath sounds occurring on inspiration and expiration. Rhonchi are associated with secretions in the larger airways and improve or resolve with cough or suctioning. Crackles are discontinuous and are heard on inspiration. Early crackles, heard during the first half of inspiration, are suggestive of atelectasis, whereas late crackles appreciated in the second half of inspiration suggest alveolar air trapping. Wheezes are continuous high-pitched musical sounds heard best on expiration and are caused by air passing at high velocity through a narrowed airway. Stridor is described as a rough or harsh sound and that is associated with narrowing of the upper airways. Stridor can be heard during inspiration and expiration.

References: Gardner SL, Enzman-Hines M, Nyp M. Respiratory diseases. In: Gardner SL, Carter BS, Niermeyer S, eds. *Merenstein & Gardner's Handbook of Neonatal Intensive Care: An Interprofessional Approach*. 9th ed. St. Louis, MO: Elsevier; 2021:759-784.

Wilson J, Snapp B, Walters M. The pulmonary system. In: Koehn A, ed. *Neonatal Nurse Practitioner Certification Intensive Review: Fast Facts and Practice Questions*. New York: Springer Publishing Company, LLC; 2020:235-260.

22. **(D)** Direct sunlight, phototherapy lights, and procedure lights can interfere with sensor function and SpO_2 accuracy and give falsely reassuring readings. Shielding the probe from external light by use of an opaque wrap is recommended. Pulse oximetry allows for rapid response to changes in oxygen saturation. Pulse oximetry provides a less precise estimation of PaO_2 at higher, not lower, saturations. Sensor reliability can be verified by comparing the heart rate displayed from pulse oximetry with the heart rate displayed from electrocardiogram monitoring.

References: Coe K, Bradshaw WT, Tanaka DT. Physiologic monitoring. In: Gardner SL, Carter BS, Niermeyer S, eds. *Merenstein & Gardner's Handbook of Neonatal Intensive Care: An Interprofessional Approach*. 9th ed. St. Louis, MO: Elsevier; 2021:165-178.

Wilson J, Snapp B, Walters M. The pulmonary system. In: Koehn A, ed. *Neonatal Nurse Practitioner Certification Intensive Review: Fast Facts and Practice Questions*. New York: Springer Publishing Company, LLC; 2020:235-260.

23. **(C)** An x-ray showing overaerated but clear lung fields is indicative of hyperinflation. Radiographic findings of a pulmonary air leak may be characterized as hyperlucent lung fields. Congenital lobar emphysema (CLE) may be seen as unequal aeration on x-ray. Opacity of lung fields may represent a hydrothorax.

Reference: Gardner SL, Enzman-Hines M, Nyp M. Respiratory diseases. In: Gardner SL, Carter BS, Niermeyer S, eds. *Merenstein & Gardner's Handbook of Neonatal Intensive Care: An Interprofessional Approach*. 9th ed. St. Louis, MO: Elsevier; 2021:796-835.

24. **(D)** Apnea causes respiratory acidosis due to insufficient alveolar ventilation, leading to carbon dioxide retention and a decrease in pH. Acetazolamide is associated with loss of bases and resulting metabolic acidosis. Maternal heroin addiction may cause hyperventilation and subsequent respiratory alkalosis. Diuretic therapy such as with loop diuretics can induce metabolic alkalosis from loss of chloride, resulting in bicarbonate retention and an increase in pH.

Reference: Barry JS, Deacon J, Hernandez C, Jones Jr D. Acid-base homeostasis and oxygenation. In: Gardner SL, Carter BS, Niermeyer S, eds. *Merenstein & Gardner's Handbook of Neonatal Intensive Care: An Interprofessional Approach*. 9th ed. St. Louis, MO: Elsevier; 2021:186-191.

25. **(B)** Normal pH ranges from 7.35 to 7.45. The pH in this scenario indicates acidosis. Abnormalities in both the metabolic (HCO_3 <22 mEq/L) and the respiratory (PCO_2 >45 mm Hg) components in combination with acidosis (pH <7.35) represent mixed acidosis. Because the pH is not normal, the blood gas is not fully compensated. To be considered partially compensated, both acid–base parameters should be abnormal in opposite directions (i.e., one

acidotic and one alkalotic). Because both parameters are acidotic, there is no compensation. The normal value for PO_2 in arterial blood gas (ABG) in the newborn is 50–80 mm Hg in room air. A PO_2 <50 mm Hg represents hypoxemia.

References: Barry JS, Deacon J, Hernandez C, Jones Jr D. Acid-base homeostasis and oxygenation. In: Gardner SL, Carter BS, Niermeyer S, eds. *Merenstein & Gardner's Handbook of Neonatal Intensive Care: An Interprofessional Approach.* 9th ed. St. Louis, MO: Elsevier; 2021:186-191.

Rhein LM. Blood gas and pulmonary function monitoring. In: Eichenwald EC, Hansen AR, Martin C, Stark AR, eds. *Cloherty and Stark's Manual of Neonatal Care.* 8th ed. Philadelphia, PA: Wolters Kluwer; 2017:420.

Travers C, Ambalavanan N. Blood gases: technical aspects and interpretation. In: Keszler M, Gautham KS, eds. *Goldsmith's Assisted Ventilation of the Neonate: An Evidence-Based Approach to Newborn Respiratory Care.* 7th ed. Philadelphia, PA: Elsevier; 2022:106-107.

26. **(C)** Heel sticks made to the curvature of the heel (calcaneus) place the infant at risk for calcaneal osteomyelitis. The posterolateral aspect of the heel is an acceptable location for obtaining capillary blood specimens. To facilitate blood flow, the puncture site should be held lower than the rest of the extremity. The nurse should avoid squeezing the extremity to prevent cell lysis.

Reference: Gardner SL, Enzman-Hines M, Agarwal R. Pain and pain relief. In: Gardner SL, Carter BS, Niermeyer S, eds. *Merenstein & Gardner's Handbook of Neonatal Intensive Care: An Interprofessional Approach.* 9th ed. St. Louis, MO: Elsevier; 2021:273-281.

27. **(C)** The resistance in the ETT is increased due to the small diameter and longer length than the trachea; therefore, work of breathing is increased. Fatigue, respiratory distress, or apnea may result. Because the ETT is in the lungs, sterile technique or use of a closed system is required when suctioning. Because pressure is delivered directly to the lungs, increased PEEP may be delivered even inadvertently, increasing the risk for air leaks. Given the drawbacks of ETT CPAP, it is not the preferred method for delivering noninvasive ventilation.

Reference: Gardner SL, Enzman-Hines M, Nyp M. Respiratory diseases. In: Gardner SL, Carter BS, Niermeyer S, eds. *Merenstein & Gardner's Handbook of Neonatal Intensive Care: An Interprofessional Approach.* 9th ed. St. Louis, MO: Elsevier; 2021:796-835.

28. **(A)** Pulmonary insufficiency is common with a large CDH defect. In CDH, bag-mask ventilation and other noninvasive modes of ventilation should be avoided because of potential gastric distension causing further compression to vital organs in the thoracic cavity. Instead, the infant should be electively intubated in the delivery room. Mechanical ventilation is also indicated for respiratory failure, pulmonary insufficiency, surfactant administration, severe apnea and bradycardia episodes, cardiovascular support, central nervous system disease, and surgery. Mechanical ventilation may be avoided with a strategy known as permissive hypercapnia. Elevated carbon dioxide levels may be accepted to minimize adverse effects of mechanical ventilation such as barotrauma. Gentle ventilation should be given using a high-frequency jet ventilator or high-frequency oscillatory ventilator. Mild-to-moderate respiratory distress and pulmonary edema may respond to noninvasive modes of ventilation such as CPAP or nasal intermittent positive pressure ventilation.

Reference: Gardner SL, Enzman-Hines M, Nyp M. Respiratory diseases. In: Gardner SL, Carter BS, Niermeyer S, eds. *Merenstein & Gardner's Handbook of Neonatal Intensive Care: An Interprofessional Approach.* 9th ed. St. Louis, MO: Elsevier; 2021:796-835.

29. **(A)** With the assist/control mode of ventilation, either a synchronized breath is delivered with each spontaneous breath that meets threshold criteria or in the absence of spontaneous respirations, mechanical breaths are delivered at a preset regular rate. Pressure support ventilation is pressure limited and flow cycled in which the ventilator supports each breath and terminates the breath when the inspiratory flow drops below a preset threshold. Neurally adjusted ventilatory assist (NAVA) uses measured diaphragmatic activity to detect the onset of a spontaneous breath to trigger ventilator support. Synchronized intermittent mandatory ventilation delivers a preset number of ventilator breaths with a preset PIP and inspiratory time synchronized with the onset of spontaneous breaths.

Reference: Gardner SL, Enzman-Hines M, Nyp M. Respiratory diseases. In: Gardner SL, Carter BS, Niermeyer S, eds. *Merenstein & Gardner's Handbook of Neonatal Intensive Care: An Interprofessional Approach.* 9th ed. St. Louis, MO: Elsevier; 2021:796-835.

30. **(A)** Closed suctioning (CS) systems use a catheter enclosed in a clear plastic sheath placed in-line with the ventilator circuit and ETT. Because the ventilator remains connected to the ETT during suctioning, there is a decreased potential loss of PEEP. While CS has been associated with a reduced number and severity of hypoxic and bradycardic events, more research is needed to compare the long-term outcomes related to open and closed suction systems in neonates. Preoxygenation prevents/reduces hypoxemia during suctioning but does not prevent loss of PEEP. Using 100% oxygen should be reserved only if indicated. To avoid exposing preterm infants to hyperoxia, it is recommended to increase oxygen by 10%–20% above baseline, or 5%–10% for extra low–birth-weight/very low–birth-weight infants. Although it is necessary to clear the artificial airway to maintain a patent airway, suctioning should be performed only when indicated. Minimizing suctioning events will not prevent loss of PEEP during the actual suctioning event.

References: Blakeman TC, Scot JB, Yoder MA, Capellari E, Strickland SL. AARC clinical practice guidelines: artificial airway suctioning. *Respir Care.* 2022;67(2):258-271.

Fraser D. Nursing care. In: Keszler M, Gautham KS, eds. *Goldsmith's Assisted Ventilation of the Neonate: An Evidence-Based Approach to Newborn Respiratory Care.* 7th ed. Philadelphia, PA: Elsevier; 2022:390-391.

Gardner SL, Enzman-Hines M, Nyp M. Respiratory diseases. In: Gardner SL, Carter BS, Niermeyer S, eds. *Merenstein & Gardner's Handbook of Neonatal Intensive Care: An Interprofessional Approach.* 9th ed. St. Louis, MO: Elsevier; 2021:749-750.

31. **(A)** Pulse oximetry relies on pulsatile flow to provide an accurate reading. In settings of vasoconstriction and poor perfusion, the pulse oximeter readings can be falsely low. Medications such as dopamine or epinephrine may affect the oxygen saturation reading due to peripheral vasoconstriction. Although pulse oximetry may reduce the number of blood gas measurements, it does not eliminate the need completely because acid–base balance and ventilation (pCO_2) must still be evaluated. The accuracy of pulse oximetry is not affected by lung function or the severity of lung disease. Pulse oximetry determines oxygen saturation quickly, although inaccurate measurements may occur with incorrect probe placement, poor perfusion, motion artifact, and in darker pigmented individuals.

References: Fraser D, Diehl-Jones W. Assisted ventilation. In: Verklan T, Walden M, Forest S, eds. *Core Curriculum for Neonatal Intensive Care Nursing.* 6th ed. St. Louis, MO: Elsevier; 2021:440.

Gallagher JJ. Impact of skin color on SpO2 detection of hypoxemia. In: *AACN Critical Care Webinar Series.* October 20, 2022. Available at: https://www.aacn.org//education/webinar-series/wb0070/impact-of-skin-color-on-spo2-detection-of-hypoxemia.

Gardner SL, Enzman-Hines M, Nyp M. Respiratory diseases. In: Gardner SL, Carter BS, Niermeyer S, eds. *Merenstein & Gardner's Handbook of Neonatal Intensive Care: An Interprofessional Approach.* 9th ed. St. Louis, MO: Elsevier; 2021:796-835.

Wilson J, Snapp B, Walters M. The pulmonary system. In: Koehn A, ed. *Neonatal Nurse Practitioner Certification Intensive Review: Fast Facts and Practice Questions.* New York: Springer Publishing Company, LLC; 2020:235-260.

32. **(B)** Rapid respiratory rates, as often occurs in infants with severe lung disease, along with small tidal volumes compromise the ability of sampled gas by the end tidal CO_2 monitor to adequately reflect alveolar gas. End-tidal CO_2 monitoring cannot be used with HFV. Transcutaneous CO_2 monitoring has a better correlation with $PaCO_2$ than end-tidal CO_2 monitoring. End-tidal CO_2 is often lower than $PaCO_2$ due to alveolar dead space ventilation. End-tidal CO_2 monitoring responds instantaneously to changes in $PaCO_2$.

Reference: Mathew B, Lakshminrusimha S. Noninvasive monitoring of gas exchange. In: Keszler M, Gautham KS, eds. *Goldsmith's Assisted Ventilation of the Neonate: An Evidence-Based Approach to Newborn Respiratory Care.* 7th ed. Philadelphia, PA: Elsevier; 2022:117-120.

33. **(D)** Evaluation for extubation should be considered when ventilator parameters are low: supplemental oxygen ranging between 21% and 30%; PIP 14–18 cm H_2O; tidal volume 3.5–5 mL/kg; and intermittent mandatory ventilation 10–20/minute.

Reference: Crowley MA. Neonatal respiratory disorders. In: Martin RJ, Fanaroff AA, Walsh MC, eds. *Fanaroff & Martin's Neonatal-Perinatal Medicine: Diseases of the Fetus and Infant.* 11th ed. Philadelphia, PA: Elsevier; 2020:1074-1086.

34. **(B)** The lecithin–sphingomyelin (L/S) ratio and the absence or presence of phosphatidylglycerol (PG) in amniotic fluid can be used to assess fetal lung maturity. The presence of PG in amniotic fluid is associated with a very low risk for the development of RDS, whereas the absence of PG is associated with RDS. PG determination is valid even in the presence of blood-contaminated amniotic fluid. An L/S ratio less than 2:1 is associated with RDS, whereas L/S ratios greater than 2:1 are generally not associated with RDS. The L/S ratio is unreliable in the presence of blood-contaminated amniotic fluid and is inaccurate for infants of diabetic mothers.

References: Gardner SL, Enzman-Hines M, Nyp M. Respiratory diseases. In: Gardner SL, Carter BS, Niermeyer S, eds. *Merenstein & Gardner's Handbook of Neonatal Intensive Care: An Interprofessional Approach.* 9th ed. St. Louis, MO: Elsevier; 2021:729-750.

Wilson J, Snapp B, Walters M. The pulmonary system. In: Koehn A, ed. *Neonatal Nurse Practitioner Certification Intensive Review: Fast Facts and Practice Questions.* New York: Springer Publishing Company, LLC; 2020:235-260.

35. **(D)** Developmental care techniques, such as providing nonnutritive sucking and body containment, are effective strategies to decrease the infant's stress response to suctioning. Saline does not thin or liquefy mucus. In addition, the instilled saline can enter the lungs and inactivate endogenous surfactant. Turning the head is an effective strategy for passing the catheter into the contralateral bronchus. The turned head position is contraindicated because of the risk for increased intracranial pressure and jugular vein occlusion in the first 3 days of life, when the risk for intraventricular hemorrhage (IVH) is highest. The infant's head should be kept in a midline position for suctioning. Every catheter passage is considered a suction event. The number of catheter passes should be limited to what is necessary to adequately remove secretions.

Reference: Gardner SL, Enzman-Hines M, Nyp M. Respiratory diseases. In: Gardner SL, Carter BS, Niermeyer S, eds. *Merenstein & Gardner's Handbook of Neonatal Intensive Care: An Interprofessional Approach.* 9th ed. St. Louis, MO: Elsevier; 2021:748-749.

36. **(D)** Studies suggest that low-dose hydrocortisone is safer for the immature brain because it has less effect on cerebral tissue volume and fewer adverse neurodevelopmental outcomes compared with dexamethasone. Unlike dexamethasone, low-dose hydrocortisone does not reduce the incidence of BPD/chronic lung disease.

Reference: Gardner SL, Enzman-Hines M, Nyp M. Respiratory diseases. In: Gardner SL, Carter BS, Niermeyer S, eds. *Merenstein & Gardner's Handbook of Neonatal Intensive Care: An Interprofessional Approach.* 9th ed. St. Louis, MO: Elsevier; 2021:784-834.

37. **(D)** The canalicular phase of fetal lung development (16–26 weeks' gestation) is characterized by the appearance of primitive gas-exchanging units, the acini. Terminal bronchioles divide, giving rise to the respiratory bronchiole, alveolar duct, and terminal sac. Pulmonary capillaries proliferate and become closer to the airways. The degree of acinus–capillary coupling will eventually have a direct effect on gas exchange capability. The embryonic foregut gives rise to the lung bud which then further divides, giving rise to the presumptive airways during the embryonic stage. Alveolar surface area and numbers increase rapidly during the alveolar stage beginning around 32 weeks' gestation, several weeks after the respiratory bronchioles have developed. The capillary network increases significantly at 30 weeks' gestation during the saccular stage.

References: Kallapur SG, Jobe AH. Lung development and maturation. In: Martin RJ, Fanaroff AA, Walsh MC, eds. *Fanaroff & Martin's Neonatal-Perinatal Medicine: Diseases of the Fetus and Infant.* 11th ed. Philadelphia, PA: Elsevier; 2020:1125-1126.

Plosa E, Guttentag SH. Lung development. In: Gleason CA, Juul SE, eds. *Avery's Diseases of the Newborn.* 10th ed. Philadelphia, PA: Elsevier; 2018:586.

38. **(C)** Pleural fluid draining from a chylothorax contains a high number of lymphocytes. Removal of these cells, which play a significant role in the immune system, places the infant at risk for infection due to lymphopenia. Continuous drainage of a chylothorax via a tube thoracotomy relieves dyspnea which may evolve to apnea. A chylothorax results from leakage of fluid from a lymphatic vessel. It does not involve air leakage as seen in a pneumothorax. Subcutaneous emphysema denotes an air leak into the subcutaneous tissue under the skin and can occur with a pneumomediastinum if air dissects through the anterior mediastinum into the neck.

Reference: Crowley MA. Neonatal respiratory disorders. In: Martin RJ, Fanaroff AA, Walsh MC, eds. *Fanaroff & Martin's Neonatal-Perinatal Medicine: Diseases of the Fetus and Infant.* 11th ed. Philadelphia, PA: Elsevier; 2020:1208-1209.

39. **(D)** Approximately 15% of alveoli are developed at term. Although there is controversy regarding when the lung ceases to add alveoli, late alveolarization is seen as late as 19–20 years of age with final vascular and alveolar growth. The potential for continued alveolar growth after birth explains why many preterm infants with interrupted lung development at birth can have relatively good lung function later in life.

References: Kallapur SG, Jobe AH. Lung development and maturation. In: Martin RJ, Fanaroff AA, Walsh MC, eds. *Fanaroff & Martin's Neonatal-Perinatal Medicine: Diseases of the Fetus and Infant.* 11th ed. Philadelphia, PA: Elsevier; 2020:1126-1128.

Plosa E, Guttentag SH. Lung development. In: Gleason CA, Juul SE, eds. *Avery's Diseases of the Newborn.* 10th ed. Philadelphia, PA: Elsevier; 2018:586.

40. **(D)** Establishing an air–liquid interface in the alveolus is one of two transitional events required for extrauterine functioning. The other is a rhythmic respiration pattern. Surfactant lowers surface tension at the air–fluid interface, reducing opening pressure, stabilizing the alveoli, and preventing alveolar collapse at end expiration. Surfactant also increases lung compliance and lowers opening pressure. Lung fluid production slows in late pregnancy and absorption commences with labor. Lung aeration, which is facilitated by surfactant, replaces lung fluid, and 80%–90% of functional residual capacity (FRC) is established within 1 hour of birth. Structural maturation is a stepwise process occurring over several years.

Reference: Kallapur SG, Jobe AH. Lung development and maturation. In: Martin RJ, Fanaroff AA, Walsh MC, eds. *Fanaroff & Martin's Neonatal-Perinatal Medicine: Diseases of the Fetus and Infant.* 11th ed. Philadelphia, PA: Elsevier; 2020:1124-1128.

41. **(C)** Increased fetal insulin production in response to maternal diabetes inhibits surfactant C (phosphatidylcholine) protein

synthesis. Surfactant deficiency is a key etiologic factor in the development of RDS. Spontaneous early fetal lung maturation may result from maternal, placental, or fetal stress-induced events. Heroin induces fetal hypoxia and stress which accelerates lung maturation. However, in utero growth restriction and preeclampisa do not facilitate lung maturation. Fetal exposure to chorioamnionitis can induce lung maturation because inflammatory mediators trigger increased surfactant lipid and protein pool sizes. Maternal administration of corticosteroids induces fetal lung maturation by increasing the surface area and lung volumes for gas exchange.

References: Kallapur SG, Jobe AH. Lung development and maturation. In: Martin RJ, Fanaroff AA, Walsh MC, eds. *Fanaroff & Martin's Neonatal-Perinatal Medicine: Diseases of the Fetus and Infant.* 11th ed. Philadelphia, PA: Elsevier; 2020:1124-1142.

Wilson J, Snapp B, Walters M. The pulmonary system. In: Koehn A, ed. *Neonatal Nurse Practitioner Certification Intensive Review: Fast Facts and Practice Questions.* New York: Springer Publishing Company, LLC; 2020:235-260.

42. **(C)** Surfactant is produced and secreted by the lamellar bodies of type II pneumocytes of the lungs. Acini are the gas-exchanging portion of lung tissue. Type I pneumocytes are thin cells of the alveoli and are responsible for gas exchange. Surfactant protein A is one of four protein components of surfactant.

Reference: Kallapur SG, Jobe AH. Lung development and maturation. In: Martin RJ, Fanaroff AA, Walsh MC, eds. *Fanaroff & Martin's Neonatal-Perinatal Medicine: Diseases of the Fetus and Infant.* 11th ed. Philadelphia, PA: Elsevier; 2020:1137-1138.

43. **(A)** Retractions are the result of increased chest wall compliance, immature intercostal muscles, and increased inspiratory pressure. Retractions indicate increased work of breathing and worsen with increasing disease. Hypotension frequently occurs with respiratory disease as a late finding due to hypoxia and acidosis caused by poor respiratory effort. Acrocyanosis is a blueness of the peripheral extremities and is normal within the first 24 hours of life. The normal respiratory rate in a newborn is 30–60 breaths per minute.

Reference: Gardner SL, Niermeyer S. Care after birth. In: Gardner SL, Carter BS, Niermeyer S, eds. *Merenstein & Gardner's Handbook of Neonatal Intensive Care: An Interprofessional Approach.* 9th ed. St. Louis, MO: Elsevier; 2021:93-98.

44. **(C)** Cerebral circulation is affected by changes in $PaCO_2$. Prolonged severe hypocapnia ($PaCO_2$ <35 mm Hg) decreases cerebral blood flow especially in premature infants in the first 3–4 days of life. Decreased cerebral blood flow induces cerebral ischemia which can lead to neuronal cell injury and death, resulting in periventricular leukomalacia. An increase in cerebral blood flow increases the risk for IVH. Hypocapnia stimulates chemoreceptors and aids in the reflexive initiation of respiration. Gastroesophageal reflux disease is a pathologic response to an incompetent lower esophageal sphincter.

References: Barry JS, Hernandez C, Jones Jr D. Acid-base homeostasis and oxygenation. In: Gardner SL, Carter BS, Niermeyer S, eds. *Merenstein & Gardner's Handbook of Neonatal Intensive Care: An Interprofessional Approach.* 9th ed. St. Louis, MO: Elsevier; 2021:186-198.

Donn SM, Attar MA. Assisted ventilation of the neonate and its complications. In: Martin RJ, Fanaroff AA, Walsh MC, eds. *Fanaroff & Martin's Neonatal-Perinatal Medicine Diseases of the Fetus and Infant.* 11th ed. Philadelphia, PA: Elsevier; 2020:1198-1199.

45. **(B)** RDS is the result of surfactant deficiency and is the most common pulmonary problem in the preterm infant. The incidence of RDS is inversely proportional to the gestational age of the infant. At 30 weeks' gestational age, surfactant production is minimal, which leads to atelectasis, hypoxia, and acidosis. The infant's attempt to increase ventilation is characterized by grunting, nasal flaring, and retractions. Preterm infants with surfactant deficiency may develop an iatrogenic air leak from excessive use of airway pressure during resuscitation. The presence of an air leak at birth

before the infant has undergone positive pressure ventilation is less likely. Air leaks can occur spontaneously, however, if there is unequal air distribution at birth. MAS occurs more commonly in term and postterm infants who passed meconium in utero. The passage of meconium was not present in this scenario and MAS rarely occurs in infants less than 36 weeks gestation. Transient tachypnea of the newborn (TTN) is due to retained fetal lung fluid and is most likely to be experienced by late preterm and full-term infants who are born by cesarean section, precipitous delivery, or spontaneous vaginal delivery without labor.

References: Gardner SL, Enzman-Hines M, Nyp M. Respiratory diseases. In: Gardner SL, Carter BS, Niermeyer S, eds. *Merenstein & Gardner's Handbook of Neonatal Intensive Care: An Interprofessional Approach.* 9th ed. St. Louis, MO: Elsevier; 2021:729-732.

Wilson J, Snapp B, Walters M. The pulmonary system. In: Koehn A, ed. *Neonatal Nurse Practitioner Certification Intensive Review: Fast Facts and Practice Questions.* New York: Springer Publishing Company, LLC; 2020:235-260.

46. **(D)** Expiratory grunting results from partial closure of the glottis during expiration. Grunting increases intrathoracic pressure in efforts to trap alveolar air, prevent alveolar collapse, and maintain FRC. Expiratory grunting reflects increased work of breathing and energy needs would be increased. Upper airway resistance is a function of nasal resistance, the cartilage, and supporting structures of the pharyngeal airway and is increased, not decreased, by expiratory grunting. Nasal flaring is a compensatory attempt to open airways and decrease upper airway resistance. Large airway obstruction is caused by mucus or congenital defects and is not relieved by expiratory grunting.

References: Lagoski M, Hamvas A, Wambach JA. Respiratory distress syndrome in the neonate. In: Martin RJ, Fanaroff AA, Walsh MC, eds. *Fanaroff & Martin's Neonatal-Perinatal Medicine: Diseases of the Fetus and Infant.* 11th ed. Philadelphia, PA: Elsevier; 2020:1159-1173.

Lopez V, Graziano P. The neonatal physical exam. In: Koehn A, ed. *Neonatal Nurse Practitioner Certification Intensive Review: Fast Facts and Practice Questions.* New York: Springer Publishing Company, LLC; 2020:27-57.

47. **(B)** The diagnosis of sepsis is hard to make based on clinical findings alone. A positive finding on cultures of the blood, cerebrospinal fluid, or urine is the gold standard. Culture of the eye is performed to diagnose suspected eye infections, such as those caused by *Neisseria gonorrhoeae*, herpes simplex virus, and *Chlamydia*. Culture of nasal secretions is a surveillance method typically used to detect methicillin-resistant *Staphylococcus aureus*. Culture of surface specimens is a surveillance method and not a definitive diagnostic method.

Reference: Polin R, Randis TM. Perinatal infection and chorioamnionitis. In: Martin RJ, Fanaroff AA, Walsh MC, eds. *Fanaroff & Martin's Neonatal-Perinatal Medicine: Diseases of the Fetus and Infant.* 11th ed. Philadelphia, PA: Elsevier; 2020:789.

48. **(D)** Classic radiographic findings of RDS include ground glass or hazy appearance, low lung volumes, air bronchograms (more prominent as disease progresses), and micro atelectasis. Air bronchograms exhibit air in the bronchial tree visualized against a background of generalized alveolar atelectasis. In pneumonia, the chest radiograph demonstrates patchy, occasionally asymmetric, radiating, bilateral interstitial infiltrates. The radiographic appearance of pulmonary edema varies from a diffuse haziness to a whiteout. In general, radiographic findings of pulmonary air leaks reveal radiolucencies or collection of air in spaces where air is not typically seen. PIE is seen as multiple small, cyst-like radiolucencies with a varying pattern. A pneumothorax appears as an air collection in the pleural space. A pneumomediastinum appears as an air collection in the mediastinum. A pneumopericardium is demonstrated by a halo of free air in the pericardial space.

References: Lagoski M, Hamvas A, Wambach JA. Respiratory distress syndrome in the neonate. In: Martin RJ, Fanaroff AA, Walsh MC, eds. *Fanaroff &*

Martin's Neonatal-Perinatal Medicine: Diseases of the Fetus and Infant. 11th ed. Philadelphia, PA: Elsevier; 2020:1159-1173.

Wilson J, Snapp B, Walters M. The pulmonary system. In: Koehn A, ed. *Neonatal Nurse Practitioner Certification Intensive Review: Fast Facts and Practice Questions*. New York: Springer Publishing Company, LLC; 2020:235-260.

49. **(C)** The pH of 7.25 indicates acidosis (normal 7.35–7.45). Respiratory acidosis is characterized by a low pH and high $PaCO_2$. The $PaCO_2$ reflects the respiratory component of acid–base balance. The normal $PaCO_2$ is 35–45 mm Hg, therefore, $PaCO_2$ of 70 indicates respiratory acidosis. In metabolic acidosis the pH and HCO_3 are both low. In this scenario, the HCO_3 is normal.

Reference: Barry JS, Hernandez C, Jones Jr D. Acid-base homeostasis and oxygenation. In: Gardner SL, Carter BS, Niermeyer S, eds. *Merenstein & Gardner's Handbook of Neonatal Intensive Care: An Interprofessional Approach*. 9th ed. St. Louis, MO: Elsevier; 2021:186-198.

50. **(D)** Criteria for endotracheal suctioning include visible secretions in the tube, coarse breath sounds, increased agitation, and changes in ABG values. After suctioning, the infant is reassessed to determine the effectiveness of the procedure. Repositioning of the infant is necessary to prevent localization of secretions in the dependent pulmonary structures. Pain management is used to improve ventilator synchrony and pulmonary function, decrease stress, and prevent complications. However, provision of an adequate airway takes precedence over either of these interventions. Equipment alarms are present to notify care providers that predetermined limits have been exceeded. Alarms require a response to determine the cause of and correct the cause of the alarm.

Reference: Gardner SL, Enzman-Hines M, Nyp M. Respiratory diseases. In: Gardner SL, Carter BS, Niermeyer S, eds. *Merenstein & Gardner's Handbook of Neonatal Intensive Care: An Interprofessional Approach*. 9th ed. St. Louis, MO: Elsevier; 2021:729-750.

51. **(D)** Clinical findings of a patent ductus arteriosus (PDA) include bounding peripheral pulses, widening pulse pressure, decreased urine output, and metabolic acidosis. A murmur is typically, although not always, present and is heard best at the second or third left intercostal space. The hemodynamic changes and the resultant clinical manifestations of a PDA depend on the magnitude of the pulmonary vascular resistance and the size of the ductal lumen. Following surfactant treatment there is an increased risk of clinically significant PDA in premature infants. The exact mechanism for this relationship needs further study. The initial signs of sepsis are nonspecific and nonlocalizing and include vital sign abnormalities, respiratory distress, lethargy, feeding problems, and metabolic acidosis. Signs of a gradual air leak include restlessness, tachypnea, and increased work of breathing. An acute air leak manifests with bradycardia and muffled heart sounds, air hunger, and cyanosis, and cardiopulmonary arrest can result. Signs and symptoms of pneumonia are nonspecific and include respiratory distress causing hypercarbia, and temperature instability.

References: Gardner SL, Enzman-Hines M, Nyp M. Respiratory diseases. In: Gardner SL, Carter BS, Niermeyer S, eds. *Merenstein & Gardner's Handbook of Neonatal Intensive Care: An Interprofessional Approach*. 9th ed. St. Louis, MO: Elsevier; 2021:729-741.

Gomella T, Eyal F, Bany-Mohammed F. *Gomella's Neonatology: Management, Procedures, On-Call Problems, Diseases, and Drugs*. 8th ed. New York: McGraw Hill; 2020:1027-1031.

Swanson T, Erickson L. Cardiovascular diseases and surgical interventions. In: Gardner SL, Carter BS, Niermeyer S, eds. *Merenstein & Gardner's Handbook of Neonatal Intensive Care: An Interprofessional Approach*. 9th ed. St. Louis, MO: Elsevier; 2021:836-860.

Weinman JP, Bronsert BM, Strain JD. Diagnostic imaging in the neonate. In: Gardner SL, Carter BS, Niermeyer S, eds. *Merenstein & Gardner's Handbook of Neonatal Intensive Care: An Interprofessional Approach*. 9th ed. St. Louis, MO: Elsevier; 2021:201-234.

52. **(B)** The inhibition of cyclooxygenase by the nonsteroidal anti-inflammatory agent indomethacin (Indocin) results in decreased prostaglandin synthesis and contributes to ductus arteriosus closure. A left-to-right shunt through the ductus arteriosus results in pulmonary edema and respiratory compromise. Restriction of fluids is an intervention implemented to reduce pulmonary symptoms. Furosemide is a known stimulant of the renal release of prostaglandin E2 which is a potent dilator of the ductus arteriosus. Therefore furosemide should not be used in PDA. Prostaglandin E1 (Alprostadil) is a vasodilator used to provide patency of the ductus arteriosus.

References: Gardner SL, Enzman-Hines M, Nyp M. Respiratory diseases. In: Gardner SL, Carter BS, Niermeyer S, eds. *Merenstein & Gardner's Handbook of Neonatal Intensive Care: An Interprofessional Approach*. 9th ed. St. Louis, MO: Elsevier; 2021:729-741.

Swanson T, Erickson L. Cardiovascular diseases and surgical interventions. In: Gardner SL, Carter BS, Niermeyer S, eds. *Merenstein & Gardner's Handbook of Neonatal Intensive Care: An Interprofessional Approach*. 9th ed. St. Louis, MO: Elsevier; 2021:836-860.

53. **(D)** The preterm infant has less pulmonary arterial musculature and immature lung parenchyma. The left-to-right shunting in PDA increases pulmonary blood flow and the chance of pulmonary hemorrhage. Because this left-to-right shunting "steals" blood from the systemic circulation (diastolic steal), hypoperfusion of the mesentery occurs and metabolic acidosis develops. Preterm infants with surfactant deficiency may develop a pulmonary air leak, which is usually iatrogenic resulting from the therapies given. Infants receiving CPAP, bag-mask ventilation, and mechanical ventilation are at increased risk of developing a pulmonary air leak due to positive pressure ventilation. Pulmonary hypoplasia results from intrinsic abnormalities in lung development, for example, from compression by abdominal contents in CDH, or from oligohydramnios as can occur with congenital renal disorders (e.g., renal agenesis).

References: Fraser D. Respiratory distress. In: Verklan T, Walden M, Forest S, eds. *Core Curriculum for Neonatal Intensive Care Nursing*. 6th ed. St. Louis, MO: Elsevier; 2021:410-411.

Gardner SL, Enzman-Hines M, Nyp M. Respiratory diseases. In: Gardner SL, Carter BS, Niermeyer S, eds. *Merenstein & Gardner's Handbook of Neonatal Intensive Care: An Interprofessional Approach*. 9th ed. St. Louis, MO: Elsevier; 2021:729-794.

54. **(C)** A neutral thermal environment maintains normal body temperature while minimizing metabolic demands and oxygen consumption. Although adequate fluid intake is necessary to meet the body's demands, excessive fluid contributes to volume overload and patency of the ductus arteriosus, which can lead to pulmonary edema and ventilation perfusion mismatching. For an acutely ill infant, minimal stimulation limits stressors that interfere with physiologic stability. Maintaining an oxygen saturation level at 88%–92% keeps the infant in a normoxemic state under most conditions.

Reference: Gardner SL, Cammack BH. Heat balance. In: Gardner SL, Carter BS, Niermeyer S, eds. *Merenstein & Gardner's Handbook of Neonatal Intensive Care: An Interprofessional Approach*. 9th ed. St. Louis, MO: Elsevier; 2021:137-158.

55. **(D)** An infant with RDS may exhibit oliguria, especially if the infant is hypoxic or renal perfusion is diminished. A natural diuresis occurs at 48–72 hours of age and precedes the onset of the recovery phase and improved pulmonary status. Renal failure results in body fluid excess. An infant with chronic lung disease exhibits fluid intolerance, including growth failure, weight gain, edema, and decreased urine output.

Reference: Cadnapaphornchai MA, Soranno DE, Bisio TJ, Woloschuk R, Kirkley M. Neonatal nephrology. In: Gardner SL, Carter BS, Niermeyer S, eds. *Merenstein & Gardner's Handbook of Neonatal Intensive Care: An Interprofessional Approach*. 9th ed. St. Louis, MO: Elsevier; 2021:886-889.

56. **(A)** Pathogens responsible for early-onset pneumonia are acquired transplacentally and from the birth canal before or during delivery. Maternal fever indicates infection; premature rupture of membranes, prolonged labor, and excessive obstetric manipulations predispose to ascending infection. The cause of RDS is surfactant deficiency. Fetal exposure to chorioamnionitis can induce lung maturation because inflammatory mediators trigger increased surfactant lipid and protein pool sizes. MAS occurs predominately in term or postterm infants who have experienced hypoxia with relaxation of the anal sphincter and the expulsion of meconium into the amniotic fluid followed by fetal gasping. TTN is delayed clearance of fetal lung fluid resulting in pulmonary edema. TTN generally occurs in term or late-preterm infants with a history of cesarean section, precipitous delivery, or spontaneous vaginal delivery without labor.

References: Gardner SL, Enzman-Hines M, Nyp M. Respiratory diseases. In: Gardner SL, Carter BS, Niermeyer S, eds. *Merenstein & Gardner's Handbook of Neonatal Intensive Care: An Interprofessional Approach.* 9th ed. St. Louis, MO: Elsevier; 2021:799-802.

Wilson J, Snapp B, Walters M. The pulmonary system. In: Koehn A, ed. *Neonatal Nurse Practitioner Certification Intensive Review: Fast Facts and Practice Questions.* New York: Springer Publishing Company, LLC; 2020:235-260.

57. **(D)** Blow by oxygen administration has relieved this infant's hypoxemia and is readily available as therapy. Supplemental oxygen will treat the problem of hypoxemia. Surfactant replacement therapy is given after surfactant deficiency is diagnosed from the history, clinical presentation, and chest radiograph. Nitric oxide is a selective pulmonary vasodilating agent used in the treatment of persistent pulmonary hypertension to relax pulmonary vasculature and enhance pulmonary blood flow. Although this infant could be developing pulmonary hypertension, nitric oxide would not be the first line of treatment for pulmonary hypertension. Intubation and mechanical ventilation are strategies used in respiratory failure or apnea. The infant's blood gas results show hypoxemia, not respiratory failure ($PaCO_2$ is within normal range), and the infant is not apneic.

Reference: Gardner SL, Enzman-Hines M, Nyp M. Respiratory diseases. In: Gardner SL, Carter BS, Niermeyer S, eds. *Merenstein & Gardner's Handbook of Neonatal Intensive Care: An Interprofessional Approach.* 9th ed. St. Louis, MO: Elsevier; 2021:729-794.

58. **(D)** TTN manifests on chest radiograph as bilateral, symmetric, perihilar streaking with fluid in the interlobar fissure, hyperaeration, and mild-to-moderate cardiomegaly. The perihilar streaking represents engorgement of the periarterial lymphatics that participate in the clearance of alveolar fluid. RDS appears on a chest radiograph as bilateral diffuse alveolar infiltrates and a reticulogranular (ground glass) appearance due to alveolar atelectasis. Additional findings include hypoinflation and air bronchograms. The chest x-ray is homogeneous in appearance. MAS manifests on a chest radiograph as bilateral, asymmetric areas of atelectasis and hyperaeration of the lungs with flattened hemidiaphragms. The chest x-ray is heterogenous in appearance. PIE appears on a chest radiograph as multiple, small, cyst-like radiolucencies caused by alveolar overdistension secondary to assisted ventilation.

Reference: Gardner SL, Enzman-Hines M, Nyp M. Respiratory diseases. In: Gardner SL, Carter BS, Niermeyer S, eds. *Merenstein & Gardner's Handbook of Neonatal Intensive Care: An Interprofessional Approach.* 9th ed. St. Louis, MO: Elsevier; 2021:729-794.

59. **(D)** Hypoxia and acidosis are endogenous mediators that increase pulmonary vascular resistance and lead to persistent pulmonary hypertension and hypoperfusion of the lungs. The increased pulmonary vascular resistance results in a right-to-left shunt through either the foramen ovale, ductus arteriosus, or both. Pneumonia results from bacterial, viral, or mycoplasmal organisms

acquired transplacentally, during delivery, or postnatally. Pneumonia is due to an immature immune system, colonization of the mother's genital and vaginal tracts with pathogens, amnionitis, prolonged rupture of membranes, and nosocomial infections acquired in the neonatal intensive care unit. TTN generally occurs in term or late-preterm infants within the first 6 hours of life with a history of cesarean section, precipitous delivery, or spontaneous vaginal delivery without labor. Without the hormonal changes that accompany spontaneous labor, the in utero secretory fetal lung fails to transition into an absorptive mode. As a result, lung fluid is retained and leads to collapse of the bronchioli.

Reference: Gardner SL, Enzman-Hines M, Nyp M. Respiratory diseases. In: Gardner SL, Carter BS, Niermeyer S, eds. *Merenstein & Gardner's Handbook of Neonatal Intensive Care: An Interprofessional Approach.* 9th ed. St. Louis, MO: Elsevier; 2021:802-811.

60. **(A)** Central apnea is the absence of spontaneous breathing effort. Without respiratory effort, there is no airflow. In obstructive apnea, breathing efforts are present but airflow is blocked. Mixed apnea is characterized by an initial central apneic episode followed by obstruction of the airway. Periodic breathing is characterized by a cyclical pattern of apnea for 5–10 seconds followed by breathing for 10–15 seconds.

Reference: Gardner SL, Enzman-Hines M, Nyp M. Respiratory diseases. In: Gardner SL, Carter BS, Niermeyer S, eds. *Merenstein & Gardner's Handbook of Neonatal Intensive Care: An Interprofessional Approach.* 9th ed. St. Louis, MO: Elsevier; 2021:734, 811-818.

61. **(C)** Responses to hypoxemia and changes in $PaCO_2$ are different in the adult and in the neonate. The adult responds with sustained increased ventilation. The neonate, however, demonstrates a brief period of increased respiration from sympathetic nervous system discharge followed by parasympathetic stimulation with resulting respiratory depression.

Reference: Gardner SL, Enzman-Hines M, Nyp M. Respiratory diseases. In: Gardner SL, Carter BS, Niermeyer S, eds. *Merenstein & Gardner's Handbook of Neonatal Intensive Care: An Interprofessional Approach.* 9th ed. St. Louis, MO: Elsevier; 2021:802-811.

62. **(B)** Weighing on a cold scale is one example of environmental stress which has been shown to precipitate apneic episodes. Limiting loud noises reduces noxious stimuli and apneic events. Abrupt changes in temperature, especially hyperthermia, trigger apnea. Maintaining thermoneutral environmental reduces apneic events. Small rolls or other positioning aids may be used to prevent airway obstruction.

Reference: Gardner SL, Enzman-Hines M, Nyp M. Respiratory diseases. In: Gardner SL, Carter BS, Niermeyer S, eds. *Merenstein & Gardner's Handbook of Neonatal Intensive Care: An Interprofessional Approach.* 9th ed. St. Louis, MO: Elsevier; 2021:802-811.

63. **(C)** Caffeine is a central nervous system stimulant which increases medullary respiratory center sensitivity to carbon dioxide, stimulates central inspiratory drive, and improves skeletal muscle contraction. Tachycardia is an adverse effect of caffeine, therefore the dose should not be administered, and the physician or neonatal nurse practitioner should be notified immediately. The nurse should monitor the infant for additional adverse effects, including ventricular ectopy, gastrointestinal upset, and central nervous system manifestations of restlessness, irritability, and agitation. Because caffeine has a half-life of 72–96 hours, it is unlikely that the heart rate would decrease in 5 minutes. Therefore, the nurse should not administer the dose after waiting 5 minutes. Although remeasuring the heart rate periodically is necessary until the heart rate returns to baseline, caffeine should be resumed at a lower dose once the heart rate is consistently below 180 beats per minute.

Reference: Ku LC, Hornik C, Buschbach D. Pharmacology in neonatal care. In: Gardner SL, Carter BS, Niermeyer S, eds. *Merenstein & Gardner's Handbook of Neonatal Intensive Care: An Interprofessional Approach.* 9th ed. St. Louis, MO: Elsevier; 2021:226-234.

64. **(C)** The use of transcutaneous oxygen and carbon dioxide monitors helps in trending an infant's oxygenation and ventilation status. Therefore the need for ABG specimens is reduced, but not eliminated. The monitor must be calibrated before use and then correlated with ABG results. The placement site must be changed frequently based on the probe temperature and the condition of the infant's skin to prevent skin burns. When the site is changed, the monitor must be recalibrated and another ABG analysis performed to determine the correlation between the monitor values and the ABG results. Transcutaneous PO_2 and PCO_2 monitors are subject to drift when left in place for longer than 4 hours or when the infant is not well perfused or has a low temperature. Arterial and transcutaneous oxygen values are not identical because of local oxygen consumption by the skin, heating of the skin, oxygen diffusion time, and the response time of the electrode. The range of accuracy of transcutaneous PO_2 monitors is limited. Values lower than 40 mm Hg and higher than 120 mm Hg are not accurately reflected. An umbilical artery catheter is removed when it is no longer required for patient care. Although the transcutaneous PO_2 and PCO_2 monitors are used as one method of assessment, they do not replace ABG analysis, and therefore the umbilical catheter cannot yet be removed.

References: Bancalari E, Claure N, Jain D. Neonatal respiratory therapy. In: Gleason CA, Juul SE, eds. *Avery's Diseases of the Newborn.* 10th ed. Philadelphia, PA: Elsevier; 2018:633.

Coe K, Bradshaw WT, Tanaka DT. Physiologic monitoring. In: Gardner SL, Carter BS, Niermeyer S, eds. *Merenstein & Gardner's Handbook of Neonatal Intensive Care: An Interprofessional Approach.* 9th ed. St. Louis, MO: Elsevier; 2021:165-180.

65. **(C)** The most common bacterial organisms causing pneumonia in the newborn period are group β-hemolytic streptococci and Gram-negative organisms. Although *Chlamydia trachomatis* can be acquired at birth, it is not among the most common etiologic agents of pneumonia. Respiratory syncytial virus is a nosocomial cause of pneumonia. Infections caused by *Candida* fungal species occur most often in neonates requiring prolonged hospitalization. These organisms are another nosocomial cause of pneumonia.

Reference: Pammi M, Brand MC, Weisman LE. Infection in the neonate. In: Gardner SL, Carter BS, Niermeyer S, eds. *Merenstein & Gardner's Handbook of Neonatal Intensive Care: An Interprofessional Approach.* 9th ed. St. Louis, MO: Elsevier; 2021:692-701.

66. **(C)** Fetuses with in utero hypoxemia and acidosis often pass meconium and initiate respiratory efforts that increase the risk of meconium aspiration. If meconium is retrieved from the trachea during resuscitation after birth, vigilance is required to monitor for the development of MAS. Mild MAS can show a normal lung pattern on chest radiograph. Pulmonary edema is associated with a high fluid intake and significant PDA, congenital heart defects that increase pulmonary blood flow, and lung injury. It rarely manifests at birth unless the infant has experienced heart failure in utero. Although respiratory distress has multiple causes, the risk of MAS is primary due to the history and presentation at birth. In the absence of indications for MAS, the care provider would proceed with differential diagnosis. TTN is caused by retained fetal lung fluid and is most likely to be experienced by late preterm or full-term infants with a history of cesarean section, precipitous delivery, or spontaneous vaginal delivery without labor. The history of thick meconium stained fluid suggests a more likely condition.

Reference: Gardner SL, Enzman-Hines M, Nyp M. Respiratory diseases. In: Gardner SL, Carter BS, Niermeyer S, eds. *Merenstein & Gardner's Handbook of Neonatal Intensive Care: An Interprofessional Approach.* 9th ed. St. Louis, MO: Elsevier; 2021:794-808.

67. **(B)** MAS places the infant at risk for air leak due to the ball-valve phenomenon in which air enters the alveoli but cannot escape. Distended alveoli rupture, resulting in an air leak. A tension pneumothorax occurs as air builds up under pressure in the pleural space. The affected lung collapses and forces the mediastinum toward the contralateral side. Signs and symptoms of tension pneumothorax are acute respiratory decompensation with cyanosis, apnea, and bradycardia. On examination, the affected lung will exhibit diminished breath sounds. Increased anteroposterior diameter of the chest will be noted on visualization. A pleural effusion is not an acute event but rather occurs over time. Normally there is a small amount of fluid present in between the visceral and parietal pleura. The fluid is reabsorbed into the parietal pleural lymphatics. Production and absorption of serous fluid are constant. In disease states, production may increase, which results in a pleural effusion. A pulmonary hemorrhage manifests with sudden, severe respiratory distress accompanied by bright-red blood or frothy pink secretions from the trachea. It is usually due to increased pulmonary capillary hydrostatic pressure, resulting in capillary rupture. PIE is an air leak syndrome that can occur after vigorous resuscitation efforts or can accompany assisted ventilation. Air dissects around blood vessels or along lymphatics. PIE manifests with hypoxia and hypercapnia. It may progress to pneumothorax or pneumomediastinum.

Reference: Gardner SL, Enzman-Hines M, Nyp M. Respiratory diseases. In: Gardner SL, Carter BS, Niermeyer S, eds. *Merenstein & Gardner's Handbook of Neonatal Intensive Care: An Interprofessional Approach.* 9th ed. St. Louis, MO: Elsevier; 2021:768-771.

68. **(C)** CDH is a herniation of abdominal organs into the thoracic cavity through a diaphragmatic defect. Clinical signs include respiratory distress and cyanosis at birth or shortly thereafter. The infant deteriorates, rather than improves, with bag-and-mask ventilation because the intestines distend with air and further compromise lung function. Breath sounds are diminished, point of maximal impulse may be shifted, the chest is barrel shaped, and the abdomen is scaphoid. A radiograph taken immediately after birth may not demonstrate intestine in the thorax, but later images will clearly demonstrate air-filled bowel. The survival rate is 50%. A tension pneumothorax occurs as air builds up under pressure in the pleural space. The affected lung collapses and forces the mediastinum toward the contralateral side, which results in decompensation. In the case of a tension pneumothorax on the left side, breath sounds would be diminished on the left, and heart sounds heard on the right. Chest x-ray findings include accumulation of air in the pleural space, an outline of the collapsed lung, and mediastinal shift. Assisted ventilation generally precedes pneumothorax. In this situation, the infant exhibited acute distress before any resuscitation efforts. A pneumomediastinum results from air that leaks into the mediastinal space. Air travels via vascular sheaths to the lining of the lung and moves into the mediastinum, which results in a pneumomediastinum. Signs include increased anteroposterior diameter of the chest and indistinct heart sounds. The characteristic x-ray finding is a "sail sign," which results from free air lifting the thymus gland. Like pneumothorax, pneumomediastinum is generally preceded by assisted ventilation. Congenital pulmonary airway malformation (CPAM), formerly known as cystic adenomatoid malformation, results from an abnormal branching of the fetal bronchial tree during the pseudoglandular phase of lung development. Respiratory symptoms vary from none to distress at birth. Chest x-ray findings in CPAM vary but usually include lesions that are multicystic air-filled, solid, or with air–fluid levels. The survival rate is 90%.

References: Gardner SL, Enzman-Hines M, Nyp M. Respiratory diseases. In: Gardner SL, Carter BS, Niermeyer S, eds. *Merenstein & Gardner's Handbook of Neonatal Intensive Care: An Interprofessional Approach.* 9th ed. St. Louis, MO: Elsevier; 2021:729-835.

Trotter CW. Radiologic evaluation. In: Verklan T, Walden M, Forest S, eds. *Core Curriculum for Neonatal Intensive Care Nursing.* 6th ed. St. Louis, MO: Elsevier; 2021:226-227.

69. (C) The pathogenesis of BPD is multifactorial. Causes include immaturity, infection, oxygen toxicity, lung damage (volutrauma or barotrauma) from mechanical ventilation, increased left-to-right shunting across a PDA, excessive fluid intake, and nutritional deficits. The incidence of BPD is inversely proportional to gestational age, occurring predominately in extreme preterm infants. TTN is due to retained fetal lung fluid and is predominately seen in term or near-term infants born by cesarean section, precipitous delivery, or spontaneous vaginal delivery without labor. Tachypnea is present, but these infants seldom require mechanical ventilation, recover rapidly, and have no residual effects.

References: Fraser D. Respiratory distress. In: Verklan T, Walden M, Forest S, eds. *Core Curriculum for Neonatal Intensive Care Nursing.* 6th ed. St. Louis, MO: Elsevier; 2021:406-407.

Gardner SL, Enzman-Hines M, Nyp M. Respiratory diseases. In: Gardner SL, Carter BS, Niermeyer S, eds. *Merenstein & Gardner's Handbook of Neonatal Intensive Care: An Interprofessional Approach.* 9th ed. St. Louis, MO: Elsevier; 2021:771-784.

70. (D) In BPD, by the end of the first or second week of life, the chest radiograph shows haziness of vessel margins progressing to linear densities representing alveolar collapse. This is followed by a bubbly appearance with hyperaeration, especially at the lung bases. In pleural effusion, pleural fluid gathers at the base of the lungs forming a meniscus, which is a concave line obscuring the costophrenic angle on x-ray. Patchy alveolar infiltrates are present in pneumonia and bilateral diffuse alveolar infiltrates are present in RDS. The absence of parenchymal markings denotes diminished pulmonary blood flow and is consistent with right-sided heart and outflow tract obstruction or persistent pulmonary hypertension.

Reference: Gardner SL, Enzman-Hines M, Nyp M. Respiratory diseases. In: Gardner SL, Carter BS, Niermeyer S, eds. *Merenstein & Gardner's Handbook of Neonatal Intensive Care: An Interprofessional Approach.* 9th ed. St. Louis, MO: Elsevier; 2021:771-784.

71. (B) Minute ventilation is the product of respiratory rate multiplied by tidal volume. Increasing minute ventilation decreases $PaCO_2$, whereas decreasing minute ventilation increases $PaCO_2$. In respiratory alkalosis, the pH is high due to a low $PaCO_2$. Decreasing minute ventilation will increase $PaCO_2$, helping to correct respiratory alkalosis. Increasing the ventilator rate will increase minute ventilation, and further reduce $PaCO_2$ levels, contributing to worsening alkalosis. Increasing the PIP or decreasing the PEEP without decreasing the PIP will increase tidal volume and minute ventilation, further reducing the $PaCO_2$ value and worsening the alkalosis.

Reference: Gardner SL, Enzman-Hines M, Nyp M. Respiratory diseases. In: Gardner SL, Carter BS, Niermeyer S, eds. *Merenstein & Gardner's Handbook of Neonatal Intensive Care: An Interprofessional Approach.* 9th ed. St. Louis, MO: Elsevier; 2021:754-760.

72. (C) Gas remaining in the lungs after a normal expiration is known as FRC. FRC is approximately 30 mL/kg. FRC is important because it keeps small airways open and prevents collapse during expiration, allowing alveolar gas exchange to occur during both inspiration and expiration. Tidal volume is the amount of air that moves in and out of the lungs with a normal breath. Vital capacity is the volume of air maximally inhaled and forcefully exhaled. Physiologic dead space is the total volume of gas not involved in gas exchange. Physiologic dead space is the sum of anatomic and alveolar dead space. Anatomic dead space is the volume of air in the conducting airways, including the nose, mouth, pharynx, larynx, trachea, and bronchi. Alveolar dead space is the volume of air in nonperfused alveoli that does not participate in gas exchange.

Reference: Fraser D, Diehl-Jones W. Assisted ventilation. In: Verklan T, Walden M, Forest S, eds. *Core Curriculum for Neonatal Intensive Care Nursing.* 6th ed. St. Louis, MO: Elsevier; 2021:425.

73. (D) An important aspect of chest tube care is the frequent monitoring and documentation of tube patency, oscillation of fluid within the drainage system, and presence or absence of bubbling in the water seal chamber. Continuous bubbling in the water seal chamber indicates an air leak; the source may be either the patient or the system. Milking and stripping of the chest tube are not necessary. If visible clots and debris are seen in the chest tube and are not free flowing, gentle kneading, not stripping, of the chest tube may be indicated. Developmentally appropriate positioning is not contraindicated in the infant with a chest tube. The infant should be maintained in a tucked midline position with care taken not to kink or dislodge the chest tube.

Reference: Gardner SL, Enzman-Hines M, Nyp M. Respiratory diseases. In: Gardner SL, Carter BS, Niermeyer S, eds. *Merenstein & Gardner's Handbook of Neonatal Intensive Care: An Interprofessional Approach.* 9th ed. St. Louis, MO: Elsevier; 2021:771-772.

74. (B) Pneumopericardium is characterized by cyanosis, muffled heart sounds, hypotension, and bradycardia. The chest radiograph reveals a "halo" around the heart. Management ranges from monitoring for deterioration in the case of a mild pneumopericardium to pericardiocentesis and placement of a pericardial tube for symptomatic cases. In pneumothorax the chest radiograph reveals accumulation of air in the pleural space. A collection of air in the mediastinum with air outlining the under surface of the thymus (sail sign) indicates a pneumomediastinum. Although heart sounds may be distant, infants with pneumomediastinum are usually asymptomatic. PIE is characterized by overdistended alveoli that appear as cyst-like radiolucencies. With ruptured alveoli, air intravasates into interstitial lung tissue.

References: Gardner SL, Enzman-Hines M, Nyp M. Respiratory diseases. In: Gardner SL, Carter BS, Niermeyer S, eds. *Merenstein & Gardner's Handbook of Neonatal Intensive Care: An Interprofessional Approach.* 9th ed. St. Louis, MO: Elsevier; 2021:767-770.

Gomella T, Eyal F, Bany-Mohammed F. *Gomella's Neonatology: Management, Procedures, On-Call Problems, Diseases, and Drugs.* 8th ed. New York: McGraw Hill; 2020:685.

75. (D) Inhaled nitric oxide (iNO) has been proven to be a selective and potent pulmonary vasodilator, decreasing pulmonary vascular resistance and increasing pulmonary blood flow. iNO prolongs clotting time but has no known myocardial effects. Although iNO plays a role in bronchodilation, its primary use is as a major mediator of endothelial function resulting in pulmonary vascular dilation. iNO is rapidly inactivated with a half-life of 3–5 seconds. For this reason, it exerts no effect on systemic blood pressure.

Reference: Gardner SL, Enzman-Hines M, Nyp M. Respiratory diseases. In: Gardner SL, Carter BS, Niermeyer S, eds. *Merenstein & Gardner's Handbook of Neonatal Intensive Care: An Interprofessional Approach.* 9th ed. St. Louis, MO: Elsevier; 2021:762.

76. (D) Immediate treatment of CDH focuses on management of pulmonary hypoplasia and hypertension. Surgical repair of a CDH is performed once pulmonary and cardiovascular stabilization has been achieved. Early management includes gentle mechanical ventilation, sedation and chemical paralysis, frequent monitoring of ABG values, inotropic support for systemic hypotension, and correction of metabolic acidosis. Extracorporeal membrane oxygenation (ECMO) and iNO may be indicated in severe cases. Immediate surgical repair is associated with a higher mortality rate. An immediate repair precludes stabilization and evaluation for associated conditions that may require iNO or ECMO. Use of surfactant is controversial, with some research showing a benefit and other studies indicating no benefit. Overall stability of the patient's condition contributes to a successful outcome. iNO may be given to promote pulmonary vasculature relaxation and help to increase pulmonary blood flow and gas exchange. This therapy is used to stabilize the infant's condition before and after surgery.

Reference: Gardner SL, Enzman-Hines M, Nyp M. Respiratory diseases. In: Gardner SL, Carter BS, Niermeyer S, eds. *Merenstein & Gardner's Handbook of Neonatal Intensive Care: An Interprofessional Approach.* 9th ed. St. Louis, MO: Elsevier; 2021:996-1000.

77. **(C)** Long-term complications associated with CDH repair include chronic lung disease, recurrent diaphragmatic hernia, gastroesophageal reflux, growth restriction, and neurodevelopmental delay. A chylothorax may be a complication of thoracic surgery evidenced shortly after surgery. Potter syndrome is the consequence of multifactorial inherence pattern, characterized by bilateral renal agenesis. It is not a complication of CDH repair. NEC is predominately a disease of prematurity with a multifactorial etiology. Mechanisms thought to be involved in the genesis of NEC include intestinal ischemia, bacterial colonization, and enteral feedings. CDH is primarily a disease of the term infant.

References: Bhandari J, Thada PK, Sergent SR. In: Potter syndrome. In: *StatPearls [Internet].* Treasure Island, FL: StatPearls Publishing; 2022. https://pubmed-ncbi-nlm-nih-gov.foyer.swmed.edu/32809693/.

Bradshaw WT. Gastrointestinal disorders. In: Verklan T, Walden M, Forest S, eds. *Core Curriculum for Neonatal Intensive Care Nursing.* 6th ed. St. Louis, MO: Elsevier; 2021:522.

Gardner SL, Enzman-Hines M, Nyp M. Respiratory diseases. In: Gardner SL, Carter BS, Niermeyer S, eds. *Merenstein & Gardner's Handbook of Neonatal Intensive Care: An Interprofessional Approach.* 9th ed. St. Louis, MO: Elsevier; 2021:996-1005.

78. **(C)** Tidal volume is directly proportional to $PaCO_2$. Increasing tidal volume increases minute ventilation which will decrease $PaCO_2$. Conversely, decreasing tidal volume will increase $PaCO_2$. Increasing PIP will increase tidal volume, thereby decreasing $PaCO_2$. Decreasing the inspiratory time and increasing PEEP will decrease tidal volume, thereby increasing $PaCO_2$. Decreasing the ventilator rate will decrease minute ventilation, leading to a further rise in $PaCO_2$.

Reference: Donn SM, Attar MA. Assisted ventilation of the neonate and its complications. In: Martin RJ, Fanaroff AA, Walsh MC, eds. *Fanaroff & Martin's Neonatal-Perinatal Medicine: Diseases of the Fetus and Infant.* 11th ed. Philadelphia, PA: Elsevier; 2020:1174-1202.

79. **(B)** Cyanosis with vigorous respirations could be indicative of an obstructed ETT. Airway clearance is the initial action the nurse should take. Once obstruction of the ETT has been excluded, chest radiography would be indicated. Although vecuronium could be administered, airway patency should be confirmed and other causes of agitation identified and managed prior to initiating paralysis. Various modes of ventilation can be considered with asynchronous respirations. However, an obstructed ETT must be excluded first.

Reference: Crowley MA. Neonatal respiratory disorders. In: Martin RJ, Fanaroff AA, Walsh MC, eds. *Fanaroff & Martin's Neonatal-Perinatal Medicine: Diseases of the Fetus and Infant.* 11th ed. Philadelphia, PA: Elsevier; 2020:1222-1223.

80. **(A)** The oxygen–hemoglobin disassociation curve is a graphical representation of the relationship between oxygen saturation of hemoglobin and the partial pressure of oxygen. Factors that affect the affinity of hemoglobin to oxygen include pH, $PaCO_2$, temperature, hemoglobin structure, and 2,3-diphosphoglycerate. Factors that increase hemoglobin's affinity to oxygen shift the curve to the left and include increased pH, decreased temperature, decreased $PaCO_2$, fetal hemoglobin, and decreased 2,3-diphosphoglycerate. Factors that decrease hemoglobin's affinity to oxygen shift the curve to the right and include decreased pH, increased temperature, increased $PaCO_2$, and increased 2,3-diphosphoglycerate. A right shift of the oxyhemoglobin curve increases oxygen availability to the tissues.

References: Di Fiore JM, Carlo WA. Assessment of neonatal pulmonary function. In: Martin RJ, Fanaroff AA, Walsh MC, eds. *Fanaroff & Martin's Neonatal-Perinatal Medicine: Diseases of the Fetus and Infant.* 11th ed. Philadelphia, PA: Elsevier; 2020:1145.

Wilson J, Snapp B, Walters M. The hematopoietic system. In: Koehn A, ed. *Neonatal Nurse Practitioner Certification Intensive Review: Fast Facts and Practice Questions.* New York: Springer Publishing Company, LLC; 2020:319.

81. **(A)** A pathologic condition in the mother or infant should be highly suspected when a full-term infant has apnea in the first 24 hours of life. Nonrespiratory issues causing apnea include systemic infections, metabolic disorders, and hypothermia. Placing infants on the back to sleep has led to a 40% reduction in cases of SIDS. Hyperglycemia can lead to an increased respiratory rate in infants. Apnea after the first 24 hours of life not associated with another pathologic condition in a preterm infant can be classified as apnea of prematurity.

References: Pammi M, Brand MC, Weisman LE. Infection in the neonate. In: Gardner SL, Carter BS, Niermeyer S, eds. *Merenstein & Gardner's Handbook of Neonatal Intensive Care: An Interprofessional Approach.* 9th ed. St. Louis, MO: Elsevier; 2021:692-714.

Polin R, Randis TM. Perinatal infections and chorioamnionitis. In: Martin RJ, Fanaroff AA, Walsh MC, eds. *Fanaroff & Martin's Neonatal-Perinatal Medicine: Diseases of the Fetus and Infant.* 11th ed. Philadelphia, PA: Elsevier; 2020:1145.

Wilson J, Snapp B, Walters M. The pulmonary system. In: Koehn A, ed. *Neonatal Nurse Practitioner Certification Intensive Review: Fast Facts and Practice Questions.* New York: Springer Publishing Company, LLC; 2020:235-260.

82. **(A)** Severe BPD is characterized by right ventricular hypertrophy and right axis deviation on electrocardiogram (due to cor pulmonale), respiratory wheezing (due to increased airway resistance), hepatomegaly from heart failure, and cystic lesions on chest radiograph. RDS is characterized by radiographic findings of bilateral diffuse alveolar infiltrates and a reticulogranular (ground-glass) appearance due to alveolar atelectasis. Additional findings include hypoinflation and air bronchograms. Clinical findings include tachypnea, an expiratory grunt, decreased breath sounds, crackles, and tachycardia. MAS is characterized by hyperinflated lungs with coarse patchy infiltrates, increased anteroposterior diameter, and respiratory distress. PIE is radiographically characterized by hyperinflated lungs with coarse nonbranching linear or cyst-like radiolucencies extending from the pleura to the hilum. Infants with PIE typically demonstrate a progressive deterioration of blood gas values. Right ventricular hypertrophy, right axis deviation, wheezing, and hepatomegaly are not pathognomonic of PIE.

References: Bancalari EH, Jain D. Bronchopulmonary dysplasia in the neonate. In: Martin RJ, Fanaroff AA, Walsh MC, eds. *Fanaroff & Martin's Neonatal-Perinatal Medicine: Diseases of the Fetus and Infant.* 11th ed. Philadelphia, PA: Elsevier; 2020:1256-1269.

Crowley M. Neonatal respiratory disorders. In: Martin RJ, Fanaroff AA, Walsh MC, eds. *Fanaroff & Martin's Neonatal-Perinatal Medicine: Diseases of the Fetus and Infant.* 11th ed. Philadelphia, PA: Elsevier; 2020:1203-1230.

Fraser D. Respiratory distress. In: Verklan T, Walden M, Forest S, eds. *Core Curriculum for Neonatal Intensive Care Nursing.* 6th ed. St. Louis, MO: Elsevier; 2021:408.

Gardner SL, Enzman-Hines M, Nyp M. Respiratory diseases. In: Gardner SL, Carter BS, Niermeyer S, eds. *Merenstein & Gardner's Handbook of Neonatal Intensive Care: An Interprofessional Approach.* 9th ed. St. Louis, MO: Elsevier; 2021:772-784.

83 **(B)** The history and clinical findings suggest that this infant has MAS. Hyperinflation occurs due to ball-valve air trapping. Lower inspiratory time will allow adequate exhalation time to

prevent air trapping. Infants with MAS require higher tidal volume and minute ventilation to achieve alveolar ventilation. A low ventilator rate would produce a low minute ventilation. Because of the resulting atelectasis, higher PIP is indicated for adequate lung expansion. Severe persistent pulmonary hypertension often complicates MAS. Therefore, adequate oxygen saturation should be maintained to prevent hypoxia-induced pulmonary vasoconstriction while not inducing hyperoxic injury. Lower PEEP is indicated to prevent air trapping.

References: Crowley M. Neonatal respiratory disorders. In: Martin RJ, Fanaroff AA, Walsh MC, eds. *Fanaroff & Martin's Neonatal-Perinatal Medicine: Diseases of the Fetus and Infant.* 11th ed. Philadelphia, PA: Elsevier; 2020: 1203-1230.

Donn SM, Attar MA. Assisted ventilation of the neonate and its complications. In: Martin RJ, Fanaroff AA, Walsh MC, eds. *Fanaroff & Martin's Neonatal-Perinatal Medicine: Diseases of the Fetus and Infant.* 11th ed. Philadelphia, PA: Elsevier; 2020:1174-1202.

Gardner SL, Enzman-Hines M, Nyp M. Respiratory diseases. In: Gardner SL, Carter BS, Niermeyer S, eds. *Merenstein & Gardner's Handbook of Neonatal Intensive Care: An Interprofessional Approach.* 9th ed. St. Louis, MO: Elsevier; 2021:755-757.

84. **(C)** Preterm infants are expected to lose 10% of their birth weight in the first week of life. This weight loss is the result of excretion of extracellular fluid. In the absence of weight loss, there is a normal total body sodium level in the presence of extra body water, which causes hyponatremia. Excessive evaporative losses lead to hypernatremia. Increased urine output results in either normal serum sodium values or hypernatremia and weight loss.

References: Dell KM. Fluid, electrolytes, and acid-base homeostasis. In: Martin RJ, Fanaroff AA, Walsh MC, eds. *Fanaroff & Martin's Neonatal-Perinatal Medicine: Diseases of the Fetus and Infant.* 11th ed. Philadelphia, PA: Elsevier; 2020:1854-1862.

Nyp M, Brunkhorst JL, Reavey D, Pallotto EK. Fluid and electrolyte management. In: Gardner SL, Carter BS, Niermeyer S, eds. *Merenstein & Gardner's Handbook of Neonatal Intensive Care: An Interprofessional Approach.* 9th ed. St. Louis, MO: Elsevier; 2021:407-415.

85. **(B)** After 3 days of life, normal fluid intake is approximately 120 mL/kg/day. Fluid restriction to 100 mL/kg/day has been found to decrease the incidence of PDA, NEC, and death. The preferable way to obtain laboratory specimens in an infant with RDS is via central umbilical arterial or venous access. If central access is unattainable, laboratory draws should be clustered. Suctioning has been shown to increase oxygen consumption and raise arterial blood pressure, thus placing the infant at risk for IVH. Suctioning is performed when indicated based on physical assessment; it is not scheduled. Surfactant administration is most effective when given in the first few hours after birth.

References: Agren J. Thermal environment of the intensive care nursery. In: Martin RJ, Fanaroff AA, Walsh MC, eds. *Fanaroff & Martin's Neonatal-Perinatal Medicine: Diseases of the Fetus and Infant.* 11th ed. Philadelphia, PA: Elsevier; 2020:566-567.

Gardner SL, Cammack BH. Heat balance. In: Gardner SL, Carter BS, Niermeyer S, eds. *Merenstein & Gardner's Handbook of Neonatal Intensive Care: An Interprofessional Approach.* 9th ed. St. Louis, MO: Elsevier; 2021:137-154.

86. **(A)** Once nitric oxide enters the pulmonary circulation it binds to hemoglobin and is biologically inactivated. Thus iNO has no direct effects on systemic blood pressure. iNO has a half-life of 3–5 seconds. The exact dosage of iNO has not been established. However, research supports initiation at 20 ppm with specific decreases over subsequent days. Weaning from iNO should be regulated in a stepwise fashion. Abrupt cessation can result in rebound elevated pulmonary vascular resistance.

References: Lagoski M, Hamvas A, Wambach JA. Respiratory distress syndrome in the neonate. In: Martin RJ, Fanaroff AA, Walsh MC, eds. *Fanaroff & Martin's Neonatal-Perinatal Medicine: Diseases of the Fetus and Infant.* 11th ed. Philadelphia, PA: Elsevier; 2020:1166-1167.

Plosa EJ. Meconium aspiration. In: Eichenwald EC, Hansen AR, Martin C, Stark AR, eds. *Cloherty and Stark's Manual of Neonatal Care.* 8th ed. Philadelphia, PA: Wolters Kluwer; 2017:472.

Stork EK. Therapy for cardiorespiratory failure in the neonate. In: Martin RJ, Fanaroff AA, Walsh MC, eds. *Fanaroff & Martin's Neonatal-Perinatal Medicine: Diseases of the Fetus and Infant.* 11th ed. Philadelphia, PA: Elsevier; 2020: 1270-1279.

87. **(C)** Prophylactic administration of surfactant occurs within the first 15 minutes of life. While early studies of prophylactic administration demonstrated benefits such as a decreased incidence and of severity of RDS, more recent studies do not support these benefits. Infants selected for prophylactic therapy should be carefully chosen because of increased risks associated with endotracheal intubation. Surfactant administered as rescue therapy is given within 1–6 hours of life to infants with progressive oxygen requirements in the first day of life and may consist of multiple doses. Assisted ventilation is any pulmonary support that fosters alveolar gas exchange and normal pulmonary function. It ranges from oxygen supplementation to mechanical ventilation. Medications used in resuscitative efforts are termed resuscitation drugs. These chemical agents increase the rate and strength of cardiac contractions and cause peripheral vasoconstriction, channeling circulatory volume centrally.

References: Fraser D. Respiratory distress. In: Verklan T, Walden M, Forest S, eds. *Core Curriculum for Neonatal Intensive Care Nursing.* 6th ed. St. Louis, MO: Elsevier; 2021:398.

Gardner SL, Enzman-Hines M, Nyp M. Respiratory diseases. In: Gardner SL, Carter BS, Niermeyer S, eds. *Merenstein & Gardner's Handbook of Neonatal Intensive Care: An Interprofessional Approach.* 9th ed. St. Louis, MO: Elsevier; 2021:744-758.

Lagoski M, Hamvas A, Wambach JA. Respiratory distress syndrome in the neonate. In: Martin RJ, Fanaroff AA, Walsh MC, eds. *Fanaroff & Martin's Neonatal-Perinatal Medicine: Diseases of the Fetus and Infant.* 11th ed. Philadelphia, PA: Elsevier; 2020:1164-1166.

Stork EK. Therapy for cardiorespiratory failure in the neonate. In: Martin RJ, Fanaroff AA, Walsh MC, eds. *Fanaroff & Martin's Neonatal-Perinatal Medicine: Diseases of the Fetus and Infant.* 11th ed. Philadelphia, PA: Elsevier; 2020:1270-1290.

88. **(C)** Because indomethacin inhibits platelet aggregation, the platelet count must be normal before administration to prevent unintended blood loss. The minimum acceptable platelet count is 60,000/mm³. A serum creatinine level of 2.0 mg/dL is a contraindication to the administration of indomethacin because it indicates impaired renal function. Indomethacin has vasoconstrictive effects on the renal artery. Decreased renal blood flow due to indomethacin administration would further compromise renal function. A low urine output can be symptomatic of decreased renal function. Indomethacin administration is contraindicated in a patient with a urine output of less than 0.6 mL/kg/h. Radiographic evidence of NEC is a contraindication to indomethacin administration because indomethacin impairs blood flow to the mesentery and intestines.

References: Basu SK, Dobrolet NC. Congenital defects of the cardiovascular system. In: Martin RJ, Fanaroff AA, Walsh MC, eds. *Fanaroff & Martin's Neonatal-Perinatal Medicine: Diseases of the Fetus and Infant.* 11th ed. Philadelphia, PA: Elsevier; 2020:1358-1359.

Ku LC, Hornik C, Buschbach D. Pharmacology in neonatal care. In: Gardner SL, Carter BS, Niermeyer S, eds. *Merenstein & Gardner's Handbook of Neonatal Intensive Care: An Interprofessional Approach.* 9th ed. St. Louis, MO: Elsevier; 2021:226-237.

89. **(B)** Laryngomalacia (weakening of larynx above the vocal cords) is the leading cause of stridor in the infant due to collapse of the airway. An infant with choanal atresia will have varying degrees of cyanosis at rest and with sucking based on the severity of the lesion. Symptoms improve with crying. Clinically, the infant with vocal cord paralysis has a weak cry but may develop stridor when stressed. Vocal cord paralysis is second to laryngomalacia as

the cause of stridor in the infant. Congenital subglottic stenosis is characterized by croup like episodes.

Reference: Otteson TD, Wang T. Upper airway lesions in the neonate. In: Martin RJ, Fanaroff AA, Walsh MC, eds. *Fanaroff & Martin's Neonatal-Perinatal Medicine: Diseases of the Fetus and Infant.* 11th ed. Philadelphia, PA: Elsevier; 2020:1250-1251.

90. **(D)** Secondary apnea is a result of prolonged asphyxia. It is marked by gasping respirations and a decrease in blood pressure and heart rate that is not responsive to stimulation and/or oxygen supplementation. Idiopathic apnea is also known as apnea of prematurity. This particular infant is full-term. In obstructive apnea, the infant has spontaneous respiratory effort, but airflow is absent. Primary apnea is the absence of respirations after a period of rapid respiratory effort that is associated with asphyxia during the delivery process. Oxygen supplementation and/or stimulation will help to initiate spontaneous respirations.

References: Goldsmith JP. Overview and initial management of delivery room resuscitation. In: Martin RJ, Fanaroff AA, Walsh MC, eds. *Fanaroff & Martin's Neonatal-Perinatal Medicine: Diseases of the Fetus and Infant.* 11th ed. Philadelphia, PA: Elsevier; 2020:521.

Niermeyer S, Clarke SB. Care at birth. In: Gardner SL, Carter BS, Niermeyer S, eds. *Merenstein & Gardner's Handbook of Neonatal Intensive Care: An Interprofessional Approach.* 9th ed. St. Louis, MO: Elsevier; 2021:67-70.

91. **(D)** The immediate initial step after determining the absence of respirations is to provide gentle tactile stimulation. This is all the infant may require to resume spontaneous respirations. Although assessing breath sounds is important, the initiation of respirations must take precedence. If apnea persists despite tactile stimulation, supplemental oxygen can be administered. If oxygen supplementation and tactile stimulation have not produced spontaneous respirations, positive pressure ventilation is indicated. Physical assessment of breath sounds can be completed after spontaneous respirations have been achieved.

Reference: Gardner SL, Enzman-Hines M, Nyp M. Respiratory diseases. In: Gardner SL, Carter BS, Niermeyer S, eds. *Merenstein & Gardner's Handbook of Neonatal Intensive Care: An Interprofessional Approach.* 9th ed. St. Louis, MO: Elsevier; 2021:813-817.

92. **(B)** Doxapram is a respiratory stimulant used to treat apnea that is refractory to methylxanthine therapy. Caffeine, theophylline, and aminophylline are methylxanthines used to treat apnea.

References: Gardner SL, Enzman-Hines M, Nyp M. Respiratory diseases. In: Gardner SL, Carter BS, Niermeyer S, eds. *Merenstein & Gardner's Handbook of Neonatal Intensive Care: An Interprofessional Approach.* 9th ed. St. Louis, MO: Elsevier; 2021:815-816.

Patrinos ME. Neonatal apnea and the foundation of respiratory control. In: Martin RJ, Fanaroff AA, Walsh MC, eds. *Fanaroff & Martin's Neonatal-Perinatal Medicine: Diseases of the Fetus and Infant.* 11th ed. Philadelphia, PA: Elsevier; 2020:1239.

93. **(C)** Apnea can be induced by a multitude of causes, including iatrogenic factors. Maintaining the environmental temperature in a neutral thermal range can help to alleviate temperature stress which can lead to iatrogenic apnea. A vagal response secondary to procedures such as suctioning stimulates apnea. Sudden environmental changes, such as the change from a warm incubator to a cold scale, also can induce apnea. Tapping on the outside of the incubator is an example of a noxious stimulus that can lead to apnea.

References: Gardner SL, Enzman-Hines M, Nyp M. Respiratory diseases. In: Gardner SL, Carter BS, Niermeyer S, eds. *Merenstein & Gardner's Handbook of Neonatal Intensive Care: An Interprofessional Approach.* 9th ed. St. Louis, MO: Elsevier; 2021:815-816.

Patrinos ME. Neonatal apnea and the foundation of respiratory control. In: Martin RJ, Fanaroff AA, Walsh MC, eds. *Fanaroff & Martin's Neonatal-Perinatal Medicine: Diseases of the Fetus and Infant.* 11th ed. Philadelphia, PA: Elsevier; 2020:1235.

94. **(D)** Caffeine has a longer half-life than theophylline, which results in smaller changes in plasma concentration. Caffeine is formulated for oral or parenteral administration, administered once a day to neonates, and is not known to be excreted more rapidly by the kidneys.

References: Gardner SL, Enzman-Hines M, Nyp M. Respiratory diseases. In: Gardner SL, Carter BS, Niermeyer S, eds. *Merenstein & Gardner's Handbook of Neonatal Intensive Care: An Interprofessional Approach.* 9th ed. St. Louis, MO: Elsevier; 2021:815-816.

Patrinos ME. Neonatal apnea and the foundation of respiratory control. In: Martin RJ, Fanaroff AA, Walsh MC, eds. *Fanaroff & Martin's Neonatal-Perinatal Medicine: Diseases of the Fetus and Infant.* 11th ed. Philadelphia, PA: Elsevier; 2020:1234-1235.

95. **(C)** CPAP ventilation is therapeutic in the treatment of an infant with laryngomalacia because it prevents collapse of poorly formed cartilage structures. It is a conservative therapy. Supraglottoplasty is a surgical intervention resulting in 71% resolution of symptoms. CPAP ventilation is seldom used in an infant with a cleft palate because of the limited ability to secure a seal that allows delivery of airway pressure. Nasal CPAP will not be effective in an infant with choanal atresia because of blockage of the posterior nares. CPAP ventilation is contraindicated in an infant with tracheoesophageal fistula because distending pressure would cause tracheal air to take the path of least resistance and enter the distal esophagus; this would cause gastric distention and possible rupture.

References: Gardner SL, Enzman-Hines M, Nyp M. Respiratory diseases. In: Gardner SL, Carter BS, Niermeyer S, eds. *Merenstein & Gardner's Handbook of Neonatal Intensive Care: An Interprofessional Approach.* 9th ed. St. Louis, MO: Elsevier; 2021:811-816.

Keller RL, Ballard RA. Bronchopulmonary dysplasia. In: Gleason CA, Juul SE, eds. *Avery's Diseases of the Newborn.* 10th ed. Philadelphia, PA: Elsevier; 2018:696-697.

Patrinos ME. Neonatal apnea and the foundation of respiratory control. In: Martin RJ, Fanaroff AA, Walsh MC, eds. *Fanaroff & Martin's Neonatal-Perinatal Medicine: Diseases of the Fetus and Infant.* 11th ed. Philadelphia, PA: Elsevier; 2020:1250-1251.

96. **(D)** A nasogastric tube should receive the least consideration. Infants are obligate nose breathers, and maximum CPAP needs to be maintained. Gastric overdistention can be managed by using a larger-bore orogastric tube. $PaCO_2$ retention at increased levels of CPAP has been documented due to alveolar overdistention. Monitoring of $PaCO_2$ levels is thus warranted. Decreased glomerular filtration rate has been documented in infants undergoing CPAP ventilation. Urine output should be monitored carefully. Vital signs and pulse oximetry readings must be monitored to determine oxygen saturation and detect complications early.

References: Brown LD, Hendrickson K, Evans R, Davis R, Davis J, William Jr WH. Enteral nutrition. In: Gardner SL, Carter BS, Niermeyer S, eds. *Merenstein & Gardner's Handbook of Neonatal Intensive Care: An Interprofessional Approach.* 9th ed. St. Louis, MO: Elsevier; 2021:511-513.

Donn SM, Attar MA. Assisted ventilation of the neonate and its complications. In: Martin RJ, Fanaroff AA, Walsh MC, eds. *Fanaroff & Martin's Neonatal-Perinatal Medicine: Diseases of the Fetus and Infant.* 11th ed. Philadelphia, PA: Elsevier; 2020:1174-1175.

97. **(D)** Full-term infants with a small CDH without liver herniation have a good prognosis and therefore meet the criteria for management using ECMO. Infants with severe lung hypoplasia are excluded from treatment with ECMO because the disease is irreversible. The gestational age requirement for ECMO is 34 weeks or older. Normal findings on cranial ultrasonography are required for treatment with ECMO. Some centers have been able to manage infants with bilateral grade I intracranial hemorrhage with lower dosages of heparin; however, infants with bilateral grade IV intracranial hemorrhages are excluded from ECMO at all centers.

References: Gallagher ME, Pacetti AS, Lovvorn III HN, Carter BS. Neonatal surgery. In: Gardner SL, Carter BS, Niermeyer S, eds. *Merenstein & Gardner's Handbook of Neonatal Intensive Care: An Interprofessional Approach*. 9th ed. St. Louis, MO: Elsevier; 2021:996-999.

Stork EK. Therapy for cardiorespiratory failure in the neonate. In: Martin RJ, Fanaroff AA, Walsh MC, eds. *Fanaroff & Martin's Neonatal-Perinatal Medicine: Diseases of the Fetus and Infant*. 11th ed. Philadelphia, PA: Elsevier; 2020: 1270-1279.

98. **(A)** Usual criteria for ECMO include the following: an oxygen index of 35–60 for 30 minutes to 6 hours, an alveolar-arterial difference in partial pressure of oxygen of 600–620 mm Hg for 4–12 hours at sea level, a PaO_2 less than 60 mm Hg for 2–12 hours, and a pH $\leq$7.25 for 2 hours or more or with hypotension. Criteria may vary by ECMO center. pCO_2 values are not included in the inclusion criteria for ECMO.

References: Cates-McGlinn LA. Extracorporeal membrane oxygenation. In: Verklan T, Walden M, Forest S, eds. *Core Curriculum for Neonatal Intensive Care Nursing*. 6th ed. St. Louis, MO: Elsevier; 2021:447.

Stork EK. Therapy for cardiorespiratory failure in the neonate. In: Martin RJ, Fanaroff AA, Walsh MC, eds. *Fanaroff & Martin's Neonatal-Perinatal Medicine: Diseases of the Fetus and Infant*. 11th ed. Philadelphia, PA: Elsevier; 2020: 1270-1279.

99. **(C)** BPD is more common in infants who have undergone mechanical ventilation. This is due to the associated barotrauma and oxygen toxicity. The incidence of BPD is inversely proportional to gestational age. Excessive fluid administration places an infant at high risk for BPD. Mechanical ventilation and oxygen supplementation provided to overcome impaired alveolar gas exchange result in damage to the lung and the development of BPD. Twenty-one percent oxygen is room air and would not cause oxygen toxicity.

References: Bancalari EH, Jain D. Bronchopulmonary dysplasia in the neonate. In: Martin RJ, Fanaroff AA, Walsh MC, eds. *Fanaroff & Martin's Neonatal-Perinatal Medicine: Diseases of the Fetus and Infant*. 11th ed. Philadelphia, PA: Elsevier; 2020:1256-1269.

Gardner SL, Enzman-Hines M, Nyp M. Respiratory diseases. In: Gardner SL, Carter BS, Niermeyer S, eds. *Merenstein & Gardner's Handbook of Neonatal Intensive Care: An Interprofessional Approach*. 9th ed. St. Louis, MO: Elsevier; 2021:772-784.

100. **(A)** Furosemide can damage the stria vascularis, part of the cochlear duct. Hearing impairment may be temporary or permanent. Furosemide is a loop diuretic which inhibits reabsorption of sodium and chloride in the ascending limb of the loop of Henle which can lead to hyponatremia and hypochloremia. Water passively follows the movement of sodium and thus allows diuresis. Furosemide-induced diuresis also results in enhanced excretion of potassium leading to hypokalemia. Metabolic alkalosis is associated with furosemide use. Loss of acid from the extracellular fluid volume creates a relative elevated bicarbonate level to maintain acid–base balance.

References: Bancalari EH, Jain D. Bronchopulmonary dysplasia in the neonate. In: Martin RJ, Fanaroff AA, Walsh MC, eds. *Fanaroff & Martin's Neonatal-Perinatal Medicine: Diseases of the Fetus and Infant*. 11th ed. Philadelphia, PA: Elsevier; 2020:1256-1269.

Burchum JR, Rosenthal LD. *Lehne's Pharmacology for Nursing Care*. 11th ed. St. Louis, MO: Elsevier; 2022:535.

Gardner SL, Enzman-Hines M, Nyp M. Respiratory diseases. In: Gardner SL, Carter BS, Niermeyer S, eds. *Merenstein & Gardner's Handbook of Neonatal Intensive Care: An Interprofessional Approach*. 9th ed. St. Louis, MO: Elsevier; 2021:772-784.

101. **(D)** Infants with BPD have increased caloric needs due to their increased metabolic expenditure associated with increased respiratory effort. The recommended caloric intake for infants with BPD is 150–180 kcal/kg/day. While caloric requirements are increased, fluid intake is generally restricted, requiring feeding with a higher caloric density.

Reference: Fraser D. Respiratory distress. In: Verklan MT, Walden M, Forest S, eds. *Core Curriculum for Neonatal Intensive Care Nursing*. 6th ed. St. Louis, MO: Elsevier; 2021:406-409.

102. **(C)** An increased incidence of neurodevelopmental dysfunction, including cerebral palsy, has been widely associated with high dose dexamethasone use for a prolonged period of time among infants less than 1-week-old. However, low-dose dexamethasone therapy is associated with fewer side effects and has been shown to be beneficial but should be used to treat only those infants at highest risk of chronic lung disease. Dexamethasone use has not been associated with an increased incidence of pulmonary air leak, pulmonary hypertension, or severe retinopathy of prematurity.

References: Bancalari EH, Jain D. Bronchopulmonary dysplasia in the neonate. In: Martin RJ, Fanaroff AA, Walsh MC, eds. *Fanaroff & Martin's Neonatal-Perinatal Medicine: Diseases of the Fetus and Infant*. 11th ed. Philadelphia, PA: Elsevier; 2020:1256-1269.

Gardner SL, Enzman-Hines M, Nyp M. Respiratory diseases. In: Gardner SL, Carter BS, Niermeyer S, eds. *Merenstein & Gardner's Handbook of Neonatal Intensive Care: An Interprofessional Approach*. 9th ed. St. Louis, MO: Elsevier; 2021:772-784.

103. **(D)** A PEEP of 5–8 cm H_2O is often required in infants with severe BPD with bronchomalacia. The higher PEEP helps to improve alveolar ventilation and may reduce expiratory airway resistance. Unlike management in the early stages of BPD, infants with progressive severe BPD require longer inspiratory times to overcome the increased dead space, heterogenous area of different lung compliance, and airway resistance. In infants with BPD lung compliance is dynamic resulting in airway obstruction and decreased compliance at higher respiratory rates. Therefore, a high rate such as 50 breaths per minute would cause breath stacking asynchrony. Serving as a potent vasodilator, oxygen should be provided to maintain saturations above 90% to prevent pulmonary hypertension from chronic hypoxemia associated with severe BPD. A PaO_2 of 30 corresponds to an oxygen saturation of approximately 60%.

References: Bancalari EH, Jain D. Bronchopulmonary dysplasia in the neonate. In: Martin RJ, Fanaroff AA, Walsh MC, eds. *Fanaroff & Martin's Neonatal-Perinatal Medicine: Diseases of the Fetus and Infant*. 11th ed. Philadelphia, PA: Elsevier; 2020:1256-1269.

Wilson J, Snapp B, Walters M. The pulmonary system. In: Koehn A, ed. *Neonatal Nurse Practitioner Certification Intensive Review: Fast Facts and Practice Questions*. New York: Springer Publishing Company, LLC; 2020:235-260.

104. **(D)** The low pH indicates acidosis. The elevated $PaCO_2$ indicates the primary problem is respiratory. In primary respiratory problems, the pH and $PaCO_2$ change in opposite directions. The elevated HCO_3 suggests compensation is occurring. The low oxygen level indicates hypoxemia.

Reference: Barry JS, Deacon J, Hernandez C, Jones Jr MD. Acid-base homeostasis and oxygenation. In: Gardner SL, Carter BS, Niermeyer S, eds. *Merenstein & Gardner's Handbook of Neonatal Intensive Care: An Interprofessional Approach*. 9th ed. St. Louis, MO: Elsevier; 2021:186-190.

105. **(A)** One of the adverse effects of corticosteroids is hypertension which is due to overstimulation of mineralocorticoid receptors, resulting in sodium retention in the kidney, which causes volume expansion and subsequent increase in blood pressure. Corticosteroids improve lung compliance, dilate airways, and enhance the synthesis of surfactant. Corticosteroid use has been shown to promote rapid ventilatory weaning, not increase the need for ventilator support. An adverse effect of corticosteroid is hyperglycemia not hypoglycemia. Biventricular hypertrophy, not atrophy, has been associated with dexamethasone use.

References: Keller RL, Ballard RA. Bronchopulmonary dysplasia. In: Gleason CA, Juul SE, eds. *Avery's Disease of the Newborn*. 10th ed. Philadelphia, PA: Elsevier Saunders; 2018:689-690.

McClary JD. Therapeutic agents. In: Martin RJ, Fanaroff AA, Walsh MC, eds. *Fanaroff & Martin's Neonatal-Perinatal Medicine: Diseases of the Fetus and Infant.* 11th ed. Philadelphia, PA: Elsevier; 2020:2018t–2027t.

106. **(C)** Albuterol is a bronchodilator—specifically, a β_2-adrenergic agent—that within minutes effectively increases compliance and decreases airway resistance. Caffeine and theophylline are methylxanthines that are used in patients with BPD to decrease airway resistance. However, they are not used as a first-line treatment for an acute bronchospastic episode. Furosemide is a loop diuretic used to treat pulmonary edema in infants with BPD. It does not relieve bronchospasm.

References: Gardner SL, Enzman-Hines M, Nyp M. Respiratory diseases. In: Gardner SL, Carter BS, Niermeyer S, eds. *Merenstein & Gardner's Handbook of Neonatal Intensive Care: An Interprofessional Approach.* 9th ed. St. Louis, MO: Elsevier; 2021:779t-781t.

McClary JD. Therapeutic agents. In: Martin RJ, Fanaroff AA, Walsh MC, eds. *Fanaroff & Martin's Neonatal-Perinatal Medicine: Diseases of the Fetus and Infant.* 11th ed. Philadelphia, PA: Elsevier; 2020:2018t-2027t.

107. **(D)** Pink-tinged secretions are indicative of a pulmonary hemorrhage with minimal bleeding. Treatment of a pulmonary hemorrhage in an intubated patient is to increase PEEP to tamponade the bleeding at the site. Suctioning should be limited in infants with pulmonary hemorrhage. Neither a platelet nor red blood cell transfusion is indicated.

Reference: Crowley MA. Neonatal respiratory disorders. In: Martin RJ, Fanaroff AA, Walsh MC, eds. *Fanaroff & Martin's Neonatal-Perinatal Medicine: Diseases of the Fetus and Infant.* 11th ed. Philadelphia, PA: Elsevier; 2020:1220.

108. **(D)** Patient selection criteria for ECMO include gestational age of more than 34 weeks, birth weight of more than 2 kg, presence of grade II or less intracranial hemorrhage, absence of complex congenital heart disease or lethal malformations, and reversible lung disease. Persistent pulmonary hypertension of the newborn (PPHN) is an acute and reversible cardiorespiratory disease. ECMO is warranted if standard therapies fail to reverse PPHN. Pulmonary hypoplasia does not meet inclusion criteria because it is an irreversible condition. ECMO is not indicated in infants with BPD. The initial pulmonary damage is irreversible and maintaining the patient on ECMO until new lung growth occurs is not feasible. TTN is a mild, self-limiting disease that does not warrant invasive ECMO therapy.

Reference: Steinhorn RH. Pulmonary vascular development. In: Martin RJ, Fanaroff AA, Walsh MC, eds. *Fanaroff & Martin's Neonatal-Perinatal Medicine: Diseases of the Fetus and Infant.* 11th ed. Philadelphia, PA: Elsevier; 2020: 1312-1315.

109. **(D)** CPAM is the most common congenital cystic lung disease in the neonate. The cysts are either macrocystic or microcystic and can affect all lobes of the lung. The malformation results from an abnormal branching of the fetal bronchial tree during the pseudoglandular phase of lung development. The lesion is connected to the tracheobronchial tree and has a pulmonary blood supply. The entity was first described as congenital cystic adenomatoid malformation but is now referred to as CPAM to reflect the site of the malformation in the tracheobronchial tree. Fetal and neonatal complications from CPAM include nonimmune hydrops and lung hypoplasia due to compression of the developing lung. Antenatal steroids may reduce the size of microcystic lesions and resolve hydrops if present. Approximately 75% of newborns with a prenatal diagnose of CPAM are asymptomatic at birth. However, surgical resection of the lesion is recommended to avoid potential infection and later malignancy. Bronchopulmonary sequestration (BPS) consists of microcystic masses of nonfunctioning lung tissue that do not attach to the bronchopulmonary tree. The lesion can be intralobar or extralobar and has a systemic arterial blood supply. BPS can be identified antenatally and may look similar to CPAM.

CLE is a rare anomaly characterized by postnatal overdistension of one or more segments or lobes of the lung with subsequent emphysema. Although no underlying pathology is identified, proposed mechanisms include dysplastic bronchial cartilage formation, inspissated mucus, aberrant cardiopulmonary vasculature, and infection. The obstructive lesion causes overinflation and air trapping because air can pass into the effected bronchus but is unable to leave. The severity of respiratory distress is dictated by the size of the lesion, compression of the surrounding tissue, and the extent of mediastinal shift. Thoracotomy and resecting the affected lung lobe are recommended if the lesion is severe. Long-term prognosis is good once the affected segment is removed. CDH is a defect in the diaphragm allowing herniation of abdominal contents into the chest cavity, rather than a cystic malformation of the lung. As air enters the gastrointestinal tract and proceeds to the intestine, intraluminal bowel gas is visible in the chest on the radiograph.

References: Crowley MA. Neonatal respiratory disorders. In: Martin RJ, Fanaroff AA, Walsh MC, eds. *Fanaroff & Martin's Neonatal-Perinatal Medicine: Diseases of the Fetus and Infant.* 11th ed. Philadelphia, PA: Elsevier; 2020: 1209-1213.

Wilson J, Snapp B, Walters M. The pulmonary system. In: Koehn A, ed. *Neonatal Nurse Practitioner Certification Intensive Review: Fast Facts and Practice Questions.* New York: Springer Publishing Company, LLC; 2020:235-260.

110. **(D)** Polyhydramnios suggests a condition in which the fetus does not swallow amniotic fluid normally, as with an upper gastrointestinal obstruction. In esophageal atresia with tracheoesophageal fistula, the esophagus ends in a blind pouch and there is a connection between the esophagus and trachea. In 85% of cases, the fistula is distal to the blind pouch. Attempts to feed and the accumulation of oropharyngeal secretions result in respiratory distress and the need for suctioning. Choanal atresia is a membranous or bony obstruction of one or both nares. Presentation is characterized by noisy breathing, cyanosis, and apnea if the mouth is closed. When crying, an infant with choanal atresia will be pink because the open mouth provides a patent airway. Pulmonary hypoplasia results from lung compression due to congenital anomalies or oligohydramnios. The infant usually shows severe respiratory distress soon after birth not intermittent distress. Infants with congenital heart disease may show cyanosis. Many infants with congenital heart disease have tachypnea without an increase in work of breathing. This is often referred to as comfortable tachypnea.

References: Dingeldein M. Selected gastrointestinal anomalies in the neonate. In: Martin RJ, Fanaroff AA, Walsh MC, eds. *Fanaroff & Martin's Neonatal-Perinatal Medicine: Diseases of the Fetus and Infant.* 11th ed. Philadelphia, PA: Elsevier; 2020:1541-1546.

Gallagher ME, Pacetti AS, Lovvorn III HN, Carter BS. Neonatal surgery. In: Gardner SL, Carter BS, Niermeyer S, eds. *Merenstein & Gardner's Handbook of Neonatal Intensive Care: An Interprofessional Approach.* 9th ed. St. Louis, MO: Elsevier; 2021:1000-1005.

111. **(C)** The oxygen–hemoglobin dissociation curve is a graphical representation of the relationship between oxygen saturation of hemoglobin and the partial pressure of oxygen. The curve reflects hemoglobin's affinity to oxygen and is primarily affected by the type of hemoglobin (fetal vs adult), temperature, pH, $PaCO_2$, and level of 2,3-diphosphoglycerate. Cyanosis is a late sign of respiratory insufficiency and is an unreliable assessment of oxygenation because it is visible only when deoxyhemoglobin is above 5 g/dL. Cyanosis may not be present in severe anemic states. A shift to the right on the oxygen–hemoglobin dissociation curve indicates decreased affinity of hemoglobin for oxygen.

References: Di Fiore JM, Carlo WA. Assessment of neonatal pulmonary function. In: Martin RJ, Fanaroff AA, Walsh MC, eds. *Fanaroff & Martin's Neonatal-Perinatal Medicine: Diseases of the Fetus and Infant.* 11th ed. Philadelphia, PA: Elsevier; 2020:1145-1150.

Mathew B, Lakshminrusimha S. Non-invasive monitoring of gas exchange. In: Keszler M, Gautham KS, eds. *Goldsmith's Assisted Ventilation of the Neonate: An Evidence-Based Approach to Newborn Respiratory Care*. 7th ed. Philadelphia, PA: Elsevier; 2022:111-123.

112. **(D)** Obtaining accurate pulse oximetry readings depends on adequate perfusion of the monitoring site, probe position, and the ability of the equipment to detect arterial pulsations. Gestational age does not affect the accuracy of saturation readings. Pulse oximetry is the most common noninvasive method of measuring oxygen saturation in infants, including preterm infants. The use of vasodilating drugs, particularly those that dilate the peripheral vasculature, enhances pulse oximetry accuracy because adequate perfusion of the probe site is vital to the use of this equipment. Pulse oximeters are accurate in the setting of low oxygen saturation, as may occur in cyanotic heart disease. Pulse oximetry screening is recommended for all infants to detect critical congenital heart defects.

References: Coe K, Bradshaw WT, Tanaka DT. Physiologic monitoring. In: Gardner SL, Carter BS, Niermeyer S, eds. *Merenstein & Gardner's Handbook of Neonatal Intensive Care: An Interprofessional Approach*. 9th ed. St. Louis, MO: Elsevier; 2021:178.

Lagoski M, Hamvas A, Wambach JA. Respiratory distress syndrome in the neonate. In: Martin RJ, Fanaroff AA, Walsh MC, eds. *Fanaroff & Martin's Neonatal-Perinatal Medicine: Diseases of the Fetus and Infant*. 11th ed. Philadelphia, PA: Elsevier; 2020:598-600.

113. **(C)** The flow rate through an oxygen hood must be sufficient to prevent the retention of carbon dioxide. This requires a flow meter and oxygen blender so that adequate flow is provided and the prescribed oxygen concentration is delivered. A nasal cannula is used to administer oxygen to an infant who is developing social and motor skills. Exact oxygen concentration is unknown when a nasal cannula is used because of entrainment of room air when the mouth is open. Nasal CPAP is not warranted if the infant demonstrates sufficient ventilation to maintain a normal $PaCO_2$ value. Oxygen administration requires some form of continuous monitoring.

Reference: Gardner SL, Enzman-Hines M, Nyp M. Respiratory diseases. In: Gardner SL, Carter BS, Niermeyer S, eds. *Merenstein & Gardner's Handbook of Neonatal Intensive Care: An Interprofessional Approach*. 9th ed. St. Louis, MO: Elsevier; 2021:741.

114. **(D)** Research has demonstrated that the use of heliox reduces the duration of mechanical ventilation in infants with obstructive pulmonary diseases such as reactive airway, bronchiolitis secondary to respiratory syncytial virus infection, and PIE. Only supportive care is required for a mild pneumothorax without evidence of significant respiratory failure. Controversy exists whether administering 100% oxygen to create a nitrogen washout will resolve or decrease the size of a pneumothorax. Recent retrospective reviews showed no difference in the resolution time of a pneumothorax in infants treated with 21% oxygen versus 100% oxygen versus somewhere in-between. Intracranial hemorrhage (ICH) is bleeding within the skull. Management of ICHs depends on severity and location of the hemorrhage and does not include the use of heliox. NEC is a serious inflammatory process causing necrosis of the bowel and affects primarily premature infants. Medical management of NEC does not include the use of heliox.

References: Crowley MA. Neonatal respiratory disorders. In: Martin RJ, Fanaroff AA, Walsh MC, eds. *Fanaroff & Martin's Neonatal-Perinatal Medicine: Diseases of the Fetus and Infant*. 11th ed. Philadelphia, PA: Elsevier; 2020: 1203-1230.

Gardner SL, Enzman-Hines M, Nyp M. Respiratory diseases. In: Gardner SL, Carter BS, Niermeyer S, eds. *Merenstein & Gardner's Handbook of Neonatal Intensive Care: An Interprofessional Approach*. 9th ed. St. Louis, MO: Elsevier; 2021:729-750.

Szczapa T, Kwapien P, Merritt AP. Neonatal application of heliox: a practical review. *Front Pediatr*. 2022;10(3):855050. doi:10.3389/fped.2022.855050.

115. **(B)** Infants with Pierre Robin sequence which is characterized by micrognathia and glossoptosis are at increased risk of posterior airway obstruction resulting in obstructive apnea. Cor pulmonale is also known as right ventricular failure. It occurs with right-sided outflow tract obstruction and prolonged pulmonary vasoconstriction and remodeling as seen in BPD. Subglottic stenosis is a complication of long-term endotracheal intubation. Reactive airway disease is a pulmonary response to an antigen or substance not normally present in the tracheobronchial tree. Aspiration of formula or gastric contents is a common precipitating event.

References: Mitchell AL. Congenital anomalies. In: Martin RJ, Fanaroff AA, Walsh MC, eds. *Fanaroff & Martin's Neonatal-Perinatal Medicine: Diseases of the Fetus and Infant*. 11th ed. Philadelphia, PA: Elsevier; 2020:502.

Otteson TD, Wang T. Upper airway lesions in the neonate. In: Martin RJ, Fanaroff AA, Walsh MC, eds. *Fanaroff & Martin's Neonatal-Perinatal Medicine: Diseases of the Fetus and Infant*. 11th ed. Philadelphia, PA: Elsevier; 2020: 1244-1255.

116. **(B)** Surfactant causes a rapid decrease in intrapulmonary pressure which facilitates left to right shunting across the PDA and an increase in pulmonary blood flow, which leads to pulmonary hemorrhage. Surfactant does not increase or decrease intrathoracic or intracardiac pressures.

References: Aziz A, Ohlssonc A. Surfactant for pulmonary hemorrhage in neonates. *Cochrane Database Syst Rev*. 2020;2:1-11. doi:10.1002/14651858. CD005254.pub4.

Berlin SC. Diagnostic imaging of the neonate. In: Martin RJ, Fanaroff JM, Walsh MC, eds. *Fanaroff and Martin's Neonatal-Perinatal Medicine Diseases of the Fetus and Infant*. 11th ed. Philadelphia, PA: Elsevier; 2020:1124-1125.

117. **(D)** PIE is a result of rupture of alveoli from overdistension. Keeping the involved area of the lung down will cause partial collapse of the affected lung, and thereby reduce PIE. Conversely, keeping the involved area of the lung up will increase overdistension of the affected alveoli and worsen PIE. Increasing PEEP and tidal volume will worsen PIE.

Reference: Bancalari E, Claure N, Jain D. Neonatal respiratory therapy. In: Gleason CA, Juul SE, eds. *Avery's Diseases of the Newborn*. 10th ed. Philadelphia, PA: Elsevier; 2018:649.

118. **(C)** TTN is delayed clearance of fetal lung fluid resulting in pulmonary edema. The condition generally occurs in term or late-preterm infants with a history of cesarean section, precipitous delivery, or spontaneous vaginal delivery without labor. Without the hormonal changes that accompany spontaneous labor, the in utero secretory fetal lung mode fails to transition into an absorptive mode. As a result, lung fluid is retained and leads to collapse of the bronchioli. FRC may be reduced, and the thoracic gas volume may increase from air trapping, resulting in a barrel-shaped chest on physical exam. Symptoms of tachypnea and respiratory distress are commonly seen in the first 6 hours of life and can persist for up to 72 hours. Ball-valve obstruction of the small airways occurs in MAS leading to regional hyperinflation and atelectasis. A reduced number of lung cells, airways, blood vessels, and alveoli occur in pulmonary hypoplasia. Air within the lung parenchyma decreasing lung compliance occurs in PIE.

References: Parker TA, Kinsella JP. Respiratory disorders in the term infant. In: Gleason CA, Juul SE, eds. *Avery's Diseases of the Newborn*. 10th ed. Philadelphia, PA: Elsevier; 2018:672.

Wilson J, Snapp B, Walters M. The pulmonary system. In: Koehn A, ed. *Neonatal Nurse Practitioner Certification Intensive Review: Fast Facts and Practice Questions*. New York: Springer Publishing Company, LLC; 2020:235-260.

119. **(C)** In CDH, intestinal contents migrate into the chest cavity. X-ray findings in CDH include the presence of both a stomach bubble and bowel gas pattern in the thoracic cavity. In early onset CDH, in which the abdominal contents migrated to the thoracic cavity

early in the course of lung development, the infant will have severe respiratory distress requiring intubation in the delivery room. If CDH develops later in gestation, once the lungs have developed (late onset), the infant presents with mild tachypnea as abdominal contents start compressing the well-developed alveoli. The chest x-ray in MAS shows air trapping, hyperexpansion, and hyperinflation with bilateral coarse diffuse patchy infiltrates. Chest x-ray findings in CPAM vary but usually include lesions that are multicystic air filled, solid, or with air–fluid levels. Additionally, the infant with CPAM will demonstrate persistent atelectasis of the affected side. Pulmonary sequestration is an abnormal mass of nonfunctioning lung tissue that is formed outside (extralobar) or inside (intralobar) the lungs but is not connected directly to the tracheobronchial tree. X-ray findings vary depending on the size and condition of the lesion. The sequestration can appear as a well-defined mass or cyst.

References: Gomella T, Eyal F, Bany-Mohammed F. *Gomella's Neonatology: Management, Procedures, On-Call Problems, Diseases, and Drugs.* 8th ed. New York: McGraw Hill; 2020:184, 188-189.

Khan AN. *Pulmonary Sequestration Imaging and Diagnosis.* Medscape.com. Available at: https://emedicine.medscape.com/article/412554-overview#a2. Updated September 15, 2020; Accessed July 16, 2022.

Steinhorn RH, Abmam SH. Persistent pulmonary hypertension. In: Gleason CA, Juul SE, eds. *Avery's Diseases of the Newborn.* 10th ed. Philadelphia, PA: Elsevier; 2018:772.

120. **(B)** Normal transition occurs at birth when the umbilical cord is clamped and the infant takes the first breath of life. Oxygen levels rise and pulmonary vascular resistance drops, allowing oxygenated blood to flow left to right across the PDA and foramen ovale. Persistent pulmonary hypertension occurs when normal transition does not occur after birth, resulting in sustained elevated pulmonary vascular resistance due to hypoxia. The persistent elevated pulmonary vascular resistance prevents blood from entering the pulmonary vasculature, resulting in a right to left shunt of unoxygenated blood into the systemic circulation via the PDA and foramen ovale. The ductus venosus lies between the umbilical vein and inferior vena cava and does not play role in persistent pulmonary hypertension.

Reference: Parker TA, Kinsella JP. Respiratory disorders in the term infant. In: Gleason CA, Juul SE, eds. *Avery's Diseases of the Newborn.* 10th ed. Philadelphia, PA: Elsevier; 2018:671-672.

121. **(C)** Infants with CDH often have pulmonary vascular remodeling along with pulmonary hypoplasia, resulting in increased pulmonary vascular resistance after birth. These infants can also have structural and functional abnormalities of the left ventricle, resulting in left ventricular dysfunction. Echocardiography is noninvasive and helps to evaluate cardiac structures and ventricular function, rule out cyanotic cardiac lesions, identify right to left shunting across the foramen ovale and/or ductus arteriosus, and estimate pulmonary artery pressure. Echocardiography can also identify septal flattening and a tricuspid regurgitation jet which are markers of the severity of pulmonary hypertension. The chest x-ray of an infant with CDH may show variable pulmonary vasculature (increased, decreased, or normal) which gives information regarding pulmonary blood flow. However, x-ray is not the best way to assess pulmonary hypertension. Cardiac catheterization is invasive and used primarily as an interventional procedure, for example, to perform balloon atrial septostomy, valvuloplasty, or coil placement. Although cardiac catheterization can determine left and right ventricular function because it is invasive, it is not the preferred diagnostic procedure used. There is not a known association between 22q11.2 deletion syndrome and CDH.

References: Gardner SL, Enzman-Hines M, Nyp M. Respiratory diseases. In: Gardner SL, Carter BS, Niermeyer S, eds. *Merenstein & Gardner's Handbook of Neonatal Intensive Care: An Interdisciplinary Approach.* 9th ed. St. Louis, MO: Elsevier; 2021:804-805.

Steinhorn RH, Abmam SH. Persistent pulmonary hypertension. In: Gleason CA, Juul SE, eds. *Avery's Diseases of the Newborn.* 10th ed. Philadelphia, PA: Elsevier; 2018:772.

122. **(A)** An adequate volume of amniotic fluid allows for normal fetal breathing motion in utero. Inadequate amniotic fluid volume inhibits fetal breathing movement and chest wall expansion, restricting pulmonary growth. Severe pulmonary hypoplasia occurs when oligohydramnios is prolonged and occurs during the canalicular phase of lung development. Fetal urine constitutes a significant proportion of the amniotic fluid. Oligohydramnios is noted with congenital renal disorders (e.g., renal agenesis, polycystic kidneys, and urinary tract obstruction). Other causes of oligohydramnios include utero-placental insufficiency, maternal dehydration, and premature ruptured membranes. Space occupying lesions such as CDH can also lead to interrupted lung development and pulmonary hypoplasia. The presence of a congenital heart defect does not cause pulmonary hypoplasia. The presence of a tracheal esophageal fistula with esophageal atresia can lead to polyhydramnios due to impaired fetal swallowing, which is the predominant mechanism for removing amniotic fluid.

References: Grassham C, Jasin L. Maternal history in the antepartum. In: Koehn A, ed. *Neonatal Nurse Practitioner Certification Intensive Review: Fast Facts and Practice Questions.* New York: Springer Publishing Company, LLC; 2020:1-14.

Jackson JC. Respiratory disorders in the preterm infant. In: Gleason CA, Juul SE, eds. *Avery's Diseases of the Newborn.* 10th ed. Philadelphia, PA: Elsevier; 2018:662-665.

Wilson J, Snapp B, Walters M. The pulmonary system. In: Koehn A, ed. *Neonatal Nurse Practitioner Certification Intensive Review: Fast Facts and Practice Questions.* New York: Springer Publishing Company, LLC; 2020:235-260.

123. **(A)** The abdomen and thigh are the preferred sites because of sufficient body surface area available to maintain good contact between the electrode and the skin. Uneven areas of the skin such as over the bones and joints should be avoided because of poor contact between the membrane and the skin surface. The infant should not lay on the electrode as this increases pressure on the underlying capillaries, thus affecting the flow of blood under the probe and resulting in a drop of the transcutaneous CO_2 values. Laying on the probe can also cause pressure injury and first degree burns because of the heat generated by the electrode (43°C–44°C/109°F–111.2°F). To minimize trauma to the infant's skin, the electrode should be repositioned every 2–4 hours depending on the infant's skin sensitivity. The head or scalp has too much hair, preventing a tight seal around the skin electrode. Without a tight seal, accuracy will be diminished. The thorax has an uneven surface, making it difficult to maintain good contact between the membrane and the skin surface. The hand and wrist are not preferred sites because they have little surface area to maintain contact between the electrode unit and the skin.

References: Bancalari E, Claure N, Jain D. Neonatal respiratory therapy. In: Gleason CA, Juul SE, eds. *Avery's Diseases of the Newborn.* 10th ed. Philadelphia, PA: Elsevier; 2018:633.

Coe K, Bradshaw WT, Tanaka DT. Physiologic monitoring. In: Gardner SL, Carter BS, Niermeyer S, eds. *Merenstein & Gardner's Handbook of Neonatal Intensive Care: An Interdisciplinary Approach.* 9th ed. St. Louis, MO: Elsevier; 2021:180.

124. **(A)** Maternal corticosteroid therapy accelerates fetal lung growth and increases the proteins needed for surfactant production by type II pneumocytes, thus reducing the risk for RDS. Antenatal corticosteroid therapy is most effective when given to a pregnant woman who is between 23 and 34 weeks of gestation. Antenatal steroids should be considered when preterm delivery is anticipated in seven days and administered at least 24 hours before delivery with the maximum benefit occurring 48 hours after administration. Antenatal corticosteroid therapy is not

recommended at 18 weeks' gestation because the airways are at the canalicular phase of development and not capable of producing surfactant yet. Giving antenatal corticosteroid therapy to a woman as soon as possible after unprotected sex has no impact on fetal lung development.

References: Jackson JC. Respiratory disorders in the preterm infant. In: Gleason CA, Juul SE, eds. *Avery's Diseases of the Newborn.* 10th ed. Philadelphia, PA: Elsevier; 2018:653-662.

Wilson J, Snapp B, Walters M. The pulmonary system. In: Koehn A, ed. *Neonatal Nurse Practitioner Certification Intensive Review: Fast Facts and Practice Questions.* New York: Springer Publishing Company, LLC; 2020:235-260.

125. **(A)** Inhaled albuterol is a beta-adrenergic agonist which reduces airway reactivity and helps improve lung function. Although corticosteroids help improve lung function, they do not dilate the bronchioles. Furosemide and thiazide are diuretics which help reduce pulmonary edema.

Reference: Keller RL, Ballard RA. Bronchopulmonary dysplasia. In: Gleason CA, Juul SE, eds. *Avery's Diseases of the Newborn.* 10th ed. Philadelphia, PA: Elsevier; 2018:678-692.

126. **(A)** The recurrent laryngeal nerve supplies innervation to the larynx. Injury to the right or left branches of the recurrent laryngeal nerve can cause vocal cord paralysis on the ipsilateral side. Right-sided vocal cord paralysis has been reported as a complication of ECMO, presumably during surgical dissection for the insertion of the catheters and injury to the right recurrent laryngeal branch. Left-sided vocal cord paralysis has been reported as a complication of PDA ligation secondary to injury to the left recurrent laryngeal nerve branch during dissection. Vocal cord paralysis is not a complication of BPD. Vocal cord paralysis increases the risk of developing BPD, reactive airway disease, and feeding problems requiring gastrostomy tube. Vocal cord paralysis is not a complication of pulmonary hypertension.

References: Keller BA, Hirose S, Farmer DL. Surgical disorders of the chest and airways. In: Gleason CA, Juul SE, eds. *Avery's Diseases of the Newborn.* 10th ed. Philadelphia, PA: Elsevier; 2018:697-698.

Prazad PA, Rajpal MN, Mangurten HH, Puppala BL. Birth injuries. In: Martin RJ, Fanaroff AA, Walsh MC, eds. *Fanaroff & Martin's Neonatal-Perinatal Medicine: Diseases of the Fetus and Infant.* 11th ed. Philadelphia, PA: Elsevier; 2020:1251.

Swanson T, Erickson L. Cardiovascular diseases and surgical interventions. In: Gardner SL, Carter BS, Niermeyer S, eds. *Merenstein & Gardner's Handbook of Neonatal Intensive Care: An Interdisciplinary Approach.* 9th ed. St. Louis, MO: Elsevier; 2021:853.

127. **(C)** Bilateral vocal cord paralysis is most frequently caused by insult to the central nervous system at birth such as in hypoxic ischemic encephalopathy. Vocal cord paralysis is not a complication of tracheoesophageal fistula. Right-sided, not bilateral, vocal cord paralysis has been reported as a complication of ECMO. Vocal cord paralysis is not a complication of PDA. However, left-sided vocal cord paralysis has been reported as a complication of PDA ligation secondary to injury to the left recurrent laryngeal nerve branch during dissection.

References: Keller BA, Hirose S, Farmer DL. Surgical disorders of the chest and airways. In: Gleason CA, Juul SE, eds. *Avery's Diseases of the Newborn.* 10th ed. Philadelphia, PA: Elsevier; 2018:697-698.

Prazad PA, Rajpal MN, Mangurten HH, Puppala BL. Birth injuries. In: Martin RJ, Fanaroff AA, Walsh MC, eds. *Fanaroff & Martin's Neonatal-Perinatal Medicine: Diseases of the Fetus and Infant.* 11th ed. Philadelphia, PA: Elsevier; 2020:1251.

128. **(B)** Side lying on the same side as the paralysis may decrease the amount of stridor, as the affected vocal cord falls away from the midline. Side lying on the contralateral side of the paralysis may increase stridor as it will bring the paralyzed cord close to midline and close the airway further. The supine position may keep the vocal cords in a neutral position, thus neither increasing nor decreasing stridor. The prone position may cause the vocal cords to be compressed by the weight of surrounding structure, thus increasing stridor.

Reference: Keller BA, Hirose S, Farmer DL. Surgical disorders of the chest and airways. In: Gleason CA, Juul SE, eds. *Avery's Diseases of the Newborn.* 10th ed. Philadelphia, PA: Elsevier; 2018:697-698.

129. **(D)** Magnetic resonance imaging has proven to be most accurate in defining most vascular malformations and can give detailed information of the surrounding anatomy. Chest x-ray, barium swallow, and bronchoscopy each may provide cues to a vascular ring but are not the most accurate diagnostic modality. Chest x-ray may show tracheal narrowing. Barium swallow may show indentation of the esophagus. Bronchoscopy may reveal a pulsatile mass with narrowing near the carina.

Reference: Keller BA, Hirose S, Farmer DL. Surgical disorders of the chest and airways. In: Gleason CA, Juul SE, eds. *Avery's Diseases of the Newborn.* 10th ed. Philadelphia, PA: Elsevier; 2018:700-701.

130. **(C)** CPAM, formerly known as cystic adenoid malformation, is the most common congenital lung lesion and develops from an overgrowth of abnormal lung tissue. CPAM is a cystic lung disorder, and the cysts communicate with the airways but do not contain normal alveoli. CPAM occurs in 1 in 8300–35,000 live births and affects more male than female infants. BPS is a rare congenital malformation consisting of nonfunctional lung parenchyma that does not have a normal connection to the tracheobronchial tree. Pulmonary sequestration accounts for less than 10% of all congenital lung malformations and mostly occurs in the lower lobes. CLE occurs due to an obstructed lobar bronchus, which may be intrinsic or extrinsic in origin. These lesions are rare as well with an estimated incidence of 1 per 20,000–30,000 births. CLE is three times more common in males and most commonly involves the upper lobes; left upper lobe (43%), right middle lobe (32%), right upper lobe (21%), and lower lobe (2%) the rarest form. Pneumatocele is a thin-walled, air-containing cystic structure resulting from alveolar and bronchial necrosis. In the era of gentle ventilation, antenatal steroid, and surfactant therapy, the incidence is low in neonatal population, estimated at 1.8%.

References: Demir OF, Hangul M, Kose M. Congenital lobar emphysema: diagnosis and treatment options. *Int J Chronic Obstructive Pulm Dis.* 2019;14:921-928. doi:10.2147/COPD.S170581.

Gallagher ME, Pacetti AS, Lovvorn III HN, Carter BS. Neonatal surgery. In: Gardner SL, Carter BS, Niermeyer S, eds. *Merenstein & Gardner's Handbook of Neonatal Intensive Care: An Interdisciplinary Approach.* 9th ed. St. Louis, MO: Elsevier; 2021:1007-1008.

Kallapur SG, Jobe AH. Lung development and maturation. In: Martin RJ, Fanaroff AA, Walsh MC, eds. *Fanaroff & Martin's Neonatal-Perinatal Medicine: Diseases of the Fetus and Infant.* 11th ed. Philadelphia, PA: Elsevier; 2020:1213.

Keller BA, Hirose S, Farmer DL. Surgical disorders of the chest and airways. In: Gleason CA, Juul SE, eds. *Avery's Diseases of the Newborn.* 10th ed. Philadelphia, PA: Elsevier; 2018:708-713.

Oermann CM. *Congenital Pulmonary Airway Malformation.* Waltham, MA: UpToDate; 2021. Available at: https://www.uptodate.com/contents/congenital-pulmonary-airway-malformation.

Price TR, Miller MA, Prescott AC, Meadows JM, Tabak BD. Expanding pneumatocele in an ELBW infant. *J Pediatr Surg Case Rep.* 2021;73(10):102000. doi:10.1016/j.epsc.2021.102000.

131. **(D)** Plication of the diaphragm is performed to reshape or reposition the diaphragm, allowing for better lung expansion. Although ECMO is not the treatment of choice for eventration of the diaphragm, infants with severe ventilation and perfusion mismatch who have isolated congenital eventration of the diaphragm may benefit from ECMO. Nitric oxide, a selective pulmonary vasodilator, is used in infants with pulmonary hypertension to relax pulmonary vessels. Lobectomy is used in infants with CPAM.

Reference: Steinhorn RH, Abmam SH. Persistent pulmonary hypertension. In: Gleason CA, Juul SE, eds. *Avery's Diseases of the Newborn.* 10th ed. Philadelphia, PA: Elsevier; 2018:722.

132. **(A)** Infants with CDH have severe pulmonary hypertension due to a decreased cross-sectional area of the pulmonary vessels, structural remodeling of the pulmonary vessels, and diminished size and function of the left ventricle. Lack of surfactant in the lungs leads to RDS. Failure to transition from fetal to neonatal circulation can lead to PPHN but is not the cause of pulmonary hypertension in CDH. Accumulation of fluid in the lungs (pulmonary edema), for example, from a large PDA, could cause damage to the pulmonary vasculature resulting in pulmonary vascular disease.

Reference: Jackson JC. Respiratory disorders in the preterm infant. In: Gleason CA, Juul SE, eds. *Avery's Diseases of the Newborn.* 10th ed. Philadelphia, PA: Elsevier; 2018:662-665.

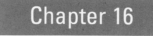

Chapter 16

Gastrointestinal Disorders

1. A term infant develops retractions, tachypnea, and cyanosis at 5 minutes of life, and positive pressure ventilation (PPV) is started. Adequate chest excursion becomes more difficult to achieve with PPV. Which of the following should be considered by the nurse as the most likely cause of the respiratory distress?
   A. Duodenal atresia
   B. Meconium ileus
   C. Congenital diaphragmatic hernia
   D. Hirschsprung disease

2. A nurse is performing a physical examination of an infant presenting with delayed respiratory distress. Which of the following diagnostic tests should the nurse anticipate as being most helpful to determine the cause of this distress?
   A. Upper gastrointestinal series
   B. Computed tomography scan
   C. Arterial blood gas
   D. Chest x-ray

3. An infant is born with an abdominal wall defect. Which of the following interventions is most important as an immediate nursing intervention postdelivery?
   A. Prepare for central line placement.
   B. Insert sump tube for gastric decompression.
   C. Place lower portion of body in sterile bowel bag.
   D. Administer intravenous antibiotics.

4. Which of the following conditions has a high association with other congenital anomalies?
   A. Malrotation
   B. Omphalocele
   C. Gastroschisis
   D. Volvulus

5. Infants with abdominal wall defects are at high risk for which of the following?
   A. Hypothermia due to excess exposed surface area
   B. Tachycardia due to fluid loss
   C. Hypotension due to blood loss
   D. Bradycardia due to low resting heart rate

6. An infant with gastroschisis is noted to have cyanotic bowel. Which of the following positions should the nurse place the infant in to promote adequate bowel perfusion?

A. Supine
B. Prone
C. Head of bed elevated
D. Lateral

7. An infant presents with bilious emesis. The nurse should suspect which of the following as a potential diagnosis?
   A. Gastroesophageal reflux disease
   B. Malrotation
   C. Necrotizing enterocolitis
   D. Tracheoesophageal fistula (TEF)

8. The nurse should anticipate an order for which of the following diagnostic studies for an infant with bilious vomiting?
   A. Hepatobiliary hepatobiliary iminodiacetic acid (HIDA) scan
   B. Magnetic resonance imaging
   C. Abdominal x-ray
   D. Upper gastrointestinal series

9. A term infant presents with flattened facies, hypotonia, low-set ears, and vomiting. Trisomy 21 is suspected. Which of the following gastrointestinal disorders or conditions is most often associated with trisomy 21?
   A. Gastroschisis
   B. Duodenal atresia
   C. Imperforate anus
   D. Constipation

10. A former 26-week-gestation infant, now 5 days old, presents with frequent bradycardic episodes, abdominal distention, and feeding intolerance. Abdominal and left lateral decubitus x-rays are positive for pneumoperitoneum. Which of the following actions by the nurse is most appropriate?
    A. Place infant on nasal continuous positive airway pressure.
    B. Insert an oral or nasogastric tube to low suction.
    C. Establish central line access.
    D. Prepare infant for magnetic resonance imaging study with contrast.

11. An infant with necrotizing enterocolitis is taken to surgery, and a bowel resection is performed. The nurse should be aware that the most common area of bowel affected is:
    A. duodenum.
    B. ileocecal valve.

C. stomach.

D. jejunum, ileum, and colon.

12. Which of the following have been shown to minimize the development of necrotizing enterocolitis?

A. Formula feedings

B. Breast milk feedings

C. Kangaroo care

D. Transpyloric or duodenal feedings

13. A term infant is put to breast for the first feeding and begins to excessively spit and cough. The nursing plan of care should include which of the following as the initial action?

A. Continuously suction infant with a catheter and wall suction.

B. Elevate head of bed and place a sump tube to low suction.

C. Intubate to protect the airway.

D. Prepare infant for upper gastrointestinal series.

14. An infant is diagnosed with TEF. Which of the following is the most commonly occurring type of TEF?

A. Esophageal atresia without TEF

B. Esophageal atresia with proximal TEF

C. Esophageal atresia with distal TEF

D. TEF without atresia

15. An infant has undergone a tracheoesophageal repair and is receiving conventional ventilation. The plan of care should include which of the following to best protect the anastomosis site?

A. Maintain infant in supine position.

B. Ventilate using high mean airway pressures.

C. Suction length of endotracheal tube only.

D. Provide bag–mask ventilation if accidental extubation occurs.

16. An infant presents with frequent, nonbilious vomiting. The parent questions the nurse as to why a reflux medication has not been started. What is the most appropriate nursing response?

A. This is a temporary issue and will resolve without medication.

B. A small percentage of infants have painful reflux.

C. Reflux medications are utilized when severe symptoms are present.

D. The medical team will discuss this during rounds tomorrow.

17. The nursing plan of care for an infant who has gastroesophageal reflux should include:

A. thickened feedings.

B. prone positioning.

C. burping every 2–3 oz.

D. large-volume feedings.

18. An upper gastrointestinal tract contrast confirms the diagnosis of malrotation and volvulus. Which of the following sequelae constitute this diagnosis as a surgical emergency in the preoperative phase?

A. Infection

B. Fluid and electrolyte imbalance

C. Intestinal ischemia and infarction

D. Disseminated intravascular coagulation

19. An infant diagnosed with malrotation and volvulus has been intubated and is being prepared for surgery. Suddenly, the infant exhibits pallor, hypotension, and tachycardia with

delayed capillary refill and diminished pulses. The nurse should anticipate which of the following as an immediate intervention for this infant?

A. Blood transfusion

B. Administration of vasopressors

C. Fluid resuscitation

D. Administration of intravenous antibiotics

20. An infant is diagnosed with esophageal atresia and TEF. The nurse should be aware that an infant with this diagnosis is at risk for having which of the following associated anomalies?

A. Omphalocele, cardiomegaly, and macroglossia

B. Vertebral anomalies, cardiac defects, and anal atresia

C. Short stature, micrognathia, hearing loss, and low-set ears

D. Cardiac defects, hypoplasia of the thymus, hypocalcemia, and microcephaly

21. Postoperative complications for repair of an esophageal atresia and a distal TEF can include which of the following?

A. Short bowel syndrome

B. Leakage or stricture at the anastomosis site

C. Renal dysfunction and urosepsis

D. Inferior vena cava compression

22. A male infant is diagnosed with imperforate anus. The parent expresses concern about bowel continence later in life. Which of the following statements should the nurse verbalize to the parent?

A. Prediction of bowel continence in infancy is difficult.

B. Females have a higher rate of bowel incontinence than males.

C. Bowel continence is not affected in the absence of urogenital fistula.

D. Low defects have a decreased incidence of bowel incontinence than high defects.

23. Hirschsprung disease should be suspected by the nurse in an infant who presents with which of the following symptoms?

A. Acholic stools

B. Projectile vomiting

C. Oliguria in the first 24 hours of life

D. Failure to pass meconium in the first 48 hours of life

24. A parent of an infant with an abdominal wall defect is confused about the difference between an omphalocele and a gastroschisis. Which of the following statements should the nurse share with the parent to provide clarification?

A. Gastroschisis has a high incidence of associated anomalies.

B. Omphalocele has a low incidence of associated anomalies.

C. Gastroschisis is enclosed in a membrane sac.

D. Gastroschisis does not usually involve the umbilical cord.

25. An infant is diagnosed with gastroschisis, and a staged reduction is planned by the surgical team. The mother questions the nurse as to why the defect can't be closed up all at once. Which of the following is the most appropriate response by the nurse?

A. A staged repair will cause the infant less pain.

B. A primary repair carries more risk of infection.

C. Staged repairs cause less stress on the cardiovascular system.

D. A primary repair will cause greater feeding intolerance.

26. An infant undergoes a primary repair for gastroschisis. A few hours postoperatively, the infant exhibits hypotension, capillary refill time of 5 seconds, decreased perfusion and temperature of lower extremities, and decreased urinary output. Given this assessment, the nurse would suspect which of the following?
    A. Development of sepsis
    B. Postoperative pain
    C. Intracranial hemorrhage
    D. Increased intraabdominal pressure

27. Infants with duodenal atresia should be assessed for which of the following conditions?
    A. Trisomy 21
    B. Trisomy 18
    C. Turner syndrome
    D. Beckwith-Wiedemann syndrome

28. An infant is diagnosed with congenital diaphragmatic hernia. The nurse should anticipate which of the following as the most likely preoperative complication?
    A. Bowel ischemia
    B. Hepatic dysfunction
    C. Pulmonary hypertension
    D. Necrotizing enterocolitis

29. The nurse should be aware that the primary risk factor for the development of necrotizing enterocolitis is which of the following?
    A. Bacterial infection
    B. Prematurity
    C. Maternal substance abuse
    D. Fungal sepsis

30. An infant has developed short bowel syndrome after surgical bowel resection, removal of ileocecal value, and creation of an ileostomy. The mother expresses concern about long-term nutritional status. Which of the following statements by the nurse is most appropriate?
    A. Constipation will be ongoing.
    B. Malabsorption will be present.
    C. Deficiency of water-soluble vitamins is common.
    D. High risk of necrotizing enterocolitis recurrence exists.

31. An infant is diagnosed with meconium ileus. The nurse should be aware that meconium ileus is commonly associated with which of the following?
    A. Trisomy 18
    B. Cystic fibrosis
    C. DiGeorge syndrome
    D. Hirschsprung disease

32. An infant presents with projectile vomiting, visible peristaltic waves at the epigastrium, and hypochloremia. The nurse should anticipate which of the following as the cause for these findings?
    A. Gastroenteritis
    B. Hiatal hernia
    C. Pyloric stenosis
    D. Duodenal atresia

33. An infant has been diagnosed with jejunal atresia. The nurse should be aware of which of the following characteristics of the defect?
    A. Apple peel deformity is the primary type.
    B. Oligohydramnios is common during pregnancy.
    C. Loose, frequent stools.
    D. Presents with abdominal distention.

34. A former 24-week infant is ordered to have a hepatobiliary HIDA scan done. The nurse should anticipate this is an imaging study for which of the following disorders?
    A. Gastroesophageal reflux
    B. Cholestasis
    C. Prune belly (Eagle-Barrett) syndrome
    D. Hydrops fetalis

35. An infant presents with acholic stools and jaundice with bronze undertones. Given these clinical findings, the nurse should suspect which of the following?
    A. Short bowel syndrome
    B. Biliary atresia
    C. Kernicterus
    D. Prune belly (Eagle-Barrett) syndrome

ANSWERS AND RATIONALES

1. **(C)** Congenital diaphragmatic hernia should be considered in any newborn infant with delayed respiratory distress due to compression of the lung by the intestines. Duodenal atresia, meconium ileus, and Hirschsprung disease do not directly or acutely affect respiratory function immediately after birth.

Reference: Kapadia V, Wyckoff M. Chest compression, medications, and special problems in neonatal resuscitation. In: Martin RJ, Fanaroff AA, Walsh MC, eds. *Fanaroff and Martin's Neonatal-Perinatal Medicine*. 11th ed. Philadelphia, PA: Elsevier; 2020:552-564.

2. **(D)** A chest x-ray can identify a number of pathologies present in the lung, including congenital defects such as diaphragmatic hernia, as well as pneumonia, respiratory distress syndrome, or transient tachypnea of the newborn. Chest radiograph shows the presence of bowel loops in the affected chest cavity that is compatible with diaphragmatic hernia. An upper gastrointestinal (GI) series is used to determine malformations in bowel structure, but not abnormalities in the chest or thorax. A computed tomography scan may assist in diagnosis but cannot be done as quickly as a chest x-ray. An arterial blood gas can be used to assess the degree of respiratory or metabolic abnormalities but will not determine the pathologic cause.

Reference: Crowley MA. Neonatal respiratory disorders. In: Martin RJ, Fanaroff AA, Walsh MC, eds. *Fanaroff and Martin's Neonatal-Perinatal Medicine*. 11th ed. Philadelphia, PA: Elsevier; 2020:1203-1230.

3. **(C)** Due to the large quantity of exposed organs, heat losses can be significant, so immediate placement of the infant in a sterile bowel bag immediately after delivery is the most important nursing intervention. Although intravenous antibiotics and placement of a sump tube will be part of the treatment plan, those interventions should be accomplished after bowel bag placement. Central line placement may be needed but will not be a first-line intervention.

Reference: Bradshaw W. Gastrointestinal disorders. In: Verklan MT, Walden W, eds. *Core Curriculum for Neonatal Intensive Care Nursing*. 6th ed. St. Louis, MO: Elsevier; 2021:504-542.

4. **(B)** Omphalocele has 45%–55% chance of being associated with other anomalies. Gastroschisis has a 10%–15% incidence. Malrotation and midgut volvulus can occur concurrently. The incidence of malrotation is 1 in 5000 births. Malrotation can be associated with omphalocele, gastroschisis, diaphragmatic hernia, or duodenal obstruction.

Reference: Ringer SA, Hansen AR. Surgical emergencies in the newborn. In: Eichenwald EC, Hansen AR, Martin CR, Stark AR, eds. *Cloherty and Stark's Manual of Neonatal Care.* 8th ed. Philadelphia, PA: Wolters Kluwer; 2017: 942-966.

5. **(A)** Infants with abdominal wall defects are at high risk for hypothermia due to an increase in exposed surface area, which subjects them to significant evaporative and convective heat loss. Infants with abdominal wall defects may occasionally have tachycardia or hypotension due to fluid loss, but more often have hypothermia. Infants with abdominal wall defects are not at high risk for bradycardia or low resting heart rate.

Reference: Ringer SA, Hansen AR. Surgical emergencies in the newborn. In: Eichenwald EC, Hansen AR, Martin CR, Stark AR, eds. *Cloherty and Stark's Manual of Neonatal Care.* 8th ed. Philadelphia, PA: Wolters Kluwer; 2017: 942-966.

6. **(D)** The optimal position of an infant with gastroschisis and cyanotic bowel is lateral or side-lying to prevent occlusion of the mesenteric arteries that supply blood flow to the bowel. Supine, prone, or elevated head of bed positions do not aid in bowel perfusion and are not recommended for infants with gastroschisis.

Reference: Bradshaw W. Gastrointestinal disorders. In: Verklan MT, Walden W, eds. *Core Curriculum for Neonatal Intensive Care Nursing.* 6th ed. St. Louis, MO: Elsevier; 2021:504-542.

7. **(B)** Malrotation should be suspected in any newborn with bilious emesis. Gastroesophageal reflux disease does not present with bilious emesis. Necrotizing enterocolitis (NEC) can present with bilious emesis but is usually associated with a host of other GI symptoms such as bloody stools, increased aspirates, metabolic acidosis, or pneumatosis on x-ray. Tracheoesophageal fistula (TEF) is accompanied by excessive secretions of a nonbilious nature.

Reference: Bradshaw W. Gastrointestinal disorders. In: Verklan MT, Walden W, eds. *Core Curriculum for Neonatal Intensive Care Nursing.* 6th ed. St. Louis, MO: Elsevier; 2021:504-542.

8. **(D)** An abdominal x-ray allows for the determination of bowel pathology such as a stricture or atresia and determines the amount of bowel gas present. It is the initial imaging study ordered. However, an upper GI radiograph is considered the gold standard to diagnose malrotation, a common cause of bilious emesis. Malrotation is considered a surgical emergency, and a magnetic resonance image may not be immediately available and is not of significant diagnostic value. A hepatobiliary scan is useful to determine cholestasis or evaluate bile flow but not of diagnostic value for bilious vomiting and malrotation.

Reference: Bradshaw W. Gastrointestinal disorders. In: Verklan MT, Walden W, eds. *Core Curriculum for Neonatal Intensive Care Nursing.* 6th ed. St. Louis, MO: Elsevier; 2021:504-542.

9. **(B)** One-third of infants with trisomy 21 have duodenal atresia. Gastroschisis, imperforate anus, and constipation are not associated with trisomy 21.

Reference: Bradshaw W. Gastrointestinal disorders. In: Verklan MT, Walden W, eds. *Core Curriculum for Neonatal Intensive Care Nursing.* 6th ed. St. Louis, MO: Elsevier; 2021:504-542.

10. **(B)** Pneumoperitoneum is free abdominal air resulting from bowel perforation. Insertion of a sump tube with low suction will continue to remove air from the bowel. Nasal continuous positive airway pressure will cause more air to be instilled into the intestines and exacerbate the pneumoperitoneum. Contrast studies should not be done because the contrast has the potential to leak into the peritoneum through the perforation. A central line may be needed but is not a first-line intervention.

Reference: Weitkamp JH, Premkumar MH, Martin CR. Necrotizing enterocolitis. In: Eichenwald EC, Hansen AR, Martin CR, Stark AR, eds. *Cloherty and Stark's Manual of Neonatal Care.* 8th ed. Philadelphia, PA: Wolters Kluwer; 2017:353-365.

11. **(D)** The jejunum, ileum, and colon are the most common sites for NEC. The duodenum is a rare NEC site. The stomach is not affected in NEC. Although the ileocecal valve can be affected in NEC, it is not the most common site.

Reference: Weitkamp JH, Premkumar MH, Martin CR. Necrotizing enterocolitis. In: Eichenwald EC, Hansen AR, Martin CR, Stark AR, eds. *Cloherty and Stark's Manual of Neonatal Care.* 8th ed. Philadelphia, PA: Wolters Kluwer; 2017:353-365.

12. **(B)** Feedings with breast milk have been shown to decrease the incidence of NEC in numerous studies. Formula feeds, kangaroo care, and transpyloric or duodenal feedings have not been shown to decrease the incidence of NEC.

Reference: Weitkamp JH, Premkumar MH, Martin CR. Necrotizing enterocolitis. In: Eichenwald EC, Hansen AR, Martin CR, Stark AR, eds. *Cloherty and Stark's Manual of Neonatal Care.* 8th ed. Philadelphia, PA: Wolters Kluwer; 2017:353-365.

13. **(B)** A normal-appearing newborn who starts to excessively spit and cough during feeds should be evaluated for TEF. Elevating the head of the bed and placing a sump tube will prevent further reflux of gastric contents into the lungs. Placing the sump tube to low wall suction will be effective in preventing the accumulation of secretions in the blind pouch. An infant should not be continuously suctioned with a catheter because that could cause tissue trauma. Unless an infant is exhibiting signs of moderate to severe respiratory distress, intubation is not needed. An upper GI study is not recommended due to risk of aspiration of contrast media.

Reference: Bradshaw W. Gastrointestinal disorders. In: Verklan MT, Walden W, eds. *Core Curriculum for Neonatal Intensive Care Nursing.* 6th ed. St. Louis, MO: Elsevier; 2021:504-542.

14. **(C)** The most common type of TEF is esophageal atresia (EA) with distal TEF (85%). This type has a blind pouch for the upper esophagus. EA without TEF only occurs in 8% of TEF. EA with proximal TEF occurs in 2% of cases. TEF without atresia occurs in 5% of cases.

Reference: Bradshaw W. Gastrointestinal disorders. In: Verklan MT, Walden W, eds. *Core Curriculum for Neonatal Intensive Care Nursing.* 6th ed. St. Louis, MO: Elsevier; 2021:504-542.

15. **(C)** By suctioning only to the end of the endotracheal tube (ETT), it will prevent suction catheter extrusion beyond the ETT. The head of the bed should be elevated to prevent aspiration. Low mean airway pressures are administered to prevent excess pressure on the anastomosis site. In the case of accidental extubation, only experienced staff such as pediatric anesthesia or a difficult airway team should attempt reintubation, and bag-and-mask ventilation should be avoided.

Reference: Bradshaw W. Gastrointestinal disorders. In: Verklan MT, Walden W, eds. *Core Curriculum for Neonatal Intensive Care Nursing.* 6th ed. St. Louis, MO: Elsevier; 2021:504-542.

16. **(C)** Reflux medicines are not needed in infants unless symptoms are severe; for example, weight loss or aspiration events and other measures have been trialed such as upright and supine positioning and/or minimizing or eliminating aggravating factors such as frequent suctioning. The majority of infants will have

spontaneous resolution of reflux over time. Pain with reflux episodes can be exhibited by some infants but nonpharmacologic methods can lessen reflux and any associated pain. Although it is acceptable to ask about reflux medications during medical rounds, nurses should know the recommended and routine treatment of reflux and when pharmacologic therapy is appropriate.

Reference: Hibbs AM. Gastrointestinal reflux and motility in the neonate. In: Martin RJ, Fanaroff AA, Walsh MC, eds. *Fanaroff and Martin's Neonatal-Perinatal Medicine.* 11th ed. Philadelphia, PA: Elsevier; 2021:1513-1521.

17. **(A)** Infants with reflux should be managed with thickened and smaller, more frequent feedings to minimize the amount in their stomachs and decrease the chance of regurgitation. Prone positioning is not recommended due to the American Academy of Pediatrics Back to Sleep initiative to prevent sudden infant death syndrome. Burping should be done every 1 ounce instead of every 2–3 oz.

Reference: Anderson DM, Poindexter BB, Martin CR. Nutrition. In: Eichenwald EC, Hansen AR, Martin CR, Stark AR, eds. *Cloherty and Stark's Manual of Neonatal Care.* 8th ed. Philadelphia, PA: Wolters Kluwer; 2017:248-283.

18. **(C)** The presence of malrotation and volvulus can result in the occlusion of intestinal blood supply, resulting in ischemia and bowel necrosis if not emergently corrected via surgical means. Although the prevention of infection is important during the postoperative course, it is not of primary concern preoperatively. Fluid and electrolytes will need to be monitored postoperatively with mL per mL of replacement for gastric losses. The development of disseminated intravascular coagulation is rare if septic or hypovolemic shock is avoided.

Reference: Bradshaw W. Gastrointestinal disorders. In: Verklan MT, Walden W, eds. *Core Curriculum for Neonatal Intensive Care Nursing.* 6th ed. St. Louis, MO: Elsevier; 2021:504-542.

19. **(C)** The infant is showing signs of significant bowel compromise resulting in shock and possible intestinal ischemia and infarction. Blood transfusion and vasopressor therapy may be required for this infant, but the priority is surgical repair and fluid resuscitation. Intravenous antibiotics are indicated as part of the medical plan, but fluid resuscitation is the most pressing concern.

Reference: Bradshaw W. Gastrointestinal disorders. In: Verklan MT, Walden W, eds. *Core Curriculum for Neonatal Intensive Care Nursing.* 6th ed. St. Louis, MO: Elsevier; 2021:504-542.

20. **(B)** Omphalocele, cardiomegaly, and macroglossia are associated with Beckwith-Wiedemann syndrome.

Associated anomalies are seen in more than half of neonates with EA and TEF. The most common are cardiac defects, which occur in approximately 20%–35% of these infants. Another common defect is VACTERL association (vertebral, anal, cardiac, tracheal esophageal, renal, and limb), which is seen in 5%–10% of cases. Short stature, micrognathia, hearing loss, and low-set ears are associated with Cornelia de Lange syndrome. Cardiac defects, hypoplasia of the thymus, hypocalcemia, and microcephaly are associated with DiGeorge syndrome.

Reference: Bradshaw W. Gastrointestinal disorders. In: Verklan MT, Walden W, eds. *Core Curriculum for Neonatal Intensive Care Nursing.* 6th ed. St. Louis, MO: Elsevier; 2021:504-542.

21. **(B)** Primary repair of EA/TEF includes a ligation of the TEF and anastomosis of the proximal and distal segments of the esophagus. Complications of the surgery include leakage at the anastomosis site, gastroesophageal reflux, and stricture. Short bowel syndrome is associated with surgical NEC or complicated jejunal or ileal atresia repair. Renal dysfunction and urosepsis are not associated complications with EA/TEF repair. Inferior vena cava compression is a more common postsurgical complication of abdominal wall defect repairs.

Reference: Bradshaw W. Gastrointestinal disorders. In: Verklan MT, Walden W, eds. *Core Curriculum for Neonatal Intensive Care Nursing.* 6th ed. St. Louis, MO: Elsevier; 2021:504-542.

22. **(D)** Infants with low imperforate anus have a rectum that descends through the puborectalis and levator ani muscles and can be expected to have normal bowel continence after repair. Higher defects may have increased frequency of incontinence due to impairment of neurologic and muscular mechanisms of bowel control. Eighty percent of females have low defects; males have an equal rate of high and low defects. Continence is determined based on the type of the defect, not gender assignment or age of infant. Bowel continence is not related to the presence or absence of urogenital fistula.

Reference: Bradshaw W. Gastrointestinal disorders. In: Verklan MT, Walden W, eds. *Core Curriculum for Neonatal Intensive Care Nursing.* 6th ed. St. Louis, MO: Elsevier; 2021:504-542.

23. **(D)** A clinical sign of Hirschsprung disease is the failure to pass meconium in the first 48 hours after birth, which may be accompanied by bilious vomiting and progressive abdominal distention. The disease is marked by a congenital absence of parasympathetic innervation to the distal intestine due to the absence of ganglionic cells. Oliguria is normal in the first 24 hours of life as the infant transitions to extrauterine life. Beyond that, renal dysfunction must be investigated. It is not a finding related to Hirschsprung. Projectile vomiting is reflective of pyloric stenosis, and acholic stools occur with biliary atresia.

Reference: Bradshaw W. Gastrointestinal disorders. In: Verklan MT, Walden W, eds. *Core Curriculum for Neonatal Intensive Care Nursing.* 6th ed. St. Louis, MO: Elsevier; 2021:504-542.

24. **(D)** The incidence of associated anomalies with omphalocele is 45%–55%; for gastroschisis the rate is 10%–15%. A gastroschisis is paraumbilical and usually located to the right of the umbilical cord. An omphalocele has a membrane covering, although the covering may be ruptured at the time of birth.

Reference: Bradshaw W. Gastrointestinal disorders. In: Verklan MT, Walden W, eds. *Core Curriculum for Neonatal Intensive Care Nursing.* 6th ed. St. Louis, MO: Elsevier; 2021:504-542.

25. **(C)** A staged repair minimizes the stress on the respiratory and vascular systems by allowing these systems to adjust slowly to the increased pressure of the organs as they gradually return to the abdominal cavity. Postoperative pain can be variable in both types of repairs. A primary repair will decrease the risk of infection and can be associated with similar rates of feeding intolerance postoperatively as a staged repair.

Reference: Bradshaw W. Gastrointestinal disorders. In: Verklan MT, Walden W, eds. *Core Curriculum for Neonatal Intensive Care Nursing.* 6th ed. St. Louis, MO: Elsevier; 2021:504-542.

26. **(D)** Although primary closure versus staged closure is preferred to reduce risk of infection, thermal losses, and exposure of abdominal organs, it is not always an option. The main risk of primary closure is increased intraabdominal pressure, which would be exhibited by decreased perfusion to the lower extremities and decreased urinary output. An increase in capillary refill time accompanied by hypotension indicates decreased blood return to the heart via the inferior vena cava. Postoperative pain and risk of infection should not cause the previously mentioned constellation of symptoms. Intracranial hemorrhage is not a factor because most infants with gastroschisis are near or at term.

Reference: Bradshaw W. Gastrointestinal disorders. In: Verklan MT, Walden W, eds. *Core Curriculum for Neonatal Intensive Care Nursing.* 6th ed. St. Louis, MO: Elsevier; 2021:504-542.

27. **(A)** Duodenal atresia is associated with trisomy 21 (30% of cases), congenital heart disease (30% of cases), intestinal malrotation (20% of cases), tracheoesophageal anomalies (10%–20% of cases, and anorectal defects (10%–20% of cases). It is not associated with Turner syndrome (sex chromosome anomaly), trisomy 18, or Beckwith-Wiedemann (congenital hyperinsulinemia) syndrome.

Reference: Bradshaw W. Gastrointestinal disorders. In: Verklan MT, Walden W, eds. *Core Curriculum for Neonatal Intensive Care Nursing.* 6th ed. St. Louis, MO: Elsevier; 2021:504-542.

28. **(C)** Congenital diaphragmatic hernia is a space-occupying lesion in that the intestinal contents fill the lung cavity to varying degrees depending on the size of the defect. This can result in pulmonary hypoplasia and pulmonary hypertension that may require mechanical/high-frequency ventilation or extracorporeal membrane oxygenation. Bowel ischemia and NEC may occur with overall hypoxia, but are not nearly as significant clinical factors as the potential for decreased pulmonary perfusion. Hepatic dysfunction is not a common sequela.

Reference: Bradshaw W. Gastrointestinal disorders. In: Verklan MT, Walden W, eds. *Core Curriculum for Neonatal Intensive Care Nursing.* 6th ed. St. Louis, MO: Elsevier; 2021:504-542.

29. **(B)** NEC is primarily a disease of the premature infant. The perfusion of the GI tract of the premature infant can be affected by hypoxia, hypotension, patent ductus arteriosus, hypothermia, and the presence of umbilical catheters. Bacterial infection of the initially sterile GI tract can lead to the development of NEC, particularly when preceded by enteral feedings in the premature infant. Fungal sepsis affects the very low–birth-weight infant and can occur concurrently or as an NEC sequela. Maternal substance abuse can compromise the intrauterine environment, but is not the primary risk factor for NEC.

Reference: Bradshaw W. Gastrointestinal disorders. In: Verklan MT, Walden W, eds. *Core Curriculum for Neonatal Intensive Care Nursing.* 6th ed. St. Louis, MO: Elsevier; 2021:504-542.

30. **(B)** Short bowel is most commonly associated with malabsorption and diarrhea and is often a sequela of surgical NEC and the loss of a significant portion of small bowel. NEC is highly unlikely to recur. Supplementation of the fat-soluble vitamins (A, D, E, and K) is required if the ileum is lost.

Reference: Bradshaw W. Gastrointestinal disorders. In: Verklan MT, Walden W, eds. *Core Curriculum for Neonatal Intensive Care Nursing.* 6th ed. St. Louis, MO: Elsevier; 2021:504-542.

31. **(B)** Approximately 10%–15% of infants with meconium ileus have cystic fibrosis. Cardiac defects are associated in 85% of infants with DiGeorge syndrome; no association with meconium ileus. Hirschsprung disease can be associated with meconium plug syndrome but not with meconium ileus. Trisomy 18 is a chromosomal syndrome most commonly exhibiting cardiac and renal defects along with multiple dysmorphic features.

Reference: Bradshaw W. Gastrointestinal disorders. In: Verklan MT, Walden W, eds. *Core Curriculum for Neonatal Intensive Care Nursing.* 6th ed. St. Louis, MO: Elsevier; 2021:504-542.

32. **(C)** Dehydration, nonbilious projectile vomiting, peristaltic waves in the epigastrium, and electrolyte imbalances, including hypochloremia, are clinical symptoms of pyloric stenosis. Bilious vomiting is associated with duodenal atresia. Hiatal hernia is associated with gastroesophageal reflux. Gastroenteritis is an infectious process and normally presents with diarrhea and nonbilious, nonprojectile vomiting.

Reference: Bradshaw W. Gastrointestinal disorders. In: Verklan MT, Walden W, eds. *Core Curriculum for Neonatal Intensive Care Nursing.* 6th ed. St. Louis, MO: Elsevier; 2021:504-542.

33. **(D)** Jejunal atresia presents with abdominal distention; the lower the obstruction, the greater the distention. The absence of stool and a history of polyhydramnios are common for infants afflicted with jejunal atresia. Apple peel deformity, or type IIIb, is considered to be a rare and more complex form of jejunal atresia.

Reference: Bradshaw W. Gastrointestinal disorders. In: Verklan MT, Walden W, eds. *Core Curriculum for Neonatal Intensive Care Nursing.* 6th ed. St. Louis, MO: Elsevier; 2021:504-542.

34. **(B)** Hepatobiliary scintigraphy scan is an imaging study to diagnose cholestasis and to evaluate bile flow. A pH probe or endoscopy is the common imaging study for gastroesophageal reflux. An ultrasound of the abdomen is the first-line imaging study for Eagle-Barrett syndrome (prune belly). Ultrasound or skeletal radiographs would be appropriate studies for the infant with hydrops.

Reference: Bradshaw W. Gastrointestinal disorders. In: Verklan MT, Walden W, eds. *Core Curriculum for Neonatal Intensive Care Nursing.* 6th ed. St. Louis, MO: Elsevier; 2021:504-542.

35. **(B)** Acholic stools, bronze undertones, dark urine, and hepatosplenomegaly are clinical manifestations of biliary atresia. Malabsorption and diarrhea are most common with short bowel syndrome but acholic stools and jaundice are not present. Kernicterus is accompanied by jaundice, but the color of the stools or urine is not affected. Prune belly (Eagle-Barrett syndrome) is an absence of abdominal musculature, genitourinary tract abnormalities, and undescended testes.

Reference: Bradshaw W. Gastrointestinal disorders. In: Verklan MT, Walden W, eds. *Core Curriculum for Neonatal Intensive Care Nursing.* 6th ed. St. Louis, MO: Elsevier; 2021:504-542.

Chapter 17

Metabolic and Endocrine Disorders

1. Which of the following infants is at lowest risk for hypoglycemia?
   A. A 32-week infant experiencing hypothermia
   B. A 36-week infant of a diabetic mother
   C. A 38-week infant with intrauterine growth restriction
   D. A 41-week infant with clubfoot deformity

2. The nurse is preparing to administer a bolus of D10W to a neonate with transient postnatal hypoglycemia. Rebound hypoglycemia can be prevented by:
   A. starting the baby on an insulin drip.
   B. repeating the bolus every 30 minutes.

C. following the bolus with a continuous intravenous (IV) infusion of D10W and feedings.

D. giving a bolus of glucagon simultaneously with the bolus of D10W.

3. What is the presumed cause of macrosomia in the infant of a diabetic mother?
   A. Fetal pancreatic beta cell hypoplasia
   B. Inherited predisposition for a larger body habitus
   C. Maternal hyperglycemia and hyperaminoacidemia, resulting in fetal hyperinsulinemia
   D. Tendency for prolonged pregnancy and postterm delivery, resulting in more weight gain

4. A 36-week-gestational-age infant of a diabetic mother has a point-of-care blood glucose level of 23 mg/dL at 6 hours of age. The infant has breastfed twice since birth. What is the best course of action under these circumstances?
   A. Draw a specimen for measurement of plasma glucose level and initiate treatment while awaiting the results.
   B. Send a blood sample to the laboratory for measurement of plasma glucose level and await the results.
   C. Have the mother breastfeed again and check the blood glucose level before the next feeding.
   D. Observe the baby for symptoms of hypoglycemia and feed or initiate IV therapy if symptoms occur.

5. An extremely premature infant nearing discharge has an elevated alkaline phosphatase level. What should the nurse include in the discharge education plan?
   A. Avoid kangaroo care.
   B. Handle the infant as carefully as possible.
   C. Recommend a soy-based formula.
   D. Limit the infant's mobility as much as possible.

6. An infant with a low thyroxine level and an elevated thyroid-stimulating hormone level is presumed to have which condition until proven otherwise?
   A. Euthyroid sick syndrome
   B. Neonatal Graves disease
   C. Congenital hypothyroidism
   D. Thyroid-binding globulin deficiency

7. What is the most prevalent thyroid disorder in preterm and low-birth-weight infants?
   A. Thyroid dysgenesis
   B. Neonatal thyrotoxicosis
   C. Transient hypothyroxinemia
   D. Central hypothyroidism

8. A 600-g neonate has a blood glucose level of 195 mg/dL. What physiologic consequence should the nurse be concerned about?
   A. Weight gain
   B. Ketonuria
   C. Hyperinsulinism
   D. Osmotic diuresis

9. Which of the following is associated with neonatal hypocalcemia?
   A. Perinatal asphyxia
   B. Hypophosphatemia

C. Hypervitaminosis D
D. Subcutaneous fat necrosis

10. The signs and symptoms of an inborn error of metabolism in a newborn infant are most likely to be associated with which other neonatal disorder?
    A. Sepsis
    B. Congenital heart defect
    C. Necrotizing enterocolitis
    D. Respiratory distress syndrome

11. Which of the following is the most important element of management when caring for a neonate with medium-chain acyl-coenzyme A dehydrogenase deficiency (MCAD), a disorder of fatty acid oxidation?
    A. Prohibit breastfeeding.
    B. Feed with a phenylalanine-free formula.
    C. Feed frequently and avoid prolonged periods of fasting.
    D. Withhold all protein sources (formula, milk, and amino acid solutions).

12. A term infant is born with a large goiter. What nursing intervention is indicated?
    A. Have a defibrillator on standby for cardioversions.
    B. Delay sending the neonatal screen until the goiter has resolved.
    C. Position the infant with the head elevated and with slight extension.
    D. Allow nothing by mouth until after surgical correction of the goiter.

13. A 35-week-gestational-age infant is born to a mother who has been receiving magnesium sulfate for gestational hypertension. What should the nurse watch for in the infant?
    A. Lethargy and apnea
    B. Hypertension and fever
    C. Jitteriness and tachycardia
    D. Tachypnea and hypoglycemia

14. The XX virilization of the neonate, the most common cause of ambiguous genitalia, is a result of which of the following?
    A. Pure gonadal dysgenesis
    B. Partial androgen insensitivity
    C. Congenital adrenal hyperplasia
    D. Prenatal exposure to progestins

15. Which of the following findings on assessment of external genitalia should prompt further investigation for possible ambiguous genitalia?
    A. Hydrocele
    B. Physiologic phimosis
    C. Inguinal hernia in a female
    D. Blood-tinged vaginal mucus

16. The parents of a baby born with ambiguous genitalia are still awaiting test results to determine the sex of their infant. Which of the following interventions by the nurse would be most helpful during this time?
    A. Telling the parents the nurse is almost certain that the baby is a boy (or girl)
    B. Suggesting that the parents choose a name suitable for either a boy or a girl

C. Arranging a meeting with a knowledgeable mental health professional

D. Advising them to keep the baby's condition a secret from all but the immediate family

17. One of the most important physiologic effects of thyroid hormones is:
    A. regulation of inflammatory responses.
    B. regulation of glucose homeostasis.
    C. mediation of gut development.
    D. support during critical periods of brain development.

18. When performing a nursing assessment, which of these observations would be of most significance for a 3-month-old infant with osteopenia of prematurity?
    A. Prominent forehead, epiphyseal widening, and a downward trend on the growth chart
    B. Internally rotated shoulders, a pronated forearm, and flexion contractures of the wrist
    C. Tenderness and crepitus at the end of the humerus with decreased movement of an arm
    D. Apnea, lethargy, and abdominal distention

19. When providing discharge education to parents of an infant who will continue receiving levothyroxine at home, the nurse should include which of these instructions?
    A. Cut the pill and encourage the infant to swallow by placing it on the back of the tongue.
    B. Follow-up with an endocrinologist is not necessary.
    C. Laboratory samples are expected to be drawn at frequent intervals.
    D. Vitamins with iron may be given at the same time as the levothyroxine.

20. Maternal Graves disease, particularly if inadequately treated, places a neonate at risk for which of the following?
    A. Hyperthyroidism
    B. Diabetes insipidus
    C. Iodine deficiency
    D. Congenital hypothyroidism

21. A nurse is caring for a newborn with a birth weight of 4.2 kg and breech presentation at delivery. On the sixth day of life the infant is noted to have a fever, pallor and jaundice, lethargy with periods of irritability, poor feeding, and vomiting. Upon notifying a physician, the nurse should first prepare for
    A. a dose of steroids.
    B. an abdominal ultrasound.
    C. an x-ray of the chest and abdomen.
    D. a blood transfusion.

22. A 3-day-old term newborn has poor feeding, vomiting, and lethargy. The mother reports that the diaper smells sweet. Laboratory results include increased levels of plasma branched-chain amino acids, metabolic acidosis, and ketonuria. What disease process is likely occurring?
    A. Maple syrup urine disease
    B. Phenylketonuria
    C. Galactosemia
    D. MCAD

23. Which of the following is the best approach for managing hyperglycemia in extremely low-birth-weight infants?
    A. Maximize IV fluid volume and IV dextrose concentration; administer insulin for blood glucose levels greater than 150 mg/dL.
    B. Maximize IV fluid volume and adjust IV dextrose concentration based on blood glucose levels; administer insulin for blood glucose levels greater than 200 mg/dL.
    C. Minimize IV fluid volume and IV dextrose concentration; administer insulin for blood glucose levels greater than 150 mg/dL.
    D. Minimize IV fluid volume and IV dextrose concentration; administer insulin for blood glucose levels greater than 200 mg/dL.

ANSWERS AND RATIONALES

1. **(D)** Although postterm birth can pose some risk of hypoglycemia, the risk is low in an infant who is feeding. Clubfoot is not a risk for alteration in blood glucose levels. Preterm infants have insufficient glycogen stores and release, as well as an immature response to counter regulation of the low glucose concentration. Hypothermia increases an infant's glucose utilization rate. An infant of a diabetic mother has an increased uptake of glucose related to hyperinsulinism, which is a result of long-term exposure to high glucose levels in utero. Intrauterine growth restriction causes an infant to have insufficient glycogen and fat stores and increased substrate utilization rate.

Reference: Armentrout D. Glucose management. In: Verklan MT, Walden M, Forest S, eds. *Core Curriculum for Neonatal Intensive Care Nursing.* 6th ed. St. Louis, MO: Elsevier; 2021:144-151.

2. **(C)** A glucose bolus induces a surge of insulin secretion in the neonate, so following the bolus with a continuous infusion of glucose or starting feedings will minimize or eliminate the insulin surge and thereby decrease the incidence-rebound hypoglycemia. Repeating glucose boluses will induce insulin surges but peaks and valleys in the blood glucose levels will continue; therefore, repeating glucose boluses probably will not solve the problem. Starting an insulin infusion would worsen hypoglycemia because the baby does not need exogenous insulin. Glucagon can have severe side effects, such as hyponatremia and thrombocytopenia, and should be used rarely in neonates.

Reference: Armentrout D. Glucose management. In: Verklan MT, Walden M, Forest S, eds. *Core Curriculum for Neonatal Intensive Care Nursing.* 6th ed. St. Louis, MO: Elsevier; 2021:144-151.

3. **(C)** Throughout pregnancy and particularly in the third trimester, the pregnant diabetic woman is increasingly insulin resistant and often has hyperglycemia and hyperaminoacidemia. The excess glucose and amino acids are transferred to the fetus and stimulate the fetal pancreas to produce insulin to use the excess fuels. The fetal hyperinsulinemia then stimulates protein, lipid, and glycogen synthesis, causing a high rate of fetal growth. The fetal pancreas may respond to excess glucose by producing more insulin, which causes beta cell hyperplasia, not hypoplasia. Although it is possible that a newborn's large size could be inherited from one or both parents, this is not the usual cause of macrosomia in infants of diabetic mothers. The pregnancy of a woman with diabetes is more likely to be end earlier, not later, and the neonate is more likely to be premature than post term.

Reference: Armentrout D. Glucose management. In: Verklan MT, Walden M, Forest S, eds. *Core Curriculum for Neonatal Intensive Care Nursing.* 6th ed. St. Louis, MO: Elsevier; 2021:144-151.

4. **(A)** An infant of a diabetic mother is at higher risk for hypoglycemia during the first 24 hours of life due to the continued hyperinsulinism occurring in utero in response to the high glucose transfer across the placenta. Therefore the plasma glucose level must be confirmed by laboratory analysis as quickly as possible and treatment be started immediately to prevent sequelae of hypoglycemia such as brain injury. Delaying treatment while awaiting test results, feeding and waiting to test before the next feeding, and observing for symptoms are all counterproductive due to the negative sequelae associated with hypoglycemia.

Reference: Armentrout D. Glucose management. In: Verklan MT, Walden M, Forest S, eds. *Core Curriculum for Neonatal Intensive Care Nursing.* 6th ed. St. Louis, MO: Elsevier; 2021:144-151.

5. **(B)** The infant's history (extreme prematurity) and laboratory findings (elevated alkaline phosphatase) suggest metabolic bone disease. The infant's bones are fragile and can be easily fractured (e.g., limbs and ribs). Kangaroo care is not contraindicated in metabolic bone disease. A soy-based formula will not positively affect metabolic bone disease and may be nutritionally inferior to what the infant is receiving. Lack of mobility contributes to metabolic bone disease.

Reference: Bell SG. Fluid and electrolyte management. In: Verklan MT, Walden M, Forest S, eds. *Core Curriculum for Neonatal Intensive Care Nursing.* 6th ed. St. Louis, MO: Elsevier; 2021:131-143.

6. **(C)** A low thyroxine (T_4) level with an elevated level of thyroid-stimulating hormone (TSH) is pathognomonic for congenital hypothyroidism (CH), because of the negative feedback control of the endocrine system. TSH level is not elevated in euthyroid sick syndrome (also called *nonthyroidal illness*). Neonatal Graves disease is associated with a high, rather than low, T_4 level. Thyroid-binding globulin deficiency does not manifest as an elevated TSH level.

Reference: Blackburn ST. Endocrine disorders. In: Verklan MT, Walden M, Forest S, eds. *Core Curriculum for Neonatal Intensive Care Nursing.* 6th ed. St. Louis, MO: Elsevier; 2021:543-567.

7. **(C)** Serum levels of thyroid hormones in preterm neonates are significantly lower and more variable than those of term neonates and usually correlate with gestational age and birth weight. Thyroid dysgenesis, neonatal thyrotoxicosis, and central hypothyroidism are each relatively uncommon or rare conditions.

Reference: Blackburn ST. Endocrine disorders. In: Verklan MT, Walden M, Forest S, eds. *Core Curriculum for Neonatal Intensive Care Nursing.* 6th ed. St. Louis, MO: Elsevier; 2021:543-567.

8. **(D)** As blood glucose level rises, glucose begins spilling into the urine, followed by water, which results in osmotic diuresis. This can be dangerous for the very low–birth-weight infant. Weight gain is unlikely, because glucose utilization is poor. Ketonuria is not expected with neonatal hyperglycemia. Very low–birth-weight infants tend to have a deficiency, not an excess, of insulin.

Reference: Polin R, Adamkin D. Glucose, calcium, and magnesium. In: Fanaroff A, Fanaroff J, eds. *Klaus and Fanaroff's Care of the High-Risk Neonate.* 7th ed. St. Louis, MO: Elsevier; 2020:227-243.

9. **(A)** Perinatal asphyxia is a significant risk factor of hypocalcemia in the neonate. Asphyxia stimulates a surge in calcitonin level, which inhibits the release of calcium from the bone. Hypophosphatemia, excessive vitamin D intake, and subcutaneous fat necrosis are all associated with hypercalcemia.

References: Bell SG. Fluid and electrolyte management. In: Verklan MT, Walden M, Forest S, eds. *Core Curriculum for Neonatal Intensive Care Nursing.* 6th ed. St. Louis, MO: Elsevier; 2021:131-143.

Polin R, Adamkin D. Glucose, calcium, and magnesium. In: Fanaroff A, Fanaroff J, eds. *Klaus and Fanaroff's Care of the High-Risk Neonate.* 7th ed. St. Louis, MO: Elsevier; 2020:227-243.

10. **(A)** Neonates have a limited repertoire of responses to illness, and the signs and symptoms of inborn errors of metabolism are often nonspecific and can mimic those of sepsis. Clinical evidence of a congenital heart defect is very different from the signs and symptoms of most inborn errors of metabolism. Clinical manifestations of necrotizing enterocolitis can include nonspecific findings, but also have a component specifically related to the abdomen and gastrointestinal tract, whereas most inborn errors of metabolism do not. The signs and symptoms of respiratory distress syndrome are fairly specific and respond to specific treatments, unlike those of most inborn errors of metabolism.

Reference: Lubbers L. Congenital anomalies. In: Verklan MT, Walden M, Forest S, eds. *Core Curriculum for Neonatal Intensive Care Nursing.* 6th ed. St. Louis, MO: Elsevier; 2021:654-677.

11. **(C)** Infants who have fatty acid oxidation defects cannot break down fatty acids to supply energy, so energy needs must be met exogenously. Long periods of fasting and other stressors lead rapidly to hypoglycemia. Breastfeeding is allowable and encouraged for infants with medium-chain acyl-coenzyme A dehydrogenase deficiency (MCAD); however, it is important to ensure the infant is getting enough milk from the breast to prevent hypoglycemia. Protein is necessary to prevent issues related to catabolism in infants with MCAD. Phenylalanine-free formula is given to infants with phenylketonuria.

References: Lubbers L. Congenital anomalies. In: Verklan MT, Walden M, Forest S, eds. *Core Curriculum for Neonatal Intensive Care Nursing.* 6th ed. St. Louis, MO: Elsevier; 2021:654-677.

McCandless S, Kripps L. Genetics, inborn errors of metabolism, and newborn screening. In: Fanaroff A, Fanaroff J, eds. *Klaus and Fanaroff's Care of the High-Risk Neonate.* 7th ed. St. Louis, MO: Elsevier; 2020:121-147.

12. **(C)** A sizable goiter can compress and obstruct the trachea, leading to airway compromise. Positioning the infant with the head of the bed elevated and head extended slightly will help maintain a patent airway. Otherwise, intubation may be necessary. If the goiter is caused by hyperthyroidism, cardiac effects are possible, but having a defibrillator on standby is not the most important intervention. The neonatal screen should be sent at the usual time to identify other potentially treatable metabolic problems. Not all goiters are corrected surgically. Many resolve spontaneously, and infants are fed as usual.

Reference: Blackburn ST. Endocrine disorders. In: Verklan MT, Walden M, Forest S, eds. *Core Curriculum for Neonatal Intensive Care Nursing.* 6th ed. St. Louis, MO: Elsevier; 2021:543-567.

13. **(A)** An infant born to a mother who received magnesium sulfate in the antepartum period is at risk of lethargy, hypotonia, and apnea. No treatment other than observation is usually necessary; however, the nurse should be prepared to resuscitate infants born to mothers receiving large doses of magnesium sulfate. Hypertension, fever, jitteriness, tachycardia, tachypnea, and hypoglycemia are not generally associated with a residual excess of magnesium.

Reference: Bell SG. Fluid and electrolyte management. In: Verklan MT, Walden M, Forest S, eds. *Core Curriculum for Neonatal Intensive Care Nursing.* 6th ed. St. Louis, MO: Elsevier; 2021:131-143.

14. **(C)** Congenital adrenal hyperplasia caused by 21-hydroxylase deficiency is the most common cause of ambiguous genitalia in the newborn and is also the most common cause of virilization, development of male characteristics in a female, in a genetically female infant. Pure gonadal dysgenesis is less common than congenital adrenal hyperplasia and genotype varies. Partial androgen insensitivity also occurs less frequently than congenital adrenal hyperplasia and the genotype is 46, XY. Prenatal exposure to progestins and synthetic steroid hormones, such as progesterone, is an uncommon cause of ambiguous genitalia.

Reference: Blackburn ST. Endocrine disorders. In: Verklan MT, Walden M, Forest S, eds. *Core Curriculum for Neonatal Intensive Care Nursing.* 6th ed. St. Louis, MO: Elsevier; 2021:543-567.

15. **(C)** An apparent female with an inguinal hernia could be an XY child with complete or partial androgen insensitivity, and the "hernia" could be a testis. A hydrocele is a collection of fluid within the scrotum and is not associated with conditions that cause ambiguous genitalia. Physiologic phimosis, congenital narrowing of the foreskin opening, is a common normal variant in male infants. Blood-tinged vaginal mucus is a common normal occurrence in female infants.

Reference: Blackburn ST. Endocrine disorders. In: Verklan MT, Walden M, Forest S, eds. *Core Curriculum for Neonatal Intensive Care Nursing.* 6th ed. St. Louis, MO: Elsevier; 2021:543-567.

16. **(C)** The birth of a baby with ambiguous genitalia raises many distressing issues for parents (such as what to tell family and friends, how to deal with registering the birth and naming the baby, etc.), and a mental health professional can help the parents deal with these and other issues. Parents should never be told with certainty that their baby is a boy (or girl) in these cases; care professionals should not attempt to guess the gender in advance of test results and should keep their opinions to themselves. Suggesting that parents choose a name suitable for either a boy or a girl is not recommended. Once the gender is established, the name is a way of reinforcing the gender for the family. Keeping secrets reinforces guilt and shame. The parents can choose how, when, and how much information will be communicated, but trying to maintain strict secrecy about the baby's condition is not recommended and can isolate the parents from supportive family and friends.

Reference: Blackburn ST. Endocrine disorders. In: Verklan MT, Walden M, Forest S, eds. *Core Curriculum for Neonatal Intensive Care Nursing.* 6th ed. St. Louis, MO: Elsevier; 2021:543-567.

17. **(D)** Thyroid hormones induce differentiation and maturation of neural circuits during critical periods of brain development. Cortisol plays a key regulatory role in inflammatory responses. Glucagon, insulin, and cortisol play major roles in glucose homeostasis. Gastrointestinal hormones, such as enteroglucagon, gastrin, motilin, and neurotensin, have a critical role in mediating gut development after birth.

Reference: Blackburn ST. Endocrine disorders. In: Verklan MT, Walden M, Forest S, eds. *Core Curriculum for Neonatal Intensive Care Nursing.* 6th ed. St. Louis, MO: Elsevier; 2021:543-567.

18. **(A)** Osteopenia manifests between 6 and 12 weeks of corrected gestational age. Growth retardation, frontal bossing (prominent forehead), craniotabes (thinning of the skull bone), prominence of the costochondral junction (rachitic rosary), and epiphyseal widening are signs of rickets, which can be a severe manifestation of osteopenia. Arthrogryposis multiplex congenital is a syndrome characterized by multiple joint contractures, including internally rotated shoulders, elbow extension, a pronated forearm, and flexion contractures of the wrist and fingers, as well as lower extremity contractures. Infants with humeral fractures will usually have pain, limitation of movements, pseudo paralysis, tenderness, and crepitus at the fractured ends of the bone. Osteopenia does not cause acute signs and symptoms such as lethargy, apnea, feeding intolerance, and abdominal distention; these are signs of hypocalcemia.

References: Abrams S, Tiosano D. Disorders of calcium, phosphorus, and magnesium metabolism in the neonate. In: Martin R, Fanraoff A, Walsh M, eds. *Fanaroff & Martin's Neonatal-Perinatal Medicine: Disease of the Fetus and Infant.* 11th ed., Vol 2. Philadelphia, PA: Elsevier; 2020:1611-1642.

Adamkin D, Radmacher P. Nutrition and selected disorders of the gastrointestinal tract; Nutrition for the high-risk neonate, part 1. In: Fanaroff A,

Fanaroff J, eds. *Klaus and Fanaroff's Care of the High-Risk Neonate.* 7th ed. St. Louis, MO: Elsevier; 2020:80-107.

19. **(C)** Frequent clinical evaluation of thyroid function, growth, and development and laboratory measurements of T_4 and TSH are required to ensure optimal treatment. Laboratory values should be obtained at 2 and 4 weeks; then every 1–2 months for 6 months; then every 3–4 months; and with every dose change, abnormal value, and with compliance concerns. Levothyroxine pills should be crushed and suspended in breast milk, formula, or a small amount of water. Placing a cut pill into an infant's mouth would put the infant at risk for choking. Consultation with a pediatric endocrinologist is recommended to aid in effective management of the disease process and treatment. Care should be taken not to give levothyroxine with soy, fiber, or iron because these products can interfere with the absorption of levothyroxine so the infant could remain hypothyroid.

Reference: Blackburn ST. Endocrine disorders. In: Verklan MT, Walden M, Forest S, eds. *Core Curriculum for Neonatal Intensive Care Nursing.* 6th ed. St. Louis, MO: Elsevier; 2021:543-567.

20. **(A)** Neonatal Graves disease (hyperthyroidism) although uncommon (occurring in approximately 1 of 70 pregnancies affected by maternal Graves disease) is typically transient, lasting approximately 3–12 weeks. Diabetes insipidus is a deficiency in antidiuretic hormone, which can be related to an abnormally functioning posterior pituitary gland (e.g., tumor, fluid, malformation). Iodine deficiency is a pathophysiologic cause of primary hypothyroidism and is not related to maternal Graves disease. CH is not caused by maternal Graves disease. The etiologies of CH include thyroid gland abnormalities, maternal autoimmune disorders that allow transplacental passage of TSH receptor-blocking antibodies, or maternal drugs that cross the placenta and affect fetal thyroid production.

Reference: Blackburn ST. Endocrine disorders. In: Verklan MT, Walden M, Forest S, eds. *Core Curriculum for Neonatal Intensive Care Nursing.* 6th ed. St. Louis, MO: Elsevier; 2021:543-567.

21. **(B)** The infant's history (macrosomia and breech presentation), along with pallor and jaundice, lethargy with periods of irritability, poor feeding, and vomiting, are signs of potential adrenal hemorrhage. The relatively large size of the adrenal gland at birth may contribute to injury. A nurse should prepare for an abdominal ultrasound before any treatments to determine the cause of the infant's signs. Steroids are indicated if the infant experiences adrenal insufficiency as a result of adrenal hemorrhage. The hemorrhage and insufficiency need to be diagnosed with diagnostic tests before treatment should be initiated. An x-ray will not aid in the identification of an adrenal hemorrhage. Although blood transfusion may be necessary in the treatment of adrenal hemorrhage, it would not be the first step at this time.

References: Berlin S, Meyers M. Neonatal imaging. In: Fanaroff A, Fanaroff J, eds. *Klaus and Fanaroff's Care of the High-Risk Neonate.* 7th ed. St. Louis, MO: Elsevier; 2020:409-436.

Blackburn ST. Endocrine disorders. In: Verklan MT, Walden M, Forest S, eds. *Core Curriculum for Neonatal Intensive Care Nursing.* 6th ed. St. Louis, MO: Elsevier; 2021:543-567.

22. **(A)** Maple syrup urine disease is an inborn error of metabolism characterized by urine that smells like maple syrup; metabolic acidosis; and elevated plasma branched-chain amino acids leucine, isoleucine, and valine. Infants are usually well at delivery, but after 2–3 days of feedings, infants begin to have poor feeding, lethargy, and vomiting that may progress to hypotonia, seizures, coma, and potentially death. Phenylketonuria is an inborn error of metabolism that is diagnosed by a newborn screen and/or persistently or gradually increasing plasma phenylalanine levels. Infants are typically asymptomatic at birth, but as an infant begins to ingest breast

milk or formula will have vomiting, poor feedings, hyperactivity, and irritability. Galactosemia is an inborn error of metabolism characterized by signs, including vomiting, diarrhea, jaundice, failure to thrive, hepatosplenomegaly, and hypoglycemia quickly appearing after milk feeding begins. Newborn screening and/or serum blood galactose levels, red blood cell 1-phosphate levels, elevated liver function tests, and urine tests are used to diagnose galactosemia. MCAD is an inborn error of metabolism that may be diagnosed in utero, during newborn screening, or with laboratory results, including hypoglycemia, absence of moderate to large ketones in urine, and elevated plasma ammonium, aspartate aminotransferase, and alanine aminotransferase levels. Symptoms typically do not appear until later in infancy and include anorexia, vomiting, diarrhea, lethargy, and hypoglycemia associated with seizures.

Reference: Lubbers L. Congenital anomalies. In: Verklan MT, Walden M, Forest S, eds. *Core Curriculum for Neonatal Intensive Care Nursing.* 6th ed. St. Louis, MO: Elsevier; 2021:654-677.

23. **(B)** Extremely low–birth-weight (ELBW) infants have insulin resistance, an immature insulin response, and are unable to stop gluconeogenesis when intravenous (IV) glucose is administered. In addition, ELBW infants require a high volume of IV fluids in efforts to meet the requirement of the immature renal function and increased sensible water loss. The increased IV fluid volume leads to an increase in the amount of glucose administered, so blood glucose levels should be monitored closely. Treatment with insulin is usually only necessary for blood glucose levels greater than 200 mg/dL. IV fluid volume should be maximized to meet the requirements of an ELBW infant's immature renal function and insensible water loss. IV dextrose should not be maximized, but instead titrated based on blood glucose levels because an ELBW infant is unable to stop the process of gluconeogenesis when IV glucose is administered. An ELBW infant has immature renal function and increased insensible water loss and therefore requires a higher amount of IV fluids. IV dextrose should not be minimized because it is necessary for growth and glucose homeostasis.

Reference: Forest S. Care of the extremely low birth weight infant. In: Verklan MT, Walden M, Forest S, eds. *Core Curriculum for Neonatal Intensive Care Nursing.* 6th ed. St. Louis, MO: Elsevier; 2021:377-387.

Chapter 18

Hematologic Disorders

1. What action improves the effectiveness of phototherapy in neonates with ABO incompatibility?
   A. Cycle phototherapy lights on and off at 4-hour intervals.
   B. Position the halogen spot phototherapy lamp 5 cm above the patient.
   C. Expose as much of the infant's skin as possible to the phototherapy source(s).
   D. Use one bank of fluorescent daylight bulbs when intensive phototherapy is required.

2. An intrauterine growth-restricted neonate born to a mother with pregnancy-induced hypertension has a venous hematocrit of 72%. This is most likely caused by:
   A. the presence of fetal hemoglobin in the neonate.
   B. a maternal–fetal hemorrhage in utero.
   C. a high level of erythropoietin in the infant's body.
   D. the sample being drawn from the vein.

3. A decision is made to perform a partial-exchange transfusion for a neonate with a venous hematocrit of 72%. After the transfusion, the neonate must be evaluated for:
   A. signs of a transfusion reaction.
   B. signs and symptoms of hypocalcemia.
   C. signs and symptoms of hyperkalemia.
   D. signs and symptoms of feeding intolerance and necrotizing enterocolitis.

4. Compared with adult red blood cells, newborn red blood cells:
   A. are more resilient.
   B. have a longer life span.
   C. have a decreased mean corpuscular volume.
   D. carry a larger amount of oxygen on the hemoglobin.

5. A neonate with a positive blood culture for *Escherichia coli* requiring ventilatory and vasopressor support has a sudden pulmonary hemorrhage. Furthermore, petechiae now covers the neonate's trunk. An examination of the maternal laboratory results shows that the platelet count is normal. Based on the history and clinical presentation of this infant, what disease process is most likely occurring?
   A. Neonatal alloimmune thrombocytopenia
   B. Maternal systemic lupus erythematosus
   C. Disseminated intravascular coagulation (DIC)
   D. Maternal idiopathic thrombocytopenic purpura

6. What are the expected laboratory results for a patient with DIC?
   A. Low platelet count, low fibrinogen level, and elevated D-dimer level
   B. Normal platelet count, low fibrinogen level, and elevated level of fibrin split products
   C. Low platelet count, prolonged prothrombin time (PT), and shortened partial thromboplastin time (PTT)
   D. Normal platelet count, prolonged PT, and prolonged PTT

7. A septic neonate in the neonatal intensive care unit (NICU) on nasal intermittent positive pressure ventilation develops sudden pulmonary hemorrhage. Immediate management of this patient consists of:
   A. administration of packed red blood cells.
   B. ensuring an open airway (through suctioning and potentially intubating the neonate) and providing positive pressure ventilation.
   C. obtaining repeat blood cultures to ensure appropriate antibiotic selection.
   D. replacement of clotting factors.

8. Fifteen minutes after an acute loss of blood, an infant will most likely display:
   A. a decreased hemoglobin, hypotension, tachycardia, and pallor.
   B. an unchanged hemoglobin, hypotension, bradycardia, and apnea.
   C. an unchanged hemoglobin, hypotension, tachycardia, and weak pulses.
   D. a decreased hemoglobin, unchanged blood pressure, unchanged heart rate, and hepatosplenomegaly.

9. The preferred first intervention for a preterm infant who has had an acute blood loss in the NICU is to:
   A. administer a rapid infusion of isotonic saline.
   B. place the infant in Trendelenburg position.
   C. give the infant 100% oxygen via nasal cannula.
   D. administer a transfusion of group O, Rh-negative whole blood.

10. A 72-day-old infant (current weight, 2.2 kg; postconceptual age, 36 weeks) with bronchopulmonary dysplasia is now receiving 100% oxygen at 1 L/min via nasal cannula, an increase of 0.5 liters per minute from before. The infant is pale, lethargic, and has had eight apneic episodes in the past 24 hours. The infant's heart rate is 176 beats/minute. Complete blood cell count results include the following: hematocrit: 21%, hemoglobin: 7.0 g/dL, and reticulocyte count: 1.8%. Based on the clinical picture and laboratory results, the appropriate action is to:
    A. continue current care.
    B. begin a course of supplemental iron with feeds.
    C. transfuse the infant with 15 mL/kg packed red blood cells.
    D. begin a course of recombinant human erythropoietin (Epogen).

11. A 5-day-old breast-feeding infant has been readmitted to the NICU for intensive phototherapy due to a total serum bilirubin level of 25 mg/dL. What potential side effect of phototherapy should the nurse be most concerned about at this time?
    A. Dehydration
    B. Constipation
    C. Retinal damage
    D. Bronze baby syndrome

12. A nurse is caring for a 4-day-old, 32-week gestation septic neonate with an indirect bilirubin level of 23.8 mg/dL despite intensive phototherapy and intravenous fluids. A double-exchange transfusion is performed. Because of potential fluid and electrolyte disturbances that are related to the blood used in exchange transfusions, the nurse should monitor for:

A. irritability, jitteriness, and tachycardia.
B. dampened T waves and cardiac dysrhythmias.
C. lethargy and poor feeding.
D. late hyperglycemia.

13. A newborn has a venous hematocrit of 62%. The newborn has shown some jitteriness and is not nipple-feeding well. The neonate is not experiencing any respiratory difficulties, and the blood glucose level is 68 mg/dL. Management at this time would most-likely include:
    A. continuing routine care.
    B. performing a partial-exchange transfusion with normal saline or 5% albumin.
    C. putting the newborn on nothing-by-mouth status and beginning maintenance intravenous fluids at 80 mL/kg/day.
    D. closely monitoring the newborn's respiratory status, glucose levels, and giving intravenous hydration while encouraging feeds.

14. After circumcision, a male newborn experiences significant bleeding. The PTT is elevated, but the PT and platelet count are normal. Upon further discussion with the mother, she states that her brother had the same problem. Based on the signs and symptoms, diagnostic test results, and history, what is the most likely cause for the bleeding?
    A. Hemophilia A
    B. Von Willebrand disease
    C. Vitamin K-dependent bleeding
    D. Idiopathic thrombocytopenia purpura

15. Which of the following statements reflects a correct understanding of ABO incompatibility?
    A. "ABO incompatibility occurs less frequently than Rh isoimmunization and is more severe."
    B. "ABO incompatibility occurs when the mother is O negative and baby is A, B, or AB positive."
    C. "Babies with ABO incompatibility have a negative direct Coombs test."
    D. "ABO incompatibility requires the mother to be exposed to fetal blood of a different type in order for her to develop antibodies."

16. A newborn is born with a subdural hematoma, petechiae over its trunk, and oozing at the umbilical cord. This is the mother's second pregnancy. Her platelet count is normal. The newborn's platelet count is 14,000. The PT and partial thromboplastic time are normal. Based on the signs and symptoms, diagnostic test results, and history, the most appropriate therapy is to:
    A. wait for the counts to normalize.
    B. transfuse with washed maternal platelets.
    C. give serial transfusions of random donor platelets.
    D. determine the presence of human platelet antigens after the first platelet transfusion.

17. If supplementary vitamin K is not given after birth, a classic vitamin K deficiency bleeding disorder will result in:
    A. decreasing fibrinogen levels.
    B. decreasing platelet levels.
    C. hemolytic anemia on a peripheral blood smear.
    D. prolonged PT and activated PTT. (aPTT)

18. A 26-week gestation neonate with O-positive blood requires a packed red blood cell transfusion. To minimize the chance of graft-versus-host disease, which of the following could be performed?
    A. Administration of packed red blood cells that are cytomegaly virus negative.
    B. Administration of packed red blood cells that are type O, either Rh positive or negative.
    C. Filtration of the packed red blood cells.
    D. Gamma irradiation of the packed red blood cells.

19. What is the primary cause of anemia of prematurity?
    A. A physiologic drop in erythropoietin
    B. Iatrogenic blood loss
    C. Iron deficiency
    D. Underlying infections

20. A 36-week gestation infant has a total serum bilirubin of 14 mg/dL at 48 hours of age. Mom is breastfeeding exclusively, but the infant is sleepy. No risk factors for hemolytic disease exist. What would be the appropriate first nursing intervention?
    A. Begin intensive phototherapy.
    B. Contact the blood bank to determine the availability of whole blood for an exchange transfusion.
    C. Continue to encourage breastfeeding and retake another total serum bilirubin level 12 hours later.
    D. Notify the physician of the bilirubin level.

ANSWERS AND RATIONALES

1. **(C)** Effectiveness of phototherapy is determined by the energy output of the light source, distance between the light source and infant, and the surface area exposed to the light. Turning the infant frequently and using more than one light source allows an increased amount of surface area to be exposed, increasing the efficacy of phototherapy to decrease unconjugated bilirubin. While the effectiveness of intermittent phototherapy is being studied for nonhemolytic and late preterm neonates, current literature still recommends that phototherapy for neonates with hemolytic disease (such as ABO incompatibility) should be maintained except for brief periods of feeding, assessment, and parental contact. Generally, fluorescent bulbs need to be positioned 10–15 cm above the patient. Halogen lights, because of the heat they generate, may need to be placed further away. Intensive phototherapy requires an irradiance of at least 30 $\mu W/cm^2/nm$ as compared to standard phototherapy which is less than 30. A single bank of fluorescent bulbs is generally used for standard phototherapy. Intensive phototherapy often requires auxiliary lights such as special blue bulbs and lights under the infant.

References: Kamath-Rayne BD, Froese PA, Thilo EH. Neonatal hyperbilirubinemia. In: Gardner SL, Carter BS, Niermeyer S, eds. *Merenstein & Gardner's Handbook of Neonatal Intensive Care: An Interprofessional Approach.* 9th ed. St. Louis, MO: Elsevier; 2021:677-683.

Bradshaw WT. Gastrointestinal disorders. In: Verklan MT, Walden M, Forest S, eds. *Core Curriculum for Neonatal Intensive Care Nursing.* 6th ed. St. Louis, MO: Elsevier; 2021:533-538.

2. **(C)** Erythropoietin levels are elevated in neonates who are intrauterine growth restricted and neonates of mothers with pregnancy-induced hypertension due to a relative amount of chronic hypoxia. High erythropoietin levels result in an increased production of erythrocytes (red blood cells [RBCs]) and polycythemia (a hematocrit of greater than 65%). While the transition to adult hemoglobin is delayed in neonates who have experienced fetal growth restriction and maternal hypoxia, this is not the cause for a significantly increased hematocrit. Fetal hemoglobin (HbF) results in a higher affinity for oxygen which is important in a low-oxygen environment. If a maternal–fetal hemorrhage occurs in utero, this can raise the hematocrit but is not the cause for polycythemia in infants born to mothers with pregnancy-induced hypertension. Venous samples can have a hematocrit that is as much as 20% lower than the hematocrit resulting from a heel stick or capillary puncture.

References: McKinney C, Warren BB, Harvey S. Newborn hematology. In: Gardner SL, Carter BS, Niermeyer S, eds. *Merenstein & Gardner's Handbook of Neonatal Intensive Care: An Interprofessional Approach.* 9th ed. St. Louis, MO: Elsevier; 2021:623-624, 636-638.

Diehl-Jones W, Fraser D. Hematologic disorders. In: Verklan MT, Walden M, Forest S, eds. *Core Curriculum for Neonatal Intensive Care Nursing.* 6th ed. St. Louis, MO: Elsevier; 2021:568–569, 581–582.

3. **(D)** Partial exchange transfusions are generally performed via an umbilical catheter and may have the risk of causing gastrointestinal symptoms such as bleeding, feeding intolerance, and necrotizing enterocolitis. This risk may be increased by the initial hyperviscosity of the neonate's blood. Because 0.9% normal saline or a colloid is generally used for the partial exchange transfusion, a transfusion reaction is not a risk factor. Hypocalcemia is a potential complication of double volume exchange transfusions due to anticoagulation citrates added to the transfused blood that bind to calcium. Hyperkalemia is a potential complication of a double volume exchange transfusion due to transfusion with blood that was obtained from the donor more than 5 days in the past.

Reference: Diehl-Jones W, Fraser D. Hematologic disorders. In: Verklan MT, Walden M, Forest S, eds. *Core Curriculum for Neonatal Intensive Care Nursing.* 6th ed. St. Louis, MO: Elsevier; 2021:583-586.

4. **(D)** Because of the increased affinity to oxygen by HbF and a lower amount of 2,3-diphosphoglycerate, newborn RBCs carry a greater amount of oxygen on the hemoglobin than do adult RBCs. Newborn RBCs are much more fragile than adult RBCs and have a life span of 60–70 days in term newborns and an even shorter life span in premature newborns. The life span of an adult RBC is 100–120 days. The mean corpuscular volume is the relative size of the RBC. Newborn RBCs are larger than adult RBCs for the first 4–5 years of life.

Reference: Diehl-Jones W, Fraser D. Hematologic disorders. In: Verklan MT, Walden M, Forest S, eds. *Core Curriculum for Neonatal Intensive Care Nursing.* 6th ed. St. Louis, MO: Elsevier; 2021:568-572.

5. **(C)** Disseminated intravascular coagulation (DIC) is an acquired hemorrhagic disorder associated with an underlying disease such as septic shock. Presenting signs of DIC include sudden hemorrhage, prolonged oozing, petechiae, and purpura. In neonatal alloimmune thrombocytopenia, although fetal platelet counts are low, maternal platelet counts are usually normal. Thrombocytopenia results from maternal antibodies that cross the placental and destroy fetal platelets. Infants show petechiae and bleeding but not sudden hemorrhage. Infants born of mothers with systemic lupus erythematosus and idiopathic (autoimmune) thrombocytopenia have thrombocytopenia because of maternal autoantibodies. Mothers of these infants typically have low platelet counts and their infants show petechiae and bleeding but not sudden hemorrhage.

References: Diehl-Jones W, Fraser D. Hematologic disorders. In: Verklan MT, Walden M, Forest S, eds. *Core Curriculum for Neonatal Intensive Care Nursing.* 6th ed. St. Louis, MO: Elsevier; 2021:577-581.

Blackburn ST. Hematologic and hemostatic systems. In: Blackburn ST, ed. *Maternal, Fetal, Neonatal Physiology: A Clinical Perspective.* 5th ed. St. Louis, MO: Elsevier; 2018:244-245.

6. **(A)** Typical laboratory results for DIC are low platelet count, low fibrinogen level, increased level of D-dimer (the marker for DIC), prolonged prothrombin time and partial thromboplastin time (although they may initially be normal), and increased level of fibrin split products.

Reference: Diehl-Jones W, Fraser D. Hematologic disorders. In: Verklan MT, Walden M, Forest S, eds. *Core Curriculum for Neonatal Intensive Care Nursing.* 6th ed. St. Louis, MO: Elsevier; 2021:578-579.

7. **(B)** The critical action for any neonate with pulmonary hemorrhage is to suction the trachea and provide assisted ventilation (generally with an advanced airway) to maintain oxygenation and ventilation. While administration of packed RBCs would provide a replacement of RBCs in the case of a sudden pulmonary hemorrhage, the provision of a secure airway and breathing support would be the priority. DIC would be on the top of the differential diagnosis for this neonate with sepsis. Aggressive treatment of the underlying disorder by selecting the appropriate antibiotic, and replacing clotting factors by administering fresh frozen plasma, platelets and potentially cryoprecipitate would be essential to control the DIC, however immediate management includes ensuring adequate cardiorespiratory support to the neonate.

References: Diehl-Jones W, Fraser D. Hematologic disorders. In: Verklan MT, Walden M, Forest S, eds. *Core Curriculum for Neonatal Intensive Care Nursing.* 6th ed. St. Louis, MO: Elsevier; 2021:578-579.

Fraser D. Respiratory disorders. In: Verklan MT, Walden M, Forest S, eds. *Core Curriculum for Neonatal Intensive Care Nursing.* 6th ed. St. Louis, MO: Elsevier; 2021:412.

8. **(C)** Immediately after an acute blood loss, the hemoglobin will be unchanged because the body has not had a chance to equilibrate. Acute blood loss results in a decreased preload leading to decreased cardiac output as evidenced by low blood pressure, tachycardia, and poor perfusion (pallor, delayed capillary refill, and weak pulses). Acute blood loss would result in tachycardia and rapid irregular respirations rather than bradycardia and apnea. A decreased hemoglobin, unchanged blood pressure and heart rate, and hepatosplenomegaly would be seen in chronic blood loss, not an acute blood loss.

Reference: Diehl-Jones W, Fraser D. Hematologic disorders. In: Verklan MT, Walden M, Forest S, eds. *Core Curriculum for Neonatal Intensive Care Nursing.* 6th ed. St. Louis, MO: Elsevier; 2021:574-577.

9. **(D)** The preferred treatment for an acute blood loss resulting in hypovolemia is transfusion of whole blood or packed RBCs, if available. In addition to increasing the volume returning to the heart, a blood transfusion increases the oxygen-carrying capacity of the body. Use of type O, Rh-negative blood does not require that typing and crossmatching be performed before the transfusion. If immediate access to whole blood or packed RBCs is not available, the next choice would be an isotonic volume expander to facilitate perfusion. Placing preterm infants in Trendelenburg position is not recommended because it changes cerebral perfusion and increases the potential for intraventricular hemorrhage. Although administration of oxygen would increase the infant's PaO_2, an increased PaO_2 by itself does not contribute significantly to oxygen content at the tissue level. Without hemoglobin to carry the oxygen, the tissues cannot be adequately perfused.

Reference: Diehl-Jones W, Fraser D. Hematologic disorders. In: Verklan MT, Walden M, Forest S, eds. *Core Curriculum for Neonatal Intensive Care Nursing.* 6th ed. St. Louis, MO: Elsevier; 2021:574-577.

10. **(C)** Because the infant is manifesting signs of hypoxemia, is requiring an increased amount of supplementary oxygen, and has an increased severity of apnea and bradycardia episodes, it would be appropriate to give a transfusion to increase oxygen delivery. The administration of 10–20 mL/kg of packed RBCs is generally recommended. Because the patient is symptomatic with anemia of prematurity, it would not be beneficial to "wait and see" at this point. Although supplemental iron is vital in RBC production once iron stores are depleted, particularly when recombinant human erythropoietin (Epogen) is being given and erythropoiesis is taking place, it is not for acute treatment of anemia of prematurity. The use of recombinant human erythropoietin (Epogen) together with more restrictive transfusion criteria has decreased the need for packed RBC transfusions related to anemia of prematurity. While treatment with Epogen stimulates erythropoiesis, this generally takes several weeks from onset of therapy.

Reference: Blackburn ST. Hematologic and hemostatic systems. In: Blackburn ST, ed. *Maternal, Fetal, Neonatal Physiology: A Clinical Perspective.* 5th ed. St. Louis, MO: Elsevier; 2018:240-243.

11. **(A)** Many infants who are readmitted to the neonatal intensive care unit from home with severe hyperbilirubinemia are already mildly dehydrated. This dehydration is then compounded by the increase in insensible water loss and possible secretory diarrhea from a temporary intestinal lactose deficiency that occurs with phototherapy. If the infant's eyes are covered during phototherapy, the risk of retinal damage is minimal. The eyes need to be inspected and cleaned on a regular basis to ensure that irritation from the eye shields is not being experienced. Bronze baby syndrome occurs as a side effect of phototherapy in infants with elevated conjugated or direct bilirubin levels. Hyperbilirubinemia related to breastfeeding is usually a result of elevated levels of indirect bilirubin.

References: Bagwell GA, Steward DK. Hematologic system. In: Kenner C, Altimier LB, Boykova MV, eds. *Comprehensive Neonatal Nursing Care.* 6th ed. New York: Springer Publishing Co.; 2020:331-333.

Kamath-Rayne BD, Froese PA, Thilo EH. Neonatal hyperbilirubinemia. In: Gardner SL, Carter BS, Niermeyer S, eds. *Merenstein & Gardner's Handbook of Neonatal Intensive Care: An Interprofessional Approach.* 9th ed. St. Louis, MO: Elsevier; 2021:665-670.

12. **(A)** Because the citrate present in common blood preservatives (acid–citrate–dextrose and citrate–phosphate–dextrose) binds calcium, the infant needs to be monitored for signs of hypocalcemia which include irritability, tachycardia, and a prolonged Q-T interval. The blood used in exchange transfusions may have high levels of sodium, potassium, and dextrose present due to common blood preservatives. Hyperkalemia would be evidenced by peaked T waves rather than dampened. Lethargy and poor feeding would be signs of hypercalcemia rather than hypocalcemia. Although the infant may have early hyperglycemia due to the dextrose in the blood preservative, late hypoglycemia will likely occur due to the infant's insulin response.

References: Kamath-Rayne BD, Froese PA, Thilo EH. Neonatal hyperbilirubinemia. In: Gardner SL, Carter BS, Niermeyer S, eds. *Merenstein & Gardner's Handbook of Neonatal Intensive Care: An Interprofessional Approach.* 9th ed. St. Louis, MO: Elsevier; 2021:685-686.

Nyp M, Brunkhorst JL, Reavey D, Pallato EK. Fluid and electrolyte management. In: Gardner SL, Carter BS, Niermeyer S, eds. *Merenstein & Gardner's Handbook of Neonatal Intensive Care: An Interprofessional Approach.* 9th ed. St. Louis, MO: Elsevier; 2021:421-424.

13. **(D)** Although this newborn does not strictly meet the criterion for polycythemia (venous hematocrit greater than 65%), the presence of jitteriness and difficulty feeding may indicate that the newborn is beginning to experience the effects of hyperviscosity. However, because the newborn's glucose and respiratory status are stable, the exchange can be delayed if the newborn is watched carefully and feeding and glucose level are monitored. Immediately performing a partial exchange transfusion increases the risk of gastrointestinal complications and is unwarranted at this time. Because the newborn is not experiencing any respiratory difficulties, the newborn can continue to feed if possible.

Reference: Diehl-Jones W, Fraser D. Hematologic disorders. In: Verklan MT, Walden M, Forest S, eds. *Core Curriculum for Neonatal Intensive Care Nursing.* 6th ed. St. Louis, MO: Elsevier; 2021:581-582.

14. **(A)** Hemophilia A is an X-linked recessive disease in which females are carriers and their sons evidence the disease. There is a 75% chance that there is another male with the disease in the family. Hemophilia A, in which factor VIII is deficient, is characterized by a normal or prolonged partial thromboplastin time and a normal prothrombin time and platelet count. Bleeding most commonly occurs at a circumcision site (50%). Von Willebrand disease has an autosomal-dominant inheritance pattern, and so men and women are affected alike. This disease affects a factor that adheres platelets to the endothelium and serves as a carrier for factor VIII. Because levels of the original factor are high at time of birth, bleeding in the neonatal period is rare. Bleeding is generally seen later in childhood and adolescence. Vitamin K deficiency results in the decreased activation of factors II, VII, IX, and X and of proteins C and S. This results in bleeding in the gastrointestinal system, umbilical cord, and circumcision site. In vitamin K–dependent bleeding, both the partial thromboplastin time and prothrombin time are prolonged. Idiopathic thrombocytopenia purpura is a condition in which autoantibodies bind to surface antigens on platelets, destroying them. Therefore the platelet count would be low.

References: Diehl-Jones W, Fraser D. Hematologic disorders. In: Verklan MT, Walden M, Forest S, eds. *Core Curriculum for Neonatal Intensive Care Nursing.* 6th ed. St. Louis, MO: Elsevier; 2021:582-583.

McKinney C, Warren BB, Harvey S. Newborn hematology. In: Gardner SL, Carter BS, Niermeyer S, eds. *Merenstein & Gardner's Handbook of Neonatal Intensive Care: An Interprofessional Approach.* 9th ed. St. Louis, MO: Elsevier; 2021:642-647.

15. **(B)** ABO incompatibility affects babies when mothers have blood group O and the babies have blood group A, B, or AB. While it occurs more frequently than Rh isoimmunization (partially because of the use of RhoGAM for Rh isoimmunization), the hemolytic disease is less severe. While not absolute, in some cases the infant will have a positive direct Coombs test or the presence of maternal antibodies on the infant's RBCs. Interestingly, maternal exposure to food, pollen and bacteria can initiate production of anti-A and anti-B antibodies so specific sensitization is not necessary. As a result, the antibodies can cross the placenta on the first pregnancy and impact the infant with type A, B, or AB blood.

Reference: Diehl-Jones W, Fraser D. Hematologic disorders. In: Verklan MT, Walden M, Forest S, eds. *Core Curriculum for Neonatal Intensive Care Nursing.* 6th ed. St. Louis, MO: Elsevier; 2021:574-577.

16. **(B)** Neonatal alloimmune thrombocytopenia has a similar pathophysiology to Rh incompatibility. It occurs when maternal platelets come into contact with fetal platelets containing an antigen lacking in the mother. Maternal antibodies cross the placenta and coat the fetal platelets—primarily on subsequent pregnancies. The maternal platelet count is normal. Neonatal partial thromboplastin time and prothrombin time are normal. Treatment of neonatal alloimmune thrombocytopenia includes giving the infant washed maternal platelets, which are free of the platelet antigen. Because the infant is symptomatic, the "wait and see" approach is not appropriate in this case. Giving serial random donor platelets rarely results in a sustained increase in platelets because of continued antibody destruction. The workup for neonatal alloimmune thrombocytopenia includes testing for human platelet antigens before the first random platelets are given.

Reference: Diehl-Jones W, Fraser D. Hematologic disorders. In: Verklan MT, Walden M, Forest S, eds. *Core Curriculum for Neonatal Intensive Care Nursing.* 6th ed. St. Louis, MO: Elsevier; 2021:580-581.

17. **(D)** Vitamin K deficiency will result in a lack of activation of factors II, VII, IX, and X as well as proteins C and S. These factors

are essential for common, intrinsic, and extrinsic coagulation pathways. aPPT represents the intrinsic and common pathway while PT reflects the extrinsic pathway. Both will be prolonged. Decreasing fibrinogen levels are classically seen in DIC and not vitamin K deficiency. Decreasing platelet levels (thrombocytopenia) is more typically seen in DIC and conditions related to impaired platelet production and destruction and not vitamin K deficiency. Because of the lysis of RBCs, hemolytic anemia on a peripheral blood smear is classically seen in DIC and not vitamin K deficiency.

References: Diehl-Jones W, Fraser D. Hematologic disorders. In: Verklan MT, Walden M, Forest S, eds. *Core Curriculum for Neonatal Intensive Care Nursing.* 6th ed. St. Louis, MO: Elsevier; 2021:577-579.

Blackburn ST. Hematologic and hemostatic systems. In: Blackburn ST, ed. *Maternal, Fetal, Neonatal Physiology: A Clinical Perspective.* 5th ed. St. Louis, MO: Elsevier; 2018:220-222, 236-240.

18. **(D)** Gamma irradiation prevents donor lymphocyte proliferation. Donor lymphocytes can proliferate in the extremely premature neonate causing graft-versus-host disease. Graft-versus-host disease may occur for an extended amount of time after administration of a nonirradiated transfusion and cause rash, diarrhea, hepatic dysfunction, and bone marrow suppression. Administering packed RBCs that are cytomegaly virus (CMV) negative will prevent the transmission of CMV to the immunodeficient, extremely premature neonate. Administration of packed RBC products that are compatible with the neonate's type and Rh will prevent a hemolytic reaction. With a neonate having O-positive blood, the blood type of the donor packed RBCs needs to be O as type A, B, or AB would have antigens that would cause a hemolytic reaction in the neonate's blood. The donor blood could either be Rh positive or negative since the neonate is Rh positive. Filtration of the packed RBCs at the time of donation or prior to the transfusion can decrease the number of leukocytes present in the aliquot. Performing this procedure may prevent a febrile reaction.

References: Diehl-Jones W, Fraser D. Hematologic disorders. In: Verklan MT, Walden M, Forest S, eds. *Core Curriculum for Neonatal Intensive Care Nursing.* 6th ed. St. Louis, MO: Elsevier; 2021:584.

Bagwell GA, Steward DK. Hematologic system. In: Kenner C, Altimier LB, Boykova MV, eds. *Comprehensive Neonatal Nursing Care.* 6th ed. New York: Springer Publishing Co.; 2020:350.

19. **(A)** Erythropoietin regulates the production of RBCs in an atmosphere of hypoxia. In utero, relative hypoxia causes erythropoietin levels to rise. After birth, erythropoietin levels gradually fall in an oxygen-rich environment resulting in a slow physiologic decrease of the neonate's hemoglobin. This is more pronounced in prematurity. The lowest point of the hemoglobin, without supplementary transfusions, is generally at about 8 weeks. Iatrogenic blood loss is a reason for anemia in many neonatal intensive care infants due to the amount of laboratory exams that are ordered. However, while it is a concern for many preterm neonates, iatrogenic blood loss is not the cause of anemia of prematurity. Iron supplementation for premature neonates beginning at about 2 months of age is essential to prevent iron deficiency anemia. This is particularly important when Epogen is being administered. While important to consider, however, iron deficiency is not the cause of anemia of prematurity. Underlying infections, both viral and bacterial, can cause chronic anemia. However, they are not the cause of anemia of prematurity.

References: Bagwell GA, Steward DK. Hematologic system. In: Kenner C, Altimier LB, Boykova MV, eds. *Comprehensive Neonatal Nursing Care.* 6th ed. New York: Springer Publishing Co.; 2020:335-342.

McKinney C, Warren BB, Harvey S. Newborn hematology. In: Gardner SL, Carter BS, Niermeyer S, eds. *Merenstein & Gardner's Handbook of Neonatal Intensive Care: An Interprofessional Approach.* 9th ed. St. Louis, MO: Elsevier; 2021:624-630.

20. **(D)** The American Academy of Pediatrics guidelines for phototherapy for infants at medium risk (35–37 6/7 weeks and well)

recommend considering phototherapy at a total serum bilirubin level of 13 mg/dL at 48 hours of age. Because phototherapy may be beneficial at this point, the nurse should notify the physician of the bilirubin level as it is not within the nurse's scope of practice to begin it. An exchange transfusion is recommended for infants at medium risk (35–37 6/7 weeks and well) at a bilirubin level of 19 mg/dL at 48 hours of age following intensive phototherapy.

Reference: Kamath-Rayne BD, Froese PA, Thilo EH. Neonatal hyperbilirubinemia. In: Gardner SL, Carter BS, Niermeyer S, eds. *Merenstein & Gardner's*

Handbook of Neonatal Intensive Care: An Interprofessional Approach. 9th ed. St. Louis, MO: Elsevier; 2021:676-678.

REFERENCE(S)

Kamath-Rayne BD, Froese PA, Thilo EH. Neonatal hyperbilirubinemia. In: Gardner SL, Carter BS, Niermeyer S, eds. *Merenstein & Gardner's Handbook of Neonatal Intensive Care: An Interprofessional Approach.* 9th ed. St. Louis: Elsevier; 2021:676-678.

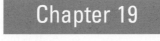

Chapter 19

Neurologic Disorders

1. A 6-hour-old, 24-week-gestation infant requires a blood gas drawn from the umbilical arterial catheter. Which statement voiced by the nurse best indicates why this infant is at risk for intracranial hemorrhage (ICH)?
   A. Umbilical arterial catheters do not allow for rapid infusions of fluid.
   B. Fluctuating cerebral blood flow velocity results in ICH.
   C. Rapid aspiration of arterial blood does not affect cerebral blood flow.
   D. Abundant and well-supported blood vessels exist in the center of the brain.

2. An infant has been diagnosed with a grade III intraventricular hemorrhage. Based on the Papile grading system, the nurse should describe grade III as:
   A. blood within the ventricles and an echogenic focus within the periventricular tissue.
   B. bleeding confined to the germinal matrix.
   C. blood within the ventricles and associated dilation of the ventricle.
   D. blood within the ventricle and no associated dilatation of the ventricle.

3. A 3-day-old, 25-week-gestational-age infant has a sudden drop in hematocrit. The nurse should initially assess for:
   A. anemia of prematurity.
   B. intracranial hemorrhage.
   C. bloody drainage from the nasogastric tube.
   D. iatrogenic blood loss from laboratory testing.

4. Which of the following nursing strategies is most beneficial to reduce the incidence of ICH?
   A. Placement of snug phototherapy mask
   B. Delaying transfer of infant from radiant warmer bed to incubator for 24 hours
   C. Positioning of bed flat for the first 72 hours of life
   D. Administration of diluted sodium bicarbonate over 30 minutes

5. Which of the following best describes periventricular leukomalacia (PVL)?
   A. It is the least common cause of brain injury in the preterm infant.
   B. PVL is not associated with motor impairment.

C. Cystic PVL can be identified on early ultrasound.
D. Hypoxia, ischemia, and inflammation are factors for PVL development.

6. The nurse should consider which of the following statements regarding neonatal seizures as most accurate?
   A. They often are the sequela of meningitis.
   B. They mimic those of an older child.
   C. Metabolic disturbances are the most common cause.
   D. Seizures cannot be stopped with limb reposition or restraint.

7. Which historical factor should the nurse consider to be most important to determine whether an infant is at risk for seizure occurrence?
   A. Initial blood glucose of 60 mg/dL
   B. Cord blood gas with a base deficit of 8 mmol/L
   C. Primary maternal herpes simplex virus outbreak during pregnancy
   D. Pharmacologic treatment of neonatal abstinence syndrome

8. Which medication is customarily the first-line drug of choice for the treatment of neonatal seizures?
   A. Lorazepam (Ativan)
   B. Phenytoin (Dilantin)
   C. Phenobarbital (Luminal)
   D. Levetiracetam (Keppra)

9. Which nursing action is of highest priority for the infant presenting with myelomeningocele in the delivery room?
   A. Place infant in the side-lying position to prevent trauma.
   B. Wrap defect in warmed, normal saline–soaked gauze.
   C. Obtain weight and length measurements.
   D. Prevent fecal contamination of the lesion.

10. An infant has a ventriculoperitoneal (VP) shunt. Which of the following signs would indicate increasing ventricular pressure and potential shunt failure?
    A. Static occipital frontal head circumference (HC) measurements
    B. Presence of overriding cranial sutures
    C. Wet burps after enteral feeding
    D. Presence of a tense fontanelle

11. Which of the following is a risk factor for shoulder dystocia and brachial plexus injury?
    A. Birth weight less than 3500 g (7 lb, 11 oz)
    B. Absence of maternal obesity
    C. Rapid second stage of labor
    D. Maternal diabetes, poorly controlled

12. An infant is brought to the nursery to be evaluated for shoulder swelling and lack of grasp in right hand with claw hand deformity. The nurse should anticipate developing a plan of care for which of the following types of brachial plexus injury?
    A. Erb palsy
    B. Klumpke paralysis
    C. Erb-Duchenne-Klumpke paralysis
    D. Phrenic nerve paralysis

13. What is the radiologic study that would be most definitive to rule out cerebral hemorrhage in the case of depressed skull fracture in a term infant?
    A. Head ultrasound (HUS)
    B. Magnetic resonance imaging
    C. Computed tomography
    D. Skull film

14. The nurse should anticipate which of the following clinical findings in an infant with a subgaleal hemorrhage?
    A. Large, firm head mass
    B. Pallor
    C. Hypertension
    D. Polycythemia

15. The nurse is instructed to assess an infant for possible facial nerve palsy. The nurse should anticipate which of the following findings on clinical examination?
    A. The paralyzed side of the face may appear edematous.
    B. The mouth is drawn to the affected side with crying.
    C. Unaffected suck.
    D. Incomplete closure of eyelids.

16. Hypoxic ischemic encephalopathy is a stepwise process resulting in neurologic injury. Which of the following should the nurse consider as the initial pathophysiologic process?
    A. Hypoxia, anaerobic metabolism, metabolic acidosis, energy failure, and neuronal death
    B. Fetal bradycardia, reperfusion injury, release of oxygen-free radicals, and neuronal death
    C. Disruption of placental or cord blood flow, fetal bradycardia, and respiratory acidosis
    D. Hypoxia, mitochondrial energy failure, and initiation of apoptosis leading to cell death

17. Which of the following infants would meet basic criteria for therapeutic hypothermia for treatment of neonatal encephalopathy?
    A. 34-week gestation with pH 6.90, base deficit of 16 mmol/L per cord gas
    B. 34-week gestation with history of an acute perinatal event with no available blood gas
    C. 41-week gestation, now 4 hours old with cord gas pH 6.80, base deficit of 17 mmol/L
    D. 38-week gestation, now 8 hours old with abnormal neurologic examination

18. A 1-hour-old, 37-week infant with hypoxia and acidosis is delivered at a community hospital without access to whole body or head cooling. While awaiting transport to a tertiary neonatal ICU, passive cooling is initiated. Which of the following statements indicates an understanding of passive cooling by the assigned nurse?
    A. Discontinuing the external heat source and monitoring body temperature with goal of 34–35°C.
    B. Passive cooling delays initiation of whole-body cooling.
    C. Gradually lower infant core temperature to 32.4°C or less.
    D. Monitor core temperature via axillary readings.

19. Which statement best characterizes neonatal meningitis?
    A. It is more common with early-onset sepsis.
    B. Signs and symptoms are nonspecific.
    C. Signs and symptoms reflect increased intracranial pressure.
    D. Morbidity is not affected by gestational age.

20. The spectrum of bilirubin-induced neurologic dysfunction ranges from acute bilirubin encephalopathy to the irreversible syndrome of kernicterus. Which clinical symptom best characterizes kernicterus?
    A. Poor sucking
    B. Sensorineural hearing impairment
    C. Opisthotonic posturing
    D. Generalized hypertonia

21. An infant's HC is measuring more than 2 standard deviations below the mean HC for gestational age. Which of the following factors in maternal history should the nurse suspect as a possible cause of the decreased HC?
    A. Consumption of one glass of wine weekly during pregnancy
    B. History of rubella infection in the first trimester
    C. Excessive weight gain during pregnancy
    D. Limited prenatal care

22. An infant has microcephaly, seizures, chorioretinitis, and cerebral calcifications. Given these assessment findings, the nurse should consider which of the following as a possible cause?
    A. Genetic disorder
    B. Inborn error of metabolism
    C. TORCH complex infection
    D. Bacterial infection

23. An infant is delivered with anencephaly. The mother questions the nurse as to the plan of care for her infant. Which of the following statements should the nurse share with the mother as the most accurate description of anencephaly?
    A. Infants often live to 1 year of age.
    B. The infant will meet criteria for brain death.
    C. Care is supportive and palliative.
    D. Anencephaly is not a lethal condition.

24. Which of the following is the most accurate description of PVL in an infant?
    A. Elevated neutrophil count in the cerebrospinal fluid
    B. Primarily affects post-term infants
    C. Insignificant finding on HUS
    D. Loss of cerebral white matter secondary to ischemic injury

25. A parent questions a nurse regarding long-term neurologic development for her 2-month-old premature infant. Which of

the following statements regarding neurodevelopment outcome should the nurse share with the parent?
A. A child may have motor delay initially but catch up by 1–2 years of age.
B. Premature infants rarely have behavioral sequelae.
C. Diagnosis of developmental delay can be made before 12 months of age.
D. Infants with intrauterine and postnatal growth failure are at decreased risk.

26. A VP shunt performs which of the following functions?
A. Connects the pulmonary artery to the subclavian artery
B. Connects the umbilical vein to the ductus venosus
C. Allows cerebrospinal fluid to drain from lateral ventricles to peritoneal cavity
D. Drains cerebrospinal fluid from lateral ventricles to the loose connective tissue below the aponeurotic membrane

27. Which of the following is the correct statement about the clinical presentation of an infant with severe hypoxic–ischemic encephalopathy as defined by Sarnat staging?
A. Dilated pupils bilaterally
B. Weak suck
C. Lethargy
D. Flaccid muscle tone

28. Brain growth is assessed most accurately by which of the following methods?
A. Daily weight measurements
B. Weekly measurements of HC
C. Weekly head ultrasonography
D. Weekly Dubowitz assessments

29. Eliciting gag, cough, and suck reflexes are an indirect assessment of the function of the:
A. cranial nerves.
B. cerebral cortex.
C. peripheral nerves.
D. autonomic nervous system.

30. Which is the most accurate statement about neonatal cerebral metabolism?
A. Hypoglycemia is well tolerated by the premature infant.
B. The neonatal brain is dependent on glucose for substrate.
C. Blood glucose levels less than 30 mg/dL are associated with decreased cerebral blood flow.
D. Blood glucose levels more than 200 mg/dL are associated with increased cerebral blood flow.

31. An infant is born with an encephalocele. Which of the following statements by the nurse would be most accurate regarding the defect?
A. Approximately 30–40% of encephaloceles occur in the occipital region of the skull.
B. They are rarely associated with other congenital anomalies.
C. Lesions generally are covered by skin or membrane.
D. Precise mechanism of encephalocele development is known.

32. An infant diagnosed with spina bifida occulta will exhibit which of the following characteristics?
A. Presence of a meningocele
B. Have a dermal lesion in the lumbosacral area
C. High likelihood of neurologic deficits
D. Herniation of the meninges at the site of the defect

33. An infant is diagnosed with microcephaly. The nurse should be aware that this represents which characteristic regarding frontal occipital circumference (FOC) of the head?
A. Greater than or equal to 2 standard deviations below the mean for age and gender.
B. Less than or equal to 2 standard deviations below the mean for age and gender.
C. Same as the HC for a term appropriate for gestational age infant.
D. FOC does not impact brain size.

34. An infant with hydrocephalus has undergone VP shunt placement and is being prepared for discharge to home. When educating the mother, the nurse should review which of the following as signs of a blocked or obstructed shunt?
A. Decreasing head size
B. Depressed fontanel
C. Increased head size
D. Redness at the shunt site

35. An infant diagnosed with a perinatal stroke is likely to exhibit which of the following characteristics?
A. Seizure activity within the first 72 hours of life.
B. Subtle seizures as the most common type.
C. Generalized motor seizures would be more common than focal motor seizures.
D. Seizure activity is present in less than 80% of newborns.

ANSWERS AND RATIONALES

1. **(B)** Umbilical arterial catheters are not used for rapid infusion of fluid due to concurrent venous access for fluids, medications, or blood products and the potential for retrograde flow. The germinal matrix is a poorly supported structure in the center of the preterm infant's brain. It is sensitive to alterations in cerebral blood flow that can occur related to blood pressure swings and rapid withdrawal of blood from arterial lines. The highest risk for germinal matrix hemorrhage is during the first week of life, so any plan of care should endeavor to prevent episodes of hypotension, hypertension, or rapid blood withdrawal.

Reference: Ditzenberger G. Neurologic disorders. In: Verklan T, Walden M, Forest S, eds. *Core Curriculum for Neonatal Intensive Care Nursing*. 6th ed. St. Louis, MO: Elsevier; 2021:646-647.

2. **(C)** Grade I is a germinal matrix hemorrhage. Grade II is an intraventricular hemorrhage without ventricular dilation. Grade III is acute ventricular dilation (clot fills >50%). Grade IV is intraventricular hemorrhage with parenchymal hemorrhage.

Reference: Ditzenberger G. Neurologic disorders. In: Verklan T, Walden M, Forest S, eds. *Core Curriculum for Neonatal Intensive Care Nursing*. 6th ed. St. Louis, MO: Elsevier; 2021:646.

3. **(B)** Anemia of prematurity would result in a more gradual drop in hematocrit. Clinical presentation of major intraventricular hemorrhage includes a sudden drop in hematocrit or failure to respond to transfusions, full anterior fontanelle, change in activity, and decreased tone. Upper gastrointestinal bleeding is uncommon in the neonate. Iatrogenic anemia from laboratory draws would

result in a more gradual drop in hematocrit and anticipated from careful recording of intake and output.

Reference: Ditzenberger G. Neurologic disorders. In: Verklan T, Walden M, Forest S, eds. *Core Curriculum for Neonatal Intensive Care Nursing*. 6th ed. St. Louis, MO: Elsevier; 2021:646.

4. **(D)** Tight phototherapy masks place pressure on the occiput, which can impede venous drainage. Delaying transfer of infant from radiant warmer bed to incubator for 24 hours will not have any impact on intracranial hemorrhage (ICH). Intracranial pressure is lowest with the head of the bed elevated to 30 degrees. Rapid infusions of sodium bicarbonate may result in elevations of carbon dioxide, causing a rapid dilation of cerebral blood vessels, which could lead to intracerebral hemorrhage. Infusing sodium bicarbonate at 4.2% concentration over 30 minutes will avoid a rapid infusion of a hyperosmolar solution.

Reference: Ditzenberger GR, Blackburn ST. Neurologic system. In: Kenner C, Altimier L, Boykova M, eds. *Comprehensive Neonatal Nursing Care*. 6th ed. New York: Springer Publishing Co.; 2020:397.

5. **(D)** Periventricular leukomalacia (PVL) is the most common brain injury seen in the preterm infants and is usually identified after 4–6 weeks of age. PVL is also the most common cause of cerebral palsy with concurrent motor impairment due to involvement of the corticospinal tracts. Data suggest that the pathogenesis of PVL is the effect of hypoxia, ischemia, and inflammation on the oligodendrocyte progenitor cells present in the periventricular white matter of infants born between 23 and 32 weeks' gestation.

Reference: Ditzenberger GR, Blackburn ST. Neurologic system. In: Kenner C, Altimier L, Boykova M, eds. *Comprehensive Neonatal Nursing Care*. 6th ed. New York: Springer Publishing Co.; 2020:399.

6. **(D)** Meningitis can certainly cause seizures but is not the most common cause. Neonates exhibit subtle seizures most frequently, which differ from that of an older child, who exhibits more outward tonic–clonic movements. The most common cause of neonatal seizures is hypoxic ischemic encephalopathy, which accounts for two-thirds of all neonatal seizures. Jittery movements will dissipate when a limb is repositioned, but focal-clonic seizures will persist with changes in limb positioning.

Reference: Hall A, Reavey D. Neurologic disorders. In: Gardner S, Carter B, Enzman-Hines M, Niermeyer S, eds. *Merenstein's & Gardner's Handbook of Neonatal Intensive Care*. 9th ed. St. Louis, MO: Elsevier; 2021:952-953.

7. **(C)** A glucose greater than 50 mg/dL reflects normoglycemia. Increased risk for hypoxic ischemic encephalopathy–associated seizures occur with a base deficit of 14 mmol/L or greater. Nonbacterial infection, specifically herpes infection during pregnancy, can place the infant at risk for seizure activity. Untreated neonatal drug withdrawal has been associated with seizures in the newborn.

Reference: Ditzenberger GR, Blackburn ST. Neurologic system. In: Kenner C, Altimier L, Boykova M, eds. *Comprehensive Neonatal Nursing Care*. 6th ed. New York: Springer Publishing Co.; 2020:387.

8. **(C)** Lorazepam, phenytoin, and levetiracetam are also medications that can be used to treat neonatal seizures if the response to phenobarbital does not control seizure activity and a second agent is required. Phenobarbital continues to be accepted as the first-line drug of choice.

Reference: Ditzenberger GR, Blackburn ST. Neurologic system. In: Kenner C, Altimier L, Boykova M, eds. *Comprehensive Neonatal Nursing Care*. 6th ed. New York: Springer Publishing Co.; 2020:389.

9. **(B)** The infant should be positioned in the prone kneeling position. Initial delivery room management is to protect the lesion by covering with sterile gauze moistened with warm sterile saline solution. Weight and length measurements are necessary but should be subsequent to initially covering and wrapping the open defect. Place a drape over the buttocks below the lesion to protect from any fecal contamination.

Reference: Ditzenberger G. Neurologic disorders. In: Verklan T, Walden M, Forest S, eds. *Core Curriculum for Neonatal Intensive Care Nursing*. 6th ed. St. Louis, MO: Elsevier; 2021:636.

10. **(D)** With ventriculoperitoneal (VP) shunt failure, intracranial pressure rises and the occipital–frontal head circumference (OFC) will increase. Static OFC indicates the VP shunt is functional. Overriding cranial sutures indicates low intracranial pressure. Wet burps after feeding is a common finding in newborns. A tense or full fontanelle is a sign of increased intracranial pressure and potential shunt failure.

Reference: Hall A, Reavey D. Neurologic disorders. In: Gardner S, Carter B, Enzman-Hines M, Niermeyer S, eds. *Merenstein's & Gardner's Handbook of Neonatal Intensive Care*. 9th ed. St. Louis, MO: Elsevier; 2021:936.

11. **(D)** A birth weight less than 3500 g does not place the infant at increased risk for shoulder dystocia, nor does a rapid second stage of labor or a mother of normal body weight. Maternal diabetes, poorly controlled, is a risk factor for shoulder dystocia and the potential for brachial plexus injury. With maternal diabetes the fetal blood glucose level exceeds normal values. The pancreas responds to the fetal blood glucose level with increased insulin production and release. Insulin is a potent growth factor and leads to macrosomia of the fetus or a large size for gestational age. Fetal macrosomia makes delivery more difficult and prone to injury.

Reference: Ditzenberger G. Neurologic disorders. In: Verklan T, Walden M, Forest S, eds. *Core Curriculum for Neonatal Intensive Care Nursing*. 6th ed. St. Louis, MO: Elsevier; 2021:642.

12. **(B)** In Erb palsy, the affected arm is abducted and internally rotated; the Moro reflex is asymmetrical with an extended elbow and wrist flexion similar to "waiter's tip" position. Klumpe paralysis exhibits swelling in the shoulder and supraclavicular fossa, which can be accompanied by clavicle fracture. Due to intrinsic muscle involvement of the hand, there is a clawlike appearance. There will be no grasp of the affected hand. Erb-Duchenne-Klumpe paralysis presents with flaccidity of the entire affected arm; Moro and grasp reflexes are absent. The phrenic nerve controls the diaphragm and is not associated with brachial plexus injury.

Reference: Ditzenberger G. Neurologic disorders. In: Verklan T, Walden M, Forest S, eds. *Core Curriculum for Neonatal Intensive Care Nursing*. 6th ed. St. Louis, MO: Elsevier; 2021:642.

13. **(C)** Cranial ultrasound is the initial imaging modality in the preterm infant. Magnetic resonance imaging is indicated to evaluate SAH or posterior fossa hemorrhage and is superior in detecting small intra axial and extra axial bleeds. Computed tomography is preferred for acute ICH and can be accomplished rapidly. Skull films cannot adequately identify hemorrhage.

Reference: Ditzenberger GR, Blackburn ST. Neurologic system. In: Kenner C, Altimier L, Boykova M, eds. *Comprehensive Neonatal Nursing Care*. 6th ed. New York: Springer Publishing Co.; 2020:404.

14. **(B)** The mass is ballotable and fluctuant upon palpation due to the large volume of blood that can accumulate in the subgaleal space. It is not uncommon for the swelling to extend into the area surrounding the ears and nape of the neck. Infants may present with signs of shock, which include a rapidly falling hematocrit, hypovolemia, pallor, hypotension, tachycardia, tachypnea, and hypotonia.

Reference: Ditzenberger GR, Blackburn ST. Neurologic system. In: Kenner C, Altimier L, Boykova M, eds. *Comprehensive Neonatal Nursing Care*. 6th ed. New York: Springer Publishing Co.; 2020:401.

15. **(A)** Facial muscles innervated by the affected facial nerve become flaccid, and slight edema may be present due to interstitial fluid accumulation secondary to lack of muscle movement. When crying, the infant's mouth is drawn to the unaffected side, not the affected side, because the affected side fails to move. The paralysis may affect oral sucking strength. The portion of the facial nerve that innervates the forehead and eyelid is generally not affected.
Reference: Ditzenberger GR, Blackburn ST. Neurologic system. In: Kenner C, Altimier L, Boykova M, eds. *Comprehensive Neonatal Nursing Care.* 6th ed. New York: Springer Publishing Co.; 2020:405.

16. **(A)** Impaired oxygen and glucose delivery to the fetus results in decreased fetal cardiac output and brain perfusion. Brain perfusion selectively shunts to the brainstem injuring the cerebral cortex, basal ganglia, and thalami as a result of diminished blood flow. The latent phase includes reperfusion, inflammation, continued apoptosis, and nearly complete failure of mitochondrial activity. Hypoxic ischemic encephalopathy can be the result of placental or cord blood flow with fetal bradycardia. However, biochemical criteria is focused on metabolic acidosis versus respiratory acidosis. In the acute phase anaerobic metabolism is utilized, followed by energy failure, release of neurotoxic agents, and cell death by necrosis or apoptosis in the later phases.
Reference: Ditzenberger GR, Blackburn ST. Neurologic system. In: Kenner C, Altimier L, Boykova M, eds. *Comprehensive Neonatal Nursing Care.* 6th ed. New York: Springer Publishing Co.; 2020:390.

17. **(C)** Candidates for therapeutic hypothermia must be greater than or equal to 36 weeks' gestation and less than 6 hours of age. At 41 weeks gestation, this infant meets basic criteria for therapeutic hypothermia based on gestational and chronological age along with biochemical criteria per blood gas.
Reference: Ditzenberger GR, Blackburn ST. Neurologic system. In: Kenner C, Altimier L, Boykova M, eds. *Comprehensive Neonatal Nursing Care.* 6th ed. New York: Springer Publishing Co.; 2020:392.

18. **(A)** Passive cooling by discontinuing the external heat source and monitoring body temperature with a goal of 34°C–35°C allows for prompt initiation of hypothermia treatment at less than 6 hours of life. Excessive cooling reflected by a core body temperature of less than 32.5°C can result in cardiac arrhythmias, electrolyte imbalances, thrombocytopenia, and coagulopathies and is contraindicated. Rectal temperatures are most accurate during the time that passive cooling is taking place.
Reference: Beauman S, Bowles S, eds. *National Association of Neonatal Nurses policies, procedures and competencies for neonatal nursing care. Procedure for induced hypothermia.* 6th ed. Chicago, IL: National Association of Neonatal Nurses; 2019:102.

19. **(B)** Meningitis is most often associated with late-onset sepsis and can be indistinguishable from that of neonatal sepsis without meningitis in that the signs and symptoms are nonspecific. Untreated meningitis can result in increased intracranial pressure. Morbidity is greater in the preterm infant.
Reference: Bodin MB, Hoffman J. Immune system. In: Kenner C, Altimier L, Boykova M, eds. *Comprehensive Neonatal Nursing Care.* 6th ed. New York: Springer Publishing Co.; 2020:262-263.

20. **(B)** Clinical signs of acute bilirubin encephalopathy include hypotonia, poor feeding, and opisthotonos posturing in later stages. Auditory abnormalities are most apparent in kernicterus because the auditory pathway is the neuronal system most sensitive to bilirubin.
Reference: Bagwell GA, Steward D. Hematologic system. In: Kenner C, Altimier L, Boykova M, eds. *Comprehensive Neonatal Nursing Care.* 6th ed. New York: Springer Publishing Co.; 2020:330.

21. **(B)** Drinking one glass of wine per week during pregnancy is not an excessive consumption. Microcephaly may be caused by teratogens, including abuse of recreational or prescription drugs, alcohol, and/or viral infection under the TORCH (toxoplasmosis, syphilis, rubella, CMV [cytomegaly virus], or herpes) spectrum. Excessive maternal weight gain may result in macrosomia and a difficult delivery, but not microcephaly. Limited prenatal care will not result in the development of microcephaly; only early detection.
Reference: Ditzenberger G. Neurologic disorders. In: Verklan T, Walden M, Forest S, eds. *Core Curriculum for Neonatal Intensive Care Nursing.* 6th ed. St. Louis, MO: Elsevier; 2021:636-637.

22. **(C)** Bacterial infection, genetic disorder, or an inborn error of metabolism would not cause this specific constellation of manifestations. Congenital CMV (TORCH spectrum) manifestations include intrauterine growth restriction, jaundice, purpura, hepatosplenomegaly, microcephaly, seizures, intracerebral calcifications, chorioretinitis, and progressive sensorineural hearing loss.
Reference: Pammi M, Brand C, Weisman L. Infection in the neonate. In: Gardner S, Carter B, Enzman-Hines M, Niermeyer S, eds. *Merenstein's & Gardner's Handbook of Neonatal Intensive Care.* 9th ed. St. Louis, MO: Elsevier; 2021:695.

23. **(C)** Infants with anencephaly usually die within the first postnatal month and most often in the first week of life; it is a lethal condition. Anencephalic infants do not meet criteria for brain death because they have degrees of brainstem function. Care should be supportive and palliative with focus on comfort and emotional support of parents.
Reference: Ditzenberger GR, Blackburn ST. Neurologic system. In: Kenner C, Altimier L, Boykova M, eds. *Comprehensive Neonatal Nursing Care.* 6th ed. New York: Springer Publishing Co.; 2020:375.

24. **(D)** An elevated neutrophil count in the cerebrospinal fluid indicates meningitis. PVL is the necrosis and then thinning or liquefaction of cerebral white matter secondary to ischemia. It occurs primarily in the preterm infant. The finding of PVL on head ultrasound is significant because it is associated with motor deficits, visual impairment, and possibly intellectual deficits.
Reference: Ditzenberger G. Neurologic disorders. In: Verklan T, Walden M, Forest S, eds. *Core Curriculum for Neonatal Intensive Care Nursing.* 6th ed. St. Louis, MO: Elsevier; 2021:652.

25. **(A)** A diagnosis of motor delay cannot take place as catch up and normalization can occur by 1–2 years of age. Behavioral problems are common in premature infants, especially extremely low birth weights, due to a higher incidence of neurologic insults. Infants who fail to achieve adequate growth are at long-term risk for adverse neurodevelopmental outcomes.
Reference: Carter A, Carter B. Discharge planning and follow-up of the neonatal intensive care unit infant. In: Gardner S, Carter B, Enzman-Hines M, Niermeyer S, eds. *Merenstein's & Gardner's Handbook of Neonatal Intensive Care.* 9th ed. St. Louis, MO: Elsevier; 2021:1154.

26. **(D)** A Blalock-Taussig shunt surgically connects the pulmonary artery to the subclavian artery. The ductus venosus connects the umbilical vein to the inferior vena cava. Cerebrospinal fluid drains from the lateral ventricles to the peritoneal cavity. A subgaleal shunt drains cerebrospinal fluid from the lateral ventricles to the space between the periosteum of the skull and the aponeurotic membrane, where it is eventually reabsorbed.
Reference: Ditzenberger GR, Blackburn ST. Neurologic system. In: Kenner C, Altimier L, Boykova M, eds. *Comprehensive Neonatal Nursing Care.* 6th ed. New York: Springer Publishing Co.; 2020:398-399.

27. **(D)** Mildly affected infants demonstrate dilated pupils bilaterally; severely affected infants have unequal, variable pupils. Absent suck is present in severely affected infants, mildly affected infants will have a weak suck. Lethargy or an obtunded level of

conscious is noted in the moderately affected infant. Flaccid/absent muscle tone is present in the severely affected infant.

Reference: Ditzenberger G. Neurologic disorders. In: Verklan T, Walden M, Forest S, eds. *Core Curriculum for Neonatal Intensive Care Nursing.* 6th ed. St. Louis, MO: Elsevier; 2021:649-650.

28. **(B)** Daily weight is a measure of overall growth and is not specific to the brain. In the absence of pathology such as hydrocephalus or craniosynostosis, head circumference is the best measure of brain growth. Head ultrasonography details anatomic structures and measures ventricular size, but is not used to measure brain growth or size. The Dubowitz examination assesses gestational age at birth.

Reference: Tappero E. Physical assessment. In: Verklan T, Walden M, Forest S, eds. *Core Curriculum for Neonatal Intensive Care Nursing.* 6th ed. St. Louis, MO: Elsevier; 2021:105.

29. **(A)** Cranial nerve IX is responsible for taste, swallowing, and gagging. Cranial nerve XII is responsible for tongue movement and symmetric movements allowing sucking. The cerebral cortex is the seat of the intellect. Peripheral nerves support movement and sensation of the extremities. The autonomic nervous system regulates functions such as heart rate, breathing, secretions, and gastrointestinal motility.

Reference: Ditzenberger G. Neurologic disorders. In: Verklan T, Walden M, Forest S, eds. *Core Curriculum for Neonatal Intensive Care Nursing.* 6th ed. St. Louis, MO: Elsevier; 2021:633.

30. **(B)** The neonatal central nervous system is quickly and significantly affected by hypoglycemia. Glycogen stores are minimal or nonexistent in the preterm infant, and the brain requires oxygen and glucose for growth and metabolism. The neonatal brain is dependent on glucose and cannot use alternative substrate. Blood glucose levels of less than 30 mg/dL are associated with increased cerebral blood flow in an attempt to maintain glucose levels. Hyperglycemia does not have this effect on cerebral blood flow.

Reference: Ditzenberger G. Neurologic disorders. In: Verklan T, Walden M, Forest S, eds. *Core Curriculum for Neonatal Intensive Care Nursing.* 6th ed. St. Louis, MO: Elsevier; 2021:631.

31. **(C)** Approximately 70%–80% of lesions occur in the occipital area of the skull. Approximately 50% of neonates with encephaloceles have associated defects such as microcephaly, cleft lip/palate, and hydrocephalus. The lesions are usually covered by skin or membrane. Cerebral spinal fluid may leak from the lesion. The precise mechanism is unclear in terms of etiology. Genetic and environmental factors have been reported but have not been proven.

Reference: Ditzenberger G. Neurologic disorders. In: Verklan T, Walden M, Forest S, eds. *Core Curriculum for Neonatal Intensive Care Nursing.* 6th ed. St. Louis, MO: Elsevier; 2021:635.

32. **(B)** Infants with spina bifida manifesta have the presence of a meningocele or myelomeningocele. Those with spina bifida occulta do not have a meningocele or myelomeningocele. Spina bifida occulta presents with a dermal lesion in the lumbosacral area in over 80% of cases. Neurological deficits are not common in infants with spina bifida occulta. Spina bifida occulta is a separation of the overlying ectoderm from the neural tube. This will present as a cutaneous dimple, mass or hair tuft absent any herniation of the meninges.

Reference: Ditzenberger G. Neurologic disorders. In: Verklan T, Walden M, Forest S, eds. *Core Curriculum for Neonatal Intensive Care Nursing.* 6th ed. St. Louis, MO: Elsevier; 2021:635-636.

33. **(A)** Microcephaly is defined as a FOC of greater than or equal to 2 standard deviations below the mean for age and gender. It is not less than or equal to 2 standard deviations below the mean for age and gender. Microcephalic infants, do not have the same FOC as a term appropriate-for-gestational-age infant. FOC does impact brain size. With microcephaly, the brain size is reduced compared to an infant with a normal FOC circumference.

Reference: Ditzenberger G. Neurologic disorders. In: Verklan T, Walden M, Forest S, eds. *Core Curriculum for Neonatal Intensive Care Nursing.* 6th ed. St. Louis, MO: Elsevier; 2021:636.

34. **(C)** A decreasing head size and depressed fontanel would indicate the shunt is working and without any blockage or obstruction. An increased head size would indicate that the shunt may be obstructed and is not adequately draining cerebral spinal fluid. Redness at the shunt site would be an indicator or infection versus blockage, especially when associated with a febrile state.

Reference: Ditzenberger G. Neurologic disorders. In: Verklan T, Walden M, Forest S, eds. *Core Curriculum for Neonatal Intensive Care Nursing.* 6th ed. St. Louis, MO: Elsevier; 2021:638.

35. **(A)** Most infants with perinatal stroke exhibit seizures within the first 72 hours of life. It is often the earliest manifestation of a perinatal stroke in an otherwise healthy appearing newborn. Subtle seizures occur in 17% of cases, focal motor seizures occur in 50% of cases and generalized motor occur is 33% of cases. Seizure activity occurs in 85%–92% of infants who experience a perinatal stroke.

Reference: Ditzenberger GR, Blackburn ST. Neurologic system. In: Kenner C, Lott JW, eds. *Comprehensive Neonatal Nursing Care.* 6th ed. New York: Springer Publishing Co.; 2020:403.

Chapter 20

Renal and Genitourinary Disorders

1. A 14-day-old term infant is noted upon assessment to have an intact and moist umbilical cord. The nurse should perform which of the following actions?
   A. Keep the umbilical area open to air by folding down the diaper.
   B. Apply silver nitrate to the cord area.
   C. Notify the physician of this finding.
   D. Swab the cord with alcohol with each diaper change.

2. The functional unit of the kidney is the:
   A. collecting duct.
   B. ureteric bud.
   C. nephron.
   D. Bowman capsule.

3. An adult quantity of nephrons is achieved by how many weeks of gestational age?

A. 10
B. 14
C. 24
D. 34

4. A 3-month-old, former 24-week infant is scheduled for a voiding cystourethrogram. The nurse should include which of the following information statements in the parent education plan?
   A. This procedure is diagnostic for multicystic kidney disease.
   B. Results of the study will determine need for daily antibiotic prophylaxis.
   C. A nasogastric tube will be inserted for the administration of radiopaque dye.
   D. This procedure will require general anesthesia.

5. The most common renal congenital abnormality detected on prenatal ultrasound is:
   A. renal agenesis.
   B. hydronephrosis.
   C. patent urachus.
   D. hypospadias.

6. An infant is diagnosed with acute kidney injury. The nurse should anticipate which of the following clinical symptoms?
   A. Hyperkalemia
   B. Metabolic alkalosis
   C. Decreased serum blood urea nitrogen
   D. Decreased serum creatinine

7. When assessing an infant who has Potter sequence, the nurse should expect which of the following findings?
   A. Arthrogryposis
   B. Pulmonary hyperplasia
   C. Prominent chin
   D. Narrow-set eyes

8. The nurse should be aware that the highest rate of blood flow to the kidneys occurs within which of the following time frames?
   A. 23 weeks' gestation
   B. 36 weeks' gestation
   C. 1 hour after delivery
   D. 2 weeks of life

9. Which of the following findings should alert the nurse to a potential renal problem?
   A. Single umbilical artery
   B. History of polyhydramnios
   C. Bilious emesis
   D. Presence of sacral anomaly

10. A 1-day-old term male infant presents with left-sided scrotal edema that is painful on examination and bluish in color. Which of the following radiologic studies should the nurse anticipate being included in the plan of care?
    A. Renal ultrasound
    B. Voiding cystourethrogram
    C. Scrotal ultrasound
    D. Spinal ultrasound

11. The main structures of the nephron from proximal to distal are:

A. distal convoluted tubule, glomerulus, and ascending and descending loop of Henle.
B. glomerulus, descending and ascending loop of Henle, and distal convoluted tubule.
C. glomerulus, distal convoluted tubule, and ascending and descending loop of Henle.
D. descending and ascending loop of Henle, glomerulus, and distal convoluted tubule.

12. A nurse notes the presence of a chordee during an admission physical examination of a term newborn male. This finding is most commonly associated with which of the following?
    A. Cryptorchidism
    B. Hydrocele
    C. Hypospadias
    D. Ambiguous genitalia

13. During fetal development, the structure that will eventually give rise to the vas deferens is the:
    A. metanephros.
    B. mesonephros.
    C. pronephros.
    D. macronephros.

14. When assessing a 2-week-old infant who has a patent urachus, the nurse would expect to identify which of these clinical findings?
    A. A soft swelling or bulge at or near the umbilicus
    B. A transparent, membranous sac protruding from the umbilicus that contains the intestines and other abdominal organs
    C. An opening that forms next to the umbilicus allowing the intestines and other abdominal organs to pass through
    D. Excessive amounts of clear drainage from the umbilicus and retraction of the umbilical cord during urination

15. An extremely low-birth-weight, 26-weeks-gestation infant has a potassium level of 7.5 mEq/L on day 4 of life. A repeat serum potassium level is collected, and the result is verified. The nurse begins to observe tall, peaked T-waves and a wide QRS complex on the cardiorespiratory monitor. Of the following, which can the nurse anticipate the advanced practice provider to order first?
    A. Calcium gluconate
    B. Insulin and dextrose bolus
    C. Sodium bicarbonate
    D. Sodium polystyrene (Kayexalate)

16. Nephrogenesis in the neonate is complete by how many weeks gestation?
    A. 4
    B. 8
    C. 16
    D. 34

17. A term neonate is born to a mother with an unremarkable prenatal history who received adequate prenatal care. The newborn is delivered via spontaneous vaginal delivery. The infant, now 18 hours old, has failed to void. The nurse should recognize the best explanation for this finding is:
    A. the infant has a urinary tract infection.
    B. this is a normal for an infant of this age.

C. the infant is dehydrated.

D. the result of a congenital disorder.

18. The primary function of the fetal kidney is:
   A. regulation of fetal blood pressure.
   B. removal of metabolic waste.
   C. formation and excretion of urine to maintain amniotic fluid levels.
   D. maintenance of fluid and electrolyte balance.

19. A 37-week neonate is delivered by emergent cesarean delivery secondary to placental abruption. The infant required prolonged resuscitation for 15 minutes using intubation, compressions, and epinephrine. Seizures occur within 30 minutes of delivery. Therapeutic hypothermia is initiated by 2 hours of age. Immediate management of this infant would consist of:
   A. obtaining a magnetic resonance imaging.
   B. prophylactic theophylline administration.
   C. peritoneal dialysis.
   D. vasopressor support.

20. Which of these observations of an infant who has Potter sequence would be most important for a nurse to consider when planning the immediate care for infant?
   A. Arthrogryposis
   B. Delayed urine output
   C. Respiratory distress
   D. Hypotension

21. Which of the following umbilical cord situations would alert the nurse to a potential renal problem?
   A. Presence of two umbilical veins and a single umbilical artery
   B. Presence of two umbilical arteries and a single umbilical vein
   C. True knot in cord present at time of delivery
   D. Presence of prolapsed cord

22. A 1-day-old term male infant develops right-sided scrotal edema with a bluish appearance. Which of the following radiologic studies should the nurse anticipate being included in the plan of care?
   A. Radioisotopic renal scanning
   B. Abdominal x-ray
   C. Scrotal ultrasound
   D. Abdominal computed tomography

ANSWERS AND RATIONALES

1. **(C)** A patent urachus is a persistent opening of the urachus to the umbilicus, to the bladder, or to both the bladder and the umbilicus. It may warrant surgical closure, and the infant should be closely monitored for urinary tract infections. A moist umbilicus at 2 weeks of age despite appropriate cord care is not a normal finding and warrants physician evaluation for patent urachus. Silver nitrate or alcohol applications will not correct the condition.

References: Briggs KB, Rentea RM. Patent urachus. In: *StatPearls*. Treasure Island, FL: StatPearls Publishing; 2022. Available at: http://www.ncbi.nlm.nih.gov/books/NBK557723/.

Cavaliere TA. Genitourinary assessment. In: Tappero EP, Holyfield ME, eds. *Physical Assessment of the Newborn: A Comprehensive Approach to the Art of Physical Examination*. 6th ed. New York: Springer Publishing Company; 2018:121-137.

2. **(C)** The nephron is the functional unit of the kidney. The collecting duct assists in reabsorption of fluid and acid–base balance and is considered part of the nephron. The ureteric bud is an embryologic structure that expands to become the glomerulus and some elements of the nephron. Bowman capsule is a capillary bed associated with each nephron where filtration of fluid and solutes occur.

References: Maguire D. Renal and genitourinary disorders. In: Verklan T, Walden M, Forest S, eds. *Core Curriculum for Neonatal Intensive Care Nursing*. 6th ed. St. Louis, MO: Elsevier; 2021:618.

Hall JE, Hall ME. The urinary system: Functional anatomy and urine formation by the kidneys. In: Hall JE, Hall ME, eds. *Guyton and Hall Textbook of Medical Physiology*. 14th ed. Philadelphia, PA: Elsevier; 2021:321-330.

Vogt BA, Springel T. The kidney and the urinary tract of the neonate. In: Martin RJ, Fanaroff AA, Walsh MC, eds. *Fanaroff and Martin's Neonatal-Perinatal Medicine: Diseases of the Fetus and Infant*. 11th ed. Philadelphia, PA: Mosby; 2020:1871-1895.

3. **(D)** By 34 weeks' gestation nephrogenesis is complete and each kidney contains 800,000–1,200,000 nephrons.

Reference: Vogt BA, Springel T. The kidney and the urinary tract of the neonate. In: Martin RJ, Fanaroff AA, Walsh MC, eds. *Fanaroff and Martin's Neonatal-Perinatal Medicine: Diseases of the Fetus and Infant*. 11th ed. Philadelphia, PA: Mosby; 2020:1871-1895.

4. **(B)** A voiding cystourethrogram (VCUG) will evaluate for the presence of vesicoureteral reflux (VUR). If VUR is noted on VCUG, then prolonged antibiotic prophylaxis may be necessary to prevent urinary tract infections. It is performed by instilling radiopaque agent into the bladder by urinary catheter; no nasogastric tube is necessary for the study. The infant is awake for the procedure and does not require general anesthesia. It does not aid in the diagnosis of multicystic kidney disease.

Reference: Vogt BA, Springel T. The kidney and the urinary tract of the neonate. In: Martin RJ, Fanaroff AA, Walsh MC, eds. *Fanaroff and Martin's Neonatal-Perinatal Medicine: Diseases of the Fetus and Infant*. 11th ed. Philadelphia, PA: Mosby; 2020:1871-1895.

5. **(B)** Hydronephrosis is the most common congenital abnormality detected on prenatal ultrasound: 1%–5% of all pregnancies. Renal agenesis occurs in 1 in 1000 to 1 in 3000 births. Hypospadias occurs between 0.3% and 0.8% of male newborns. Patent urachus has an incidence of 2 per 100,000 live births.

References: Bates CM, Schwaderer AL. Clinical evaluation of renal and urinary tract disease. In: Gleason CA, Juul SE, eds. *Avery's Diseases of the Newborn*. 10th ed. Philadelphia, PA: Elsevier; 2018:1274-1279.

Vogt BA, Springel T. The kidney and the urinary tract of the neonate. In: Martin RJ, Fanaroff AA, Walsh MC, eds. *Fanaroff and Martin's Neonatal-Perinatal Medicine: Diseases of the Fetus and Infant*. 11th ed. Philadelphia, PA: Mosby; 2020:1871-1895.

Merguerian PA, Rowe CK. Developmental abnormalities of the genitourinary system. In: Gleason CA, Juul SE, eds. *Avery's Diseases of the Newborn*. 10th ed. Philadelphia, PA: Elsevier; 2018:1260-1273.

6. **(A)** Acute kidney injury (AKI) is associated with hyperkalemia. It is also associated with metabolic acidosis, not metabolic alkalosis. Serum creatinine and blood urea nitrogen is elevated with AKI rather than decreased.

Reference: Vogt BA, Springel T. The kidney and the urinary tract of the neonate. In: Martin RJ, Fanaroff AA, Walsh MC, eds. *Fanaroff and Martin's Neonatal-Perinatal Medicine: Diseases of the Fetus and Infant*. 11th ed. Philadelphia, PA: Mosby; 2020:1871-1895.

7. **(A)** Arthrogryposis is a common finding with Potter sequence. Pulmonary hypoplasia is common due to anhydramnios. A receding chin and wide-set eyes are other features of the syndrome.

Reference: Maguire D. Renal and genitourinary disorders. In: Verklan T, Walden M, Forest S, eds. *Core Curriculum for Neonatal Intensive Care Nursing*. 6th ed. St. Louis, MO: Elsevier; 2021:622.

8. **(C)** There is high vascular resistance in the kidneys in utero. Renal blood flow increases gradually throughout gestation, and there is a dramatic increase immediately after birth. Renal blood flow does not reach adult levels until 2 years of age.

Reference: Vogt BA, Springel T. The kidney and the urinary tract of the neonate. In: Martin RJ, Fanaroff AA, Walsh MC, eds. *Fanaroff and Martin's Neonatal-Perinatal Medicine: Diseases of the Fetus and Infant.* 11th ed. Philadelphia, PA: Mosby; 2020:1871-1895.

9. **(A)** A single umbilical artery is concerning for renal abnormalities. Polyhydramnios is associated with gastrointestinal anomalies such as tracheoesophageal fistula. Bilious emesis is a finding consistent with bowel obstruction. Sacral anomalies are not generally associated with renal abnormalities related to the timing of embryologic formation.

Reference: Palazzi DL, Brandt ML. *Care of the Umbilicus and Management of Umbilical Disorders.* Waltham, MA: UpToDate; 2022.

10. **(C)** This presentation is concerning for testicular torsion. The best evaluation tool in scrotal pathology is ultrasound. The other studies do not assist in the diagnosis of an acute scrotum.

Reference: Maguire D. Renal and genitourinary disorders. In: Verklan T, Walden M, Forest S, eds. *Core Curriculum for Neonatal Intensive Care Nursing.* 6th ed. St. Louis, MO: Elsevier; 2021:627.

11. **(B)** The nephron consists of a glomerulus, descending and ascending loops of Henle, and distal convoluted tubule.

Reference: Scanga CB, Tkacs NC. Kidneys. In: Tkacs NC, Herrmann LL, Johnson R, eds. *Advanced Physiology and Pathophysiology: Essentials for Clinical Practice.* New York: Springer Publishing; 2020:427-466.

12. **(C)** Three anomalies typically found with hypospadias are ectopic opening of the urethral meatus, chordee, and hooded foreskin. Cryptorchidism is a failure of the testes to descend into the scrotal sac. Hydrocele is a fluid collection within the scrotum. Ambiguous genitalia vary in terms of physical examination findings, depending on the specifics of the individual defect (e.g., micropenis, enlarged clitoris, or labia).

Reference: Maguire D. Renal and genitourinary disorders. In: Verklan T, Walden M, Forest S, eds. *Core Curriculum for Neonatal Intensive Care Nursing.* 6th ed. St. Louis, MO: Elsevier; 2021:627.

13. **(B)** The metanephros begins development at 5 weeks of gestation and will become the definitive kidney. By the end of the second month of gestation, most portions of the mesonephros disappear. However, a few caudal tubules remain in close proximity to the testis and ovaries, developing into the vas deferens in males and remaining as remnant tissue in females. The pronephros is a vestigial structure that disappears by the fourth week of gestation. The macronephros is not a structure.

Reference: Maguire D. Renal and genitourinary disorders. In: Verklan T, Walden M, Forest S, eds. *Core Curriculum for Neonatal Intensive Care Nursing.* 6th ed. St. Louis, MO: Elsevier; 2021:627.

14. **(D)** An umbilical hernia is a protrusion of abdominal contents into the hernia, which is soft and easily reducible. An omphalocele is an abdominal wall defect that is a herniation of abdominal contents into the umbilical cord. The hernia is contained within a translucent sac that is contiguous with the umbilical cord. Gastroschisis is a defect in the abdominal wall through which the viscera protrude. There is no sac covering this defect, and the umbilical cord is discrete from it. The gastroschisis is usually to the right of midline. The urachus is an embryologic structure that connects the fetal bladder with the umbilicus. Postnatal patency of the urachal remnant can result in a clear discharge (urine) from an otherwise normal appearing umbilical cord. Urinary drainage from an urachal remnant can lead to umbilical granuloma, redness, or swelling below the umbilicus. A sign of a persistent urachus is retraction of the umbilical cord during urination.

Reference: Tappero EP, Honeyfield ME. *Physical Assessment of the Newborn: A Comprehensive Approach to the Art of Examination.* 6th ed. New York: Springer; 2018.

15. **(A)** Given the observed electrocardiogram changes, the nurse can anticipate that calcium gluconate will be ordered first. Improvement should occur in 1–5 minutes. Insulin and glucose drive potassium into the cells which reduces serum potassium levels. Onset of action usually occurs within 15 minutes; however, correcting the cardiac arrhythmia takes precedence. Sodium bicarbonate is most effective if the infant is acidotic. However, it is no longer recommended in the management of metabolic acidosis in the neonate due to its adverse effects. Sodium polystyrene removes potassium form the gut in exchange for sodium. It should not be used in extremely low–birth-weight infants due to its adverse effects.

Reference: Gomella T, Eyal F, Bany Mohammed F. *Gomella's Neonatology: Management, Procedures, On-Call Problems, Diseases and Drugs.* 8th ed. New York: McGraw-Hill; 2020.

16. **(D)** By the fourth week of gestation, the pronephros, the primitive and nonfictional kidney, appears. By the eighth week of gestation, the first nephrons are formed. By 16 weeks' gestation, the kidneys can be visualized in most fetuses on ultrasonography. By 34 weeks' gestation, nephrogenesis is complete and each kidney contains 800,000–1.2 million nephrons. Maturation and hypertrophy of the nephrons continue into infancy.

References: Blackburn ST. *Maternal, Fetal, & Neonatal Physiology: A Clinical Perspective.* 5th ed. St. Louis, MO: Elsevier; 2018.

Vogt BA, Springel T. The kidney and the urinary tract of the neonate. In: Martin RJ, Fanaroff AA, Walsh MC, eds. *Fanaroff and Martin's Neonatal-Perinatal Medicine: Diseases of the Fetus and Infant.* 11th ed. Philadelphia, PA: Mosby; 2020:1871-1895.

17. **(B)** Urinary tract infections are very uncommon in the first few days of life. The first void following delivery usually occurs within the first 24 hours but can be delayed up to 30 hours. All infants, unless renal function is impaired, should have their initial void by 48 hours of age. Voiding that occurs in the delivery room or with parents may be missed or not recorded. Dehydration and decreased urine output can occur over the course of the first few days of life particularly in infants who are exclusively breastfed and whose mothers may experience low milk production. Prenatal ultrasounds are the primary tool to diagnosis renal and urinary track disorders. Since the mother received good prenatal care and her prenatal history was unremarkable, undiagnosed fetal congenital disorders are less likely.

References: Bates CM, Scheaderer AL. Clinical evaluation of renal and urinary tract disease. In: Gleason CA, Juul SE, eds. *Avery's Diseases of the Newborn.* 10th ed. Philadelphia, PA: Elsevier; 2018:1272-1279.

Blackburn ST. *Maternal, Fetal, & Neonatal Physiology: A Clinical Perspective.* 5th ed. St. Louis, MO: Elsevier; 2018.

Vogt BA, Springel T. The kidney and the urinary tract of the neonate. In: Martin RJ, Fanaroff AA, Walsh MC, eds. *Fanaroff and Martin's Neonatal-Perinatal Medicine: Diseases of the Fetus and Infant.* 11th ed. Philadelphia, PA: Mosby; 2020:1871-1895.

18. **(C)** Prenatally, the placenta is the primary regulator of fetal blood pressure. Postnatally, the kidney will assume the function of waste removal. The most important function of the fetal kidney is the form and excrete urine to maintain adequate amniotic fluid levels. By contributing to amniotic fluid, the fetal kidney has an essential role in the normal development of the fetus. In utero, the kidneys play only a minor role in regulating fluids and electrolytes; this function is primarily maintained by the placenta.

References: Cadnapahornchai MA, Soranno DE, Bisio TJ, Woloschuk R, Kirkley M. Neonatal nephrology. In: Gardner SL, Carter BS, Enzman-Hines M, Niermeyer S, eds. *Merenstein & Gardner's Handbook of Neonatal Intensive Care: An Interprofessional Approach.* 9th ed. St. Louis, MO: Elsevier; 2021:886-928.

Maguire D. Renal and genitourinary disorders. In: Verklan T, Walden M, Forest S, eds. *Core Curriculum of Neonatal Intensive Care Nursing*. 6th ed. St. Louis, MO: Elsevier; 2021:617-628.

19. **(B)** Once initiated, the infant should be cooled for 72 hours. A magnetic resonance imaging should be obtained after the infant has been rewarmed. The infant is at high risk of developing AKI due to perinatal asphyxia. Prophylactic theophylline has been shown to reduce the incidence of AKI in asphyxiated neonates if given within the first hour of life. Renal replacement therapy is rarely needed in neonates with AKI unless maximum management fails to maintain acceptable fluid and electrolyte levels. Vasopressor support may be needed to maintain hemodynamic stability to prevent the development of AKI but the infant's current condition does not support prophylactic treatment.

References: Maguire D. Renal and genitourinary disorders. In: Verklan T, Walden M, Forest S, eds. *Core Curriculum of Neonatal Intensive Care Nursing*. 6th ed. St. Louis, MO: Elsevier; 2021:617-628.

McEwen ST, Vogt BA. The kidney. In: Fanaroff AA, Fanaroff JM, eds. *Klaus & Fanaroff's Care of the High-Risk Neonate*. 7th ed. St. Louis, MO: Elsevier; 2020:333-351.

20. **(C)** Arthrogryposis is a common finding in infants with Potter sequence due to oligohydramnios and uterine wall compression; however, it should not be nurse's immediate concern. Potter sequence occurs in infants with bilateral renal agenesis. The nurse should not expect urine output to be delayed, but nonexistent. Oligohydramnios results in pulmonary hypoplasia and postnatal respiratory distress. High-pressure ventilatory support may be needed to ventilate and oxygenate the neonate. Chest tube placement may be required in neonates who develop a pneumothorax. Next to pulmonary hypoplasia, severe hypotension is responsible

for poor survival. However, addressing the infant's respiratory status takes precedence.

References: Engen R, Hingorani S. Developmental abnormalities of the kidneys. In: Gleason CA, Juul SE, eds. *Avery's Diseases of the Newborn*. 10th ed. Philadelphia, PA: Elsevier; 2018:1250-1259.

Maguire D. Renal and genitourinary disorders. In: Verklan T, Walden M, Forest S, eds. *Core Curriculum of Neonatal Intensive Care Nursing*. 6th ed. St. Louis, MO: Elsevier; 2021:617-628.

21. **(A)** A single umbilical artery has been associated with an increased risk of genitourinary abnormalities. Two arteries and one vein are the normal vessel configuration in the umbilical cord. A true knot in the cord can occur as a result of fetal movement in utero and may compromise overall fetal circulation. A prolapsed cord is an intrapartum complication that has the potential to compromise overall blood flow to the fetus during the delivery phase.

References: Maguire D. Renal and genitourinary disorders. In: Verklan T, Walden M, Forest S, eds. *Core Curriculum of Neonatal Intensive Care Nursing*. 6th ed. St. Louis, MO: Elsevier; 2021:617-628.

22. **(C)** This presentation is concerning for testicular torsion. Radio isotopic renal scanning is useful to determine kidney size and identify obstruction or renal scarring. An abdominal x-ray can identify masses, presence of free air and obstructions but would not be helpful in the diagnosis of scrotal pathology. The best evaluation tool in scrotal pathology is ultrasound. An abdominal computed tomography is useful in the diagnosis of renal tumors, abscesses, and nephrolithiasis.

Reference: Maguire D. Renal and genitourinary disorders. In: Verklan T, Walden M, Forest S, eds. *Core Curriculum of Neonatal Intensive Care Nursing*. 6th ed. St. Louis, MO: Elsevier; 2021:617-628.

Chapter 21

Genetics and Congenital Abnormalities

1. The parents of an infant with an isolated cardiac defect ask the nurse if either of them caused their baby to have this anomaly. The best response is based on which of the following?
   A. There is no genetic basis or inheritance pattern for cardiac defects.
   B. Most cardiac defects are inherited from paternal genes.
   C. Most cardiac defects are inherited from maternal genes.
   D. The etiology of congenital heart defects is considered multifactorial.

2. A newborn infant with suspected trisomy 21 has a protruding tongue, hypotonia, and prominent epicanthal folds. After a karyotype is sent, what should be done next?
   A. Nothing because infants with trisomy 21 have few problems.
   B. Orthopedic consult to assess for fractures/abnormalities.
   C. Echocardiogram to assess for cardiac defects.
   D. Neurology consult to assess for seizures.

3. The parents of an infant with cystic fibrosis ask the nurse if their future offspring could also have this disorder. What is the nurse's best response?

   A. Because cystic fibrosis is an autosomal dominant condition, there is a 50% chance with each pregnancy of having another affected offspring.
   B. Because cystic fibrosis is an autosomal recessive condition, there is a 25% chance with each pregnancy of having another affected offspring.
   C. Cystic fibrosis is caused by a chromosomal microdeletion, and no future offspring will have this disorder.
   D. Cystic fibrosis is an X-linked recessive disorder, and only future male offspring will have this disorder.

4. An infant is born with an amputated hand caused by amniotic bands. This defect is an example of which of the following?
   A. Sequence
   B. Disruption
   C. Deformation
   D. Malformation

5. An infant has been diagnosed with a genetic disorder. The mother of the infant does not exhibit the disorder but is a carrier. The mother's brother does have the disorder. What should the mother know about this disorder?

A. It is considered an X-linked recessive disorder.
B. It is considered an X-linked dominant disorder.
C. It is considered an autosomal recessive disorder.
D. It is considered an autosomal dominant disorder.

6. An infant is observed to have prominent epicanthal folds, a flat face, a protruding tongue, and a herniated umbilicus. What genetic disorder does this infant likely have?
A. Trisomy 13
B. Trisomy 18
C. Trisomy 21
D. Turner syndrome

7. Which of the following should be performed to confirm a diagnosis of DiGeorge syndrome?
A. Rectal biopsy
B. Electrocardiography
C. Oxygen challenge test
D. Fluorescence in situ hybridization chromosomal analysis

8. Which of the following is true of an autosomal dominant disorder?
A. There is a 25% chance with each pregnancy of having an affected offspring.
B. There is a 50% chance with each pregnancy of having an affected offspring.
C. Only female offspring are affected.
D. Only male offspring are affected.

9. An infant is transferred to a neonatal intensive care unit with multiple anomalies, including omphalocele, large tongue, and hypoglycemia. What is the suspected diagnosis?
A. Beckwith-Wiedemann syndrome
B. VATER association
C. DiGeorge syndrome
D. Turner syndrome

10. Patterns of predictable methods of inheritance include which of the following?
A. X-linked recessive
B. Deletions
C. Trisomy 21
D. Translocations

11. If a prenatal quad screen was positive for risk of trisomy 18, the next step would be to:
A. repeat the quad screen.
B. obtain a diagnostic test for trisomy 18.
C. send urine for organic acids.
D. obtain a CT scan.

12. What distinguishes a sequence from a syndrome?
A. A sequence and syndrome are the same.
B. A syndrome involves random occurrence; a sequence is always inherited.
C. A sequence is initiated by a single malformation; a syndrome has multiple anomalies occurring simultaneously.
D. A sequence cascade occurs more often than a syndrome.

13. Which of the following cases are the mostly likely causes of absent or mild symptoms of trisomy 21?

A. The extra the 21st chromosome is inherited from the mother.
B. Mosaicism for trisomy 21; translocation 14/21 or 21/22.
C. The extra 21st chromosome is inherited from the father.
D. Monosomy of the 21st chromosome.

14. Which of the following syndromes would be suspected from an infant (observed or phenotype) with the following: malformed ears, cataracts both eyes, rocker bottom feet, polydactyly, omphalocele?
A. Trisomy 13
B. Trisomy 21
C. Trisomy 18
D. VACTERL

ANSWERS AND RATIONALES

1. **(D)** The exact cause of most cardiac defects (85%) is unknown and believed to be due to a complex interaction between genetic and environmental factors. There is some genetic basis for cardiac defects. Ten to twelve percent of congenital heart defects are due to chromosomal factors, and 1%–2% are due to genetic factors. Paternal genes are not known to cause cardiac defects. Although maternal risk factors have been implicated as the cause of some congenital cardiac defects, maternal genes are not known to cause cardiac defects.

Reference: American Heart Association (AHA). *Understand Your Risk for Congenital Heart Defects.* 2022. Available at: https://www.heart.org/en/health-topics/congenital-heart-defects/understand-your-risk-for-congenital-heart-defects. Reviewed March 22, 2022; Accessed January 28, 2023.

Sadowski SL, Verklan MT. Cardiovascular disorders. In: Verklan MT, Walden M, Forest S, eds. *Core Curriculum for Neonatal Intensive Care Nursing.* 6th ed. St. Louis, MO: Elsevier; 2021:460-503.

2. **(C)** Because up to 50% of infants with trisomy 21 have some form of congenital heart disease, an echocardiogram should be done as soon as possible after birth. Additional workup is warranted, because infants with trisomy 21 are at risk for multiple problems, including cardiac, gastrointestinal, and hematologic disorders. Orthopedic problems and seizures are not common in infants with trisomy 21.

References: American Academy of Pediatrics (AAP). *Atlantoaxial Instability in Children with Down Syndrome.* Available at: https://www.healthychildren.org/English/health-issues/conditions/developmental-disabilities/Pages/Atlantoaxial-Instability-in-Children-with-Down-Syndrome.aspx. Updated February 28, 2023; Accessed Sept 25, 2023.

American Heart Association. *Complete Atrioventricular Canal Defect.* 2022. Available at: https://www.heart.org/en/health-topics/congenital-heart-defects/about-congenital-heart-defects/complete-atrioventricular-canal-defect-cavc. Reviewed March 23, 2022; Accessed January 28, 2023.

Bertolizio G, Saint-Martin C, Ingelmo P. Cervical instability in patients with trisomy 21: the eternal gamble. *Pediatr Anesth.* 2018;28(10):830-833.

Sadowski SL, Verklan MT. Cardiovascular disorders. In: Verklan MT, Walden M, Forest S, eds. *Core Curriculum for Neonatal Intensive Care Nursing.* 6th ed. St. Louis, MO: Elsevier; 2021:460-503.

3. **(B)** Cystic fibrosis is an autosomal-recessive condition, which carries a 25% chance with each pregnancy of having an affected offspring. The risk of inheriting this condition is gender neutral.

References: National Library of Medicine. *Genetics Home Reference. Deletion.* Available at: https://www.genome.gov/genetics-glossary/Deletion. Updated January 26, 2023; Accessed January 28, 2023.

National Library of Medicine Medline Plus. *What are the Different Ways A Genetic Condition Can Be Inherited?* Available at: https://medlineplus.gov/genetics/understanding/inheritance/inheritancepatterns. Updated April 19, 2021; Accessed January 28, 2023.

NSW (Australia) Government Health Centre for Genetics Education. *Autosomal Recessive Inheritance.* 2021. Available at: https://www.genetics.edu.au/SitePages/Autosomal-recessive-inheritance.aspx. Updated October 2021; Accessed January 28, 2023.

4. **(B)** A disruption is an abnormality of morphogenesis caused by disruptive forces acting on the developing structures. Defects that result from amniotic bands are an example of disruption. A sequence is a group of anomalies resulting from a cascade of events initiated by a single malformation. Pierre Robin is an example of a sequence. A deformation is an alteration of morphogenesis caused by unusual forces on previously normal tissue. Clubfoot and plagiocephaly are examples of deformations. A malformation is an abnormality of morphogenesis caused by an intrinsic abnormal developmental process. Examples are neural tube defects, cleft lip, and cleft palate.

References: Schiefelbien J. Genetics: from bench to bedside. In: Verklan MT, Walden M, Forest S, eds. *Core Curriculum for Neonatal Intensive Care Nursing.* 6th ed. St. Louis, MO: Elsevier; 2021:346-358.

Lubbers L. Congenital anomalies. In: Verklan MT, Walden M, Forest S, eds. *Core Curriculum for Neonatal Intensive Care Nursing.* 6th ed. St. Louis, MO: Elsevier; 2021:654-677.

5. **(A)** An X-linked disorder is caused by an abnormal gene on the X chromosome. In X-linked recessive disorders male offspring are affected and carrier females transmit the disorder. In almost all cases, only male offspring have the disorder. The mother will require genetic counseling with subsequent pregnancies. A dominant inheritance pattern requires that only one copy of a defective gene be present for its effect to be expressed. An individual with the faulty gene will always express the effect of the gene. An X-linked dominant disorder affects both sexes, but females have twice the risk of manifesting the disorder because their chances of receiving a mutant X chromosome are doubled. Because this mother is a carrier but does not have the disorder, the disorder cannot have a dominant inheritance pattern. An autosomal-recessive inheritance pattern requires that the corresponding genes on both chromosomes of a pair be defective for the gene's effect to be expressed. The faulty gene is on an autosome (non–sex determining chromosome) and therefore either sex can be affected. The maternal history in this case suggests that the disorder is X-linked. An autosomal-dominant inheritance pattern requires that only one copy of a defective gene be present for its effect to be expressed. An individual with the defective gene will always express the effect of the gene. Either parent can pass the gene on to sons or daughters.

Reference: Schiefelbien J. Genetics: from bench to bedside. In: Verklan MT, Walden M, Forest S, eds. *Core Curriculum for Neonatal Intensive Care Nursing.* 6th ed. St. Louis, MO: Elsevier; 2021:346-358.

6. **(C)** Additional clinical features of trisomy 21 include brachycephaly with flattened occiput, low-set and malformed ears, generalized hypotonia, hyperflexibility of the joints, clinodactyly of the fifth fingers, wide spacing between the first and second toes, and loose skinfolds in the posterior neck. Clinical features of trisomy 13 include microphthalmos, malformed ears, umbilical hernia, omphalocele, cutaneous hemangiomas, and hand deformities. Clinical features of trisomy 18 include low birth weight in a term infant, ears that are low set and/or of abnormal shape, micrognathia and microstomia, rocker-bottom feet, clenched hand with flexed fingers, and flexion contraction of the middle two fingers. Clinical features of Turner syndrome include low posterior hairline with the appearance of a short neck, small stature, low-set ears, broad chest with widely spaced nipples, limb abnormalities, and ptosis of the eyelids.

Reference: Lubbers L. Congenital anomalies. In: Verklan MT, Walden M, Forest S, eds. *Core Curriculum for Neonatal Intensive Care Nursing.* 6th ed. St. Louis, MO: Elsevier; 2021:654-677.

7. **(D)** DiGeorge syndrome is one of several velocardiofacial syndromes caused by a deletion in chromosome band 22q11. Fluorescence in situ hybridization is a genetic testing method used to detect microdeletions on chromosomes. A rectal biopsy is indicated in patients with Hirschsprung disease. Although congenital heart defects are common in infants with DiGeorge syndrome; there is no urgent need to obtain an electrocardiogram (ECG), nor would its findings be diagnostic of DiGeorge syndrome. The oxygen challenge test uses 100% oxygen to differentiate persistent pulmonary hypertension of the newborn from a congenital heart defect. Since DiGeorge syndrome involves many systems including cardiac, an oxygen challenge test would not facilitate diagnosis.

References: Sadowski SL, Verklan MT. Cardiovascular disorders. In: Verklan MT, Walden M, Forest S, eds. *Core Curriculum for Neonatal Intensive Care Nursing.* 6th ed. St. Louis, MO: Elsevier; 2021:460-503.

Schiefelbien J. Genetics: from bench to bedside. In: Verklan MT, Walden M, Forest S, eds. *Core Curriculum for Neonatal Intensive Care Nursing.* 6th ed. St. Louis, MO: Elsevier; 2021:346-358.

8. **(B)** A dominant disorder requires only one gene to be present to be expressed. In an autosomal-dominant disorder, males and females are affected equally, and there is a 50% chance with each pregnancy that the offspring will be affected. Autosomal-recessive disorders carry a 25% chance of each pregnancy producing offspring that will be affected. Disorders with an X-linked recessive pattern are characterized by only male offspring being affected.

Reference: Schiefelbien J. Genetics: from bench to bedside. In: Verklan MT, Walden M, Forest S, eds. *Core Curriculum for Neonatal Intensive Care Nursing.* 6th ed. St. Louis, MO: Elsevier; 2021:346-358.

9. **(A)** Infants with Beckwith-Wiedemann present with macroglossia and hypoglycemia. Additional findings include abdominal wall defects, renal abnormalities, Wilm's tumor, and facial nevus. Infants with VATER association present with vertebral anomalies, anal atresia, tracheoesophageal fistula, and radial and renal anomalies. Infants with DiGeorge syndrome (22q11.2 deletion) have cardiac anomalies and hypocalcemia and are often hypotonic. Girls with Turner syndrome have short stature and altered growth. About 30% have extra folds of skin on the neck or webbed neck, a low hairline at the neck, and skeletal or renal problems. One-third to one-half of infants with Turner syndrome have a heart defect such as coarctation of the aorta.

References: Blackburn ST. Endocrine disorders. In: Verklan MT, Walden M, Forest S, eds. *Core Curriculum for Neonatal Intensive Care Nursing.* 6th ed. St. Louis, MO: Elsevier; 2021:564.

Schiefelbien J. Genetics: from bench to bedside. In: Verklan MT, Walden M, Forest S, eds. *Core Curriculum for Neonatal Intensive Care Nursing.* 6th ed. St. Louis, MO: Elsevier; 2021:346-358.

10. **(A)** The current patterns of inheritance include autosomal dominant, autosomal recessive, X-linked dominant, X-linked recessive, codominant, and mitochondrial or maternal inheritance. Deletions occur when a chromosome breaks and some genetic material is lost. These occur by chance and are not inherited. Trisomies also occur randomly, but trisomy 21 can occur more often in certain aged females. Translocations are random and have no predictable pattern of inheritance.

Reference: National Library of Medicine. *Genetics Home Reference. What Are the Different Ways in Which A Genetic Condition Can Be Inherited?* Available at: https://medlineplus.gov/genetics/understanding/inheritance/inheritancepatterns/. Updated April 19, 2021; Accessed January 28, 2023.

11. **(B)** A prenatal quad screen is not diagnostic of a condition but indicates the need for additional testing to rule out abnormalities.

If trisomy 18 is suspected based on the prenatal quad screen, additional diagnostic tests are recommended, including ultrasonography, amniocentesis, and postnatal testing. Urine organic acids do not aid in the diagnosis of trisomy 18. While a computed tomography scan may aid identification of some features of trisomy 18, it would not be used for diagnostic purposes.

Reference: Schiefelbien J. Genetics: from bench to bedside. In: Verklan MT, Walden M, Forest S, eds. *Core Curriculum for Neonatal Intensive Care Nursing.* 6th ed. St. Louis, MO: Elsevier; 2021:346-358.

12. **(C)** A sequence is initiated by a single malformation, disruption, or deformation, such as mandibular hypoplasia. A syndrome involves multiple malformations that occur in different systems simultaneously. For example, in Pierre Robin sequence (also known as micrognathia), mandibular hypoplasia occurs early in the first trimester of pregnancy and results in a cascade of events including position of the tongue high in the oral cavity causing a cleft palate. Syndrome identification is more common than a sequence.

Reference: Schiefelbien J. Genetics: from bench to bedside. In: Verklan MT, Walden M, Forest S, eds. *Core Curriculum for Neonatal Intensive Care Nursing.* 6th ed. St. Louis, MO: Elsevier; 2021:346-358.

13. **(B)** The presence of mild trisomy 21 symptoms can occur if there is mosaicism where only some cells are affected. The absence of symptoms can occur when there is a translocation of an extra chromosome on chromosome 14 or 22. When a translocation occurs, the person may be unaware, but can have a child with trisomy 21 where all cells are affected. Since most cases of trisomy 21 occur randomly without a known inheritance pattern, symptom expression is not affected by either parent. Monosomy of chromosomes 1–22 results in early fetal death. Monosomy of the X chromosome results in Turner syndrome which affects many systems including webbed neck, short stature, premature ovarian failure, and can involve the kidneys and heart.

References: Schiefelbien J. Genetics: from bench to bedside. In: Verklan MT, Walden M, Forest S, eds. *Core Curriculum for Neonatal Intensive Care Nursing.* 6th ed. St. Louis, MO: Elsevier; 2021:346-358.

U.S. Department of Health and Human Services, National Institutes of Health (NIH), National Center for Advanced Translation Sciences. *Turner Syndrome.* Genetic and Rare Diseases Information Center (GARD). Available at: https://rarediseases.info.nih.gov/diseases/7831/turner-syndrome. Updated November 08, 2021; Accessed January 28, 2023.

14. **(A)** The observed phenotype for an infant with trisomy 13 includes malformed ears, eye deformities (microphthalmos, colobomas, and cataracts), and broad/flattened nose; can have cleft lip/palate, umbilical hernia/omphalocele, rocker-bottom feet, and polydactyly. Many infants with trisomy 13 also have cardiac defects including ventricular septal defect, patent ductus arteriosus, or rotational anomalies such as dextrocardia. Although these symptoms are similar to infants with trisomy 18, the differences are eye deformities, omphalocele, and polydactyly (infants with trisomy 18 often have syndactyly instead) not usually seen with trisomy 18. Infants with trisomy 21 can have small size, prematurity, eyes that are slanted upward and outward, prominent epicanthal folds, flat face, Brushfield's spots (flecks of gold or grayish spots forming a ring around the iris), protruding tongue, loose skin around neck, short fingers, single simian creases, hypotonia. Infants with VACTERAL association may have vertebral anomalies, (imperforate) anus, cardiac defects, tracheoesophageal fistula, renal anomalies, absent radii or limbs.

Reference: Schiefelbien J. Genetics: from bench to bedside. In: Verklan MT, Walden M, Forest S, eds. *Core Curriculum for Neonatal Intensive Care Nursing.* 6th ed. St. Louis, MO: Elsevier; 2021:346-358.

Chapter 22

Immunologic Disorders and Infections

1. A pregnant woman asks the nurse, "What is the most practical method for me to prevent getting a cytomegalovirus (CMV) infection while I'm pregnant?" What should the nurse tell the pregnant woman?
   A. She should avoid contact with cat feces by wearing gloves to empty the litter box.
   B. Avoiding exposure is virtually impossible.
   C. She should avoid eating raw/undercooked meat.
   D. She should avoid contact with anyone exhibiting symptoms consistent with an influenza-like illness.

2. Ganciclovir (Zirgan) is associated with which of the following side effects?
   A. Sensorineural hearing loss
   B. Thrombocytosis
   C. Neutrophilia
   D. Neutropenia

3. Which of the following statements about respiratory syncytial virus (RSV) is generally true?

A. RSV usually occurs in the spring and summer.
B. Infection is by noncontact mode of transmission (e.g., airborne or vehicle).
C. Prophylaxis with palivizumab (Synagis) decreases the risk of severe RSV disease and hospitalization.
D. Palivizumab (Synagis) is effective as a control measure for hospital outbreaks of RSV infection.

4. Which of the following interventions is mandatory for an infant suspected of having congenital syphilis?
   A. Long-bone x-ray examination
   B. Cranial ultrasound
   C. Venereal disease research laboratory (VDRL) tests on cerebrospinal fluid (CSF)
   D. Fluorescent treponemal–antibody absorption immunoglobulin M (IgM)

5. The Kaiser Neonatal Early-Onset Sepsis (EOS) Calculator has been endorsed by the American Academy of Pediatrics (AAP) for use in clinical practice to assess the risk of early-onset sepsis

among infants. Which of the following scenarios would require utilizing the calculator to determine the risk of early-onset sepsis and subsequent management?

A. 2-day-old 32-week-gestation infant presenting with clinical signs of sepsis.

B. 14-day-old 36-week-gestation infant presenting with clinical signs of sepsis.

C. 38-week-gestation infant born to a mother diagnosed with chorioamnionitis.

D. 38-week-gestation infant born to a mother with rupture of membranes for 8 hours.

6. A 1500-g preterm infant born to a hepatitis B surface antigen (HBsAg)–negative mother should receive the initial dose of hepatitis B vaccine at:

A. birth.

B. 37 weeks postmenstrual age.

C. 1 month of age or at hospital discharge (whichever is first).

D. 2000-g or at hospital discharge (whichever is first).

7. Which of the following measures is the most effective in preventing nosocomial infections in preterm infants?

A. Avoiding overcrowding in the neonatal intensive care unit (NICU)

B. Cohorting

C. Limiting parent and sibling visits

D. Proper hand hygiene

8. The newborn nursery nurse observes edematous eyelids with purulent exudate in a 1-day-old infant brought by ambulance to the hospital emergency department immediately after being born at home to a mother who had no prenatal care. The records do not indicate whether the infant received eye prophylaxis. The nurse should expect the infant to receive:

A. intravenous ceftriaxone (Zinacef).

B. erythromycin ophthalmic ointment.

C. oral erythromycin base or erythromycin ethylsuccinate.

D. tetracycline (Sumycin) ophthalmic ointment.

9. Which of the following CSF values is abnormal and could indicate meningitis?

A. CSF protein level of 50 mg/dL

B. CSF protein level of 70 mg/dL

C. CSF glucose level of 23 mg/dL with a serum glucose level of 100 mg/dL

D. CSF leukocyte count of 15/mm³ with 40% polymorphonuclear cells

10. An otherwise healthy-appearing term newborn has pustules localized to the axillae and groin. Laboratory analysis reveals Gram-positive cocci and neutrophils. The lesions most likely represent:

A. a benign newborn rash.

B. *Staphylococcus aureus* infection.

C. *Candida* diaper dermatitis.

D. *Staphylococcus epidermidis* infection.

11. A 37-week gestational age infant is born with hydrocephalus, diffuse generalized intracranial calcifications, and chorioretinitis. What congenital infection is associated with these clinical findings?

A. Herpes infection

B. Rubella

C. Toxoplasmosis

D. CMV infection

12. Which of the following antimicrobials is contraindicated for use in newborns?

A. Ticarcillin (Ticar)

B. Amikacin (Amikin)

C. Ceftazidime (Fortaz)

D. Sulfamethoxazole/trimethoprim (Bactrim)

13. A preterm infant with a birth weight of 1800-g was delivered to a mother who was not tested during pregnancy for HBsAg. A maternal blood sample was drawn at delivery for HBsAg determination. While the results are awaited, and within 12 hours of birth, the infant should receive hepatitis B vaccine. When should the nurse administer hepatitis B immune globulin?

A. Within 12 hours of age if maternal status cannot be determined or if the mother tests positive.

B. Within 7 days of age if the mother tests positive for hepatitis B.

C. According to the recommendations for term infants.

D. At 1 month of age.

14. Even with appropriate neonatal prophylaxis, breastfeeding poses additional risks for infants whose mothers test positive for:

A. human immunodeficiency virus (HIV).

B. HBsAg.

C. both HBsAg and HIV.

D. neither HBsAg nor HIV.

15. Which Ig crosses the placenta in significant amounts?

A. IgA

B. IgE

C. IgG

D. IgM

16. Which of the following sets of hematologic values best predicts infection in a 1-hour-old term neonate?

A. White blood cell (WBC) $8.25 \times 10^3/mm^3$; segs 52%; bands 12%

B. WBC $6.1 \times 10^3/mm^3$; segs 32%; bands 4%

C. WBC $15 \times 10^3/mm^3$; segs 17%; bands 3%

D. WBC $4.7 \times 10^3/mm^3$; segs 27%; bands 8%

17. The initial blood culture report on an infant with suspected sepsis reveals coagulase-positive, Gram-positive cocci. The most likely organism is:

A. *Escherichia coli.*

B. *S. aureus.*

C. *Listeria monocytogenes.*

D. *S. epidermidis.*

18. What is the organism most commonly responsible for nosocomial bloodstream infection in NICU patients?

A. *Enterococcus*

B. Group B *streptococcus*

C. *S. aureus*

D. Coagulase-negative *staphylococci*

19. An infant receiving zidovudine (Retrovir) for prevention of maternal–fetal HIV transmission should be monitored for:

A. anemia.

B. neutrophilia.

C. hypotension.

D. hypokalemia.

20. A 7-day-old infant with a postmenstrual age of 24 weeks has a history of hyperglycemia and is receiving steroids for treatment of hypotension. The nurse caring for the patient notices erosive skin lesions with serous drainage and crusting on the infant's back. Suspicion should be raised for infection with which of the following agents?

    A. *Candida*

    B. Parvovirus B19

    C. *E. coli*

    D. *S. epidermidis*

21. A woman who is 36 weeks gestation presents with rupture of membranes. Upon further investigation, her group B *Streptococcus* (GBS) screening is found to be unknown. Which of the following additional risk factors would indicate the need for intrapartum antibiotic prophylaxis in a mother with unknown GBS screening?

    A. Maternal upper respiratory infection

    B. Previous infant with GBS infection

    C. Premature rupture of membranes

    D. Maternal temperature of 37.8°C (100°F)

22. The mother of a 5-day-old 32-week-gestation infant notified the NICU nurse she was "not feeling well" with a temperature of 37.6°C (99.7°F) and a headache, which she associates with stress and lack of sleep. She reports no other symptoms. Which of the following is the best response in this situation?

    A. The nurse should notify Infection Control.

    B. The mother should continue to visit but not have any direct contact with her infant.

    C. The mother should dispose of any of her milk she pumps during this time.

    D. The mother can continue normal visitation.

23. Treatment for proven or highly probable congenital syphilis consists of:

    A. benzathine penicillin G 50,000 units/kg as a single intramuscular dose.

    B. ampicillin 50 mg/kg/dose intravenously for 48 hours followed by penicillin G 50,000 Units/kg intravenously for 8 days.

    C. no treatment, as the infant will acquire natural immunity from the mother.

    D. aqueous crystalline penicillin G 50,000 units/kg intravenously every 12 hours for the first 7 days and then every 8 hours thereafter for a total of 10 days.

24. A symptomatic infant is receiving prophylactic acyclovir (Zovirax) as a part of an evaluation for sepsis. Which diagnostic and laboratory studies should be monitored to ensure tolerance?

    A. Chest x-ray, blood gas

    B. Complete blood count, blood urea nitrogen, and serum creatinine

    C. Blood cultures for herpes simplex virus type 1 (HSV-1) and HSV-2

    D. No monitoring is indicated, as acyclovir (Zovirax) is routinely well tolerated

25. A 38-week-gestation infant is admitted to the NICU on bubble continuous positive airway pressure secondary to respiratory distress following delivery. The mother presented to labor and delivery complaining of symptoms related to severe acute respiratory syndrome coronavirus 2 (SARS-CoV-2) and later tested positive for the virus. According to the AAP, what is the current timing for utilizing infection control precautions for the infant exposed to SARS-CoV-2?

    A. The infant does not require infection control precautions or testing unless symptoms present.

    B. Infection control precautions should be used until the infant has a negative test in the first 72 hours of age.

    C. Infection control precautions should be used until the infant has a negative test at 24 and 48 hours of age.

    D. Infection control precautions should be used until the mother tests negative.

26. Antibiotics are included in the management of infants with necrotizing enterocolitis (NEC). What is the recommended duration of treatment for a critically ill infant diagnosed with medical NEC (stages II and III), including the presence of pneumatosis on serial abdominal x-rays?

    A. 48 hours

    B. 7–9 days

    C. 10–14 days

    D. 15–21 days

ANSWERS AND RATIONALES

1. **(B)** Avoiding exposure to cytomegalovirus (CMV) is virtually impossible because the virus is ubiquitous and infectious people are usually asymptomatic. Contact with cat feces and eating raw or undercooked meat increase the risk of toxoplasmosis. A pregnant woman who avoids contact with people who have symptoms of an influenza-like illness may still be exposed to the virus because of the asymptomatic nature of CMV infection.

Reference: Pammi M, Brand C, Weisman L. Infection in the neonate. In: Gardner WL, Carter BS, Enzman-Hines M, Niermeyer S, eds. *Merenstein & Gardner's Handbook of Neonatal Intensive Care: An Interprofessional Approach.* 9th ed. St. Louis, MO: Elsevier; 2021:695.

2. **(D)** Two-thirds of neonates treated with ganciclovir (Zirgan) experience neutropenia. Progressive sensorineural hearing loss is a symptom of neonatal CMV infection, and ganciclovir (Zirgan) is used to prevent hearing deterioration. Thrombocytosis and neutrophilia are not side effects of ganciclovir (Zirgan). Use of ganciclovir (Zirgan) should be considered in infants with serious end-organ disease, including thrombocytopenia.

Reference: Pammi M, Brand C, Weisman L. Infection in the neonate. In: Gardner WL, Carter BS, Enzman-Hines M, Niermeyer S, eds. *Merenstein & Gardner's Handbook of Neonatal Intensive Care: An Interprofessional Approach.* 9th ed. St. Louis, MO: Elsevier; 2021:695.

3. The risk of severe respiratory syncytial virus (RSV) disease and hospitalization is reduced by approximately 50% when prophylaxis with palivizumab (Synagis) is given. RSV usually occurs in annual fall and winter epidemics and in early spring in temperate climates. Transmission is usually by close or direct contact with contaminated secretions. Administration of palivizumab (Synagis) is not indicated as an infection control measure for hospital outbreaks of RSV. Strict observance of infection control practices (e.g., cohorting RSV–infected patients) is the best means to prevent RSV disease in the hospital.

Reference: Kilpatrick SJ, Papile LA, eds. *Guidelines for Perinatal Care.* 8th ed. Elk Grove Village, IL: American Academy of Pediatrics; 2017:517-519.

4. **(C)** Venereal disease research laboratory (VDRL) testing on cerebrospinal fluid (CSF) is mandatory in all infants suspected of congenital syphilis because treatment regimens differ depending on whether or not there is central nervous system involvement. Long-bone x-ray examination may show metaphysitis or periostitis, which may help in the diagnosis, but it is not mandatory. A cranial ultrasound is not indicated for diagnosing syphilis. A fluorescent treponemal–antibody absorption immunoglobulin M test is unreliable.

Reference: Pammi M, Brand C, Weisman L. Infection in the neonate. In: Gardner WL, Carter BS, Enzman-Hines M, Niermeyer S, eds. *Merenstein & Gardner's Handbook of Neonatal Intensive Care: An Interprofessional Approach*. 9th ed. St. Louis, MO: Elsevier; 2021:697.

5. **(C)** The Kaiser Neonatal Early-Onset Sepsis calculator should be performed on an infant greater than or equal to 34 weeks' gestation at birth with exposure to maternal chorioamnionitis as the infant is at an increased risk for early-onset sepsis. The sepsis calculator was created out of the necessity to promote antibiotic stewardship and reduce antibiotic usage in neonates early after delivery by quantifying the risk of early-onset sepsis using maternal risk factors and neonatal clinical exam findings. EOS is defined as blood and/or CSF culture-proven sepsis at less than 7 days of age, thus a 14-day-old infant does not meet the criteria for early-onset sepsis. Prolonged rupture of membranes, greater than or equal to 18 hours prior to delivery, is a maternal risk factor which predisposes the infant to potential early-onset sepsis. Although this infant is term, the timing of the rupture of membranes was not prolonged and decreases the likelihood of the infant becoming infected.

References: Gomella T, Eyal F, Bany-Mohammed F. *Gomella's Neonatology: Management, Procedures, On-Call Problems, Diseases and Drugs*. 8th ed. New York: McGraw Hill; 2020:1180-1181.

Kaiser Permanente Research. *Neonatal Early-Onset Sepsis Calculator*. 2022. Available at: https://neonatalsepsiscalculator.kaiserpermanente.org/.

Pammi M, Brand C, Weisman L. Infection in the neonate. In: Gardner WL, Carter BS, Enzman-Hines M, Niermeyer S, eds. *Merenstein & Gardner's Handbook of Neonatal Intensive Care: An Interprofessional Approach*. 9th ed. St. Louis, MO: Elsevier; 2021:711-714.

6. **(C)** For infants weighing less than 2000-g, the initial dose of hepatitis B vaccine should be delayed until 1 month of age or hospital discharge, whichever is first, because of suboptimal immune response in some preterm infants. The exception is when hospital discharge occurs in less than 1 month of age, in which case, the vaccine should be given at discharge. Administration of hepatitis B vaccine at birth is appropriate for any infant born to a hepatitis B surface antigen (HBsAg)–positive mother, any infant born to a mother whose status cannot be determined within 12 hours of birth, or for infants of HBsAg-negative mothers as long as birth weight is 2000-g or more. Gestational age (initial or corrected) is not a consideration for the timing of hepatitis B immunization.

Reference: Kilpatrick SJ, Papile LA, eds. *Guidelines for Perinatal Care*. 8th ed. Elk Grove Village, IL: American Academy of Pediatrics; 2017:380.

7. **(D)** Studies demonstrate that proper hand hygiene before and after each patient contact is the single most effective means of preventing nosocomial infections. In addition to hand washing, alcohol-based disinfectants are effective for use before and after patient contact. Overcrowding in the neonatal intensive care unit (NICU) may increase the risk for cross-contamination. Adequate spacing between patients is recommended. Cohorting during epidemics is required to limit the number of contacts of one infant with other infants and personnel. As long as visitors employ the proper precautions, limiting parent and sibling visits has not been shown to decrease the incidence of nosocomial infections.

Reference: Pammi M, Brand C, Weisman L. Infection in the neonate. In: Gardner WL, Carter BS, Enzman-Hines M, Niermeyer S, eds. *Merenstein & Gardner's*

Handbook of Neonatal Intensive Care: An Interprofessional Approach. 9th ed. St. Louis, MO: Elsevier; 2021:719.

8. **(A)** The symptoms are consistent with gonococcal conjunctivitis. Symptoms of gonococcal conjunctivitis begin 1–4 days after birth. Although chlamydial conjunctivitis is the most commonly identified infectious conjunctivitis in the United States and may present with similar symptoms, chlamydial conjunctivitis does not present until 5–14 days of age. The appropriate treatment for gonococcal conjunctivitis is a single dose of ceftriaxone (Zinacef) intravenously. Erythromycin ophthalmic ointment is used for prophylaxis at birth to prevent ophthalmia neonatorum but is insufficient once infection is present. Oral erythromycin is used to treat chlamydial conjunctivitis. Tetracycline (Sumyacin) may be used for bacterial conjunctivitis, but it is ineffective for *Neisseria gonorrhoeae*.

Reference: Permar SR. Viral infections. In: Eichenwald EC, Hansen AR, Martin CR, Stark AR, eds. *Cloherty and Stark's Manual of Neonatal Care*. 8th ed. Philadelphia, PA: Lippincott Williams & Wilkins; 2017:877-879.

9. **(C)** A CSF glucose less than 25 mg/dL is abnormal and could indicate meningitis. Normal mean serum glucose values are 79–83 mg/dL (range 64–106 mg/dL) for preterm infants, and 51–55 mg/dL (range 32–78 mg/dL) for term infants. Normal mean CSF protein values are 75–150 mg/dL (range 31–292 mg/dL) for preterm infants, and 47–67 mg/dL (range 17–240 mg/dL) for term infants. CSF cell counts are variable in the first few weeks, and interpretation is difficult, especially when blood is present in the CSF. Polymorphonuclear leukocytes are commonly present and may be as high as 70%.

References: Rudd KM. Infectious diseases in the neonate. In: Verklan MT, Walden M, Forest S, eds. *Core Curriculum for Neonatal Intensive Care Nursing*. 6th ed. St. Louis, MO: Elsevier; 2021:593.

Pammi M, Brand C, Weisman L. Infection in the neonate. In: Gardner WL, Carter BS, Enzman-Hines M, Niermeyer S, eds. *Merenstein & Gardner's Handbook of Neonatal Intensive Care: An Interprofessional Approach*. 9th ed. St. Louis, MO: Elsevier; 2021:714.

10. **(B)** Infectious pustulosis is usually caused by *Staphylococcus aureus*, a Gram-positive coccus. Lesions are commonly found in the axillae, groin, and periumbilical area. Benign rashes, such as erythema toxicum and transient pustular melanosis, typically have a generalized distribution. Cultures of benign rashes produce negative results or grow contaminating organisms such as *Staphylococcus epidermidis*. Eosinophils are seen on a Wright stain preparation of erythema toxicum. Neutrophils, but no organisms, are seen on a Gram stain preparation of neonatal pustular melanosis. The characteristic rash of *Candida* diaper dermatitis is consistent with intense inflammation that is bright red and often seen in the inguinal folds, buttocks, thighs, abdomen, and genitalia, often with satellite lesions. Laboratory analysis reveals fungal elements rather than bacteria. *S. epidermidis* infection does not present as described in the scenario, although it may be isolated as a contaminant in culture of a benign rash.

Reference: Puopolo KM. Bacterial and fungal infections. In: Eichenwald EC, Hansen AR, Martin CR, Stark AR, eds. *Cloherty and Stark's Manual of Neonatal Care*. 8th ed. Philadelphia, PA: Lippincott Williams & Wilkins; 2017:876.

11. **(C)** Hydrocephalus with generalized calcifications and chorioretinitis are clinical findings suggestive of congenital toxoplasmosis. Herpes infection is associated with keratoconjunctivitis, skin vesicles, and acute central nervous system findings. Rubella is associated with cataracts, cloudy cornea, pigmented retina, blueberry muffin syndrome, and certain cardiac abnormalities. CMV infection is associated with microcephaly, periventricular calcifications, thrombocytopenia, jaundice, and hearing loss.

References: Puopolo KM. Bacterial and fungal infections. In: Eichenwald EC, Hansen AR, Martin CR, Stark AR, eds. *Cloherty and Stark's Manual of Neonatal*

Care. 8th ed. Philadelphia, PA: Lippincott Williams & Wilkins; 2017:886.

Gomella T, Eyal F, Bany-Mohammed F. *Gomella's Neonatology: Management, Procedures, On-Call Problems, Diseases and Drugs.* 8th ed. New York: McGraw Hill; 2020:1198.

12. (D) The use of sulfonamides, such as sulfamethoxazole/trimethoprim (Bactrim), is contraindicated in newborns because these agents displace bilirubin from albumin-binding sites. Ticarcillin (Ticar) has expanded Gram-negative activity and can be used to treat susceptible pseudomonas infections in newborns. Amikacin (Amikin) is indicated for treatment of infections with aerobic Gram-negative organisms and can be used in newborns. Ceftazidime (Fortaz) is used to treat sepsis and meningitis caused by susceptible Gram-negative organisms and can be used in newborns.

References: Kamath-Rayne BD, Froese PA, Thilo EH. Neonatal hyperbilirubinemia. In: Eichenwald EC, Hansen AR, Martin CR, Stark AR, eds. *Cloherty and Stark's Manual of Neonatal Care.* 8th ed. Philadelphia, PA: Lippincott Williams & Wilkins; 2017:664.

Gomella T, Eyal F, Bany-Mohammed F. *Gomella's Neonatology: Management, Procedures, On-Call Problems, Diseases and Drugs.* 8th ed. New York: McGraw Hill; 2020:905.

13. (A) A preterm infant weighing less than 2000-g whose mother's HBsAg status is unknown should receive hepatitis B immune globulin (HBIG, 0.5 mL) within the initial 12 hours after birth if the mother's status cannot be determined within 12 hours, as the vaccine has potentially decreased immunogenicity in these infants. Term infants born to mothers not tested during pregnancy for HBsAg can receive HBIG up to 7 days after birth while maternal HBsAg results are awaited. The recommendations for term infants should be followed for preterm infants with birth weights of more than 2000-g.

Reference: Kilpatrick SJ, Papile LA, eds. *Guidelines for Perinatal Care.* 8th ed. Elk Grove Village, IL: American Academy of Pediatrics; 2017:490-492.

14. (A) Human immunodeficiency virus (HIV) has been isolated from breast milk and can be transmitted through breastfeeding. In the United States HIV-infected women should be counseled not to breastfeed even if neonatal prophylaxis is given. If the infant has been given hepatitis B vaccine and HBIG, breastfeeding by a mother positive for HBsAg poses no additional risk of hepatitis B infection for the infant. In the absence of HBsAg or HIV, there are no additional restrictions to breastfeeding.

Reference: Kilpatrick SJ, Papile L-A, eds. *Guidelines for Perinatal Care.* 8th ed. Elk Grove Village, IL: American Academy of Pediatrics; 2017: 375-376, 507.

15. (C) Immunoglobulin G (IgG) placental transport begins during fetal development, and the term infant has a complete store of maternal IgG antibodies, which protects the newborn from many infections during the first months of life. IgA is not transferred transplacentally in significant amounts. Fresh human milk contains secretory IgA. IgE normally is produced only with induction of inflammation, but maternal IgE may be acquired by the fetus via ingestion of amniotic fluid. Maternal–fetal transfer of IgM does not occur due to the large size of the IgM molecule. An elevated concentration of IgM is indicative of infection in the fetus or newborn.

Reference: Permar SR. Viral infections. In: Eichenwald EC, Hansen AR, Martin CR, Stark AR, eds. *Cloherty and Stark's Manual of Neonatal Care.* 8th ed. Philadelphia, PA: Lippincott Williams & Wilkins; 2017:789.

16. (D) The lower limit of the total neutrophil count is 1750/mm³ at birth and rises to 7200/mm³ by 12 hours of age. It then declines to approximately 1720/mm³ by 72 hours of age. The absolute neutrophil count (ANC) and immature to total neutrophils (I:T) ratio are useful neutrophil indices in the diagnosis of neonatal sepsis. Values suggestive of infection include the following:

Neutropenia: ANC of <1750/mm³. This infant's ANC is 1645/mm³.

I:T ratio of >0.2. This infant's I:T ratio is 0.23.

Calculation of the ANC: From the white blood cell (WBC) count (4.7×10^3/mm³) and differential (27% segmented neutrophils, 8% bands), the ANC is calculated as follows:

ANC = (% segmented cells + % immature cells) × WBCs

ANC = (0.27+ 0.08) × 4700

ANC = (0.35) × 4700 = 1645/mm³

Calculation of the I:T ratio:

Mature cells = segmented cells

Immature cells = bands, metamyelocytes, myelocytes, promyelocytes

I:T ratio = (% immature cells)/(% mature cells + % immature cells)

I:T ratio = (0.08)/(0.27 + 0.08)

I:T ratio = 0.08/0.35

I:T ratio = 0.23

Reference: Ferrieri P, Wallen LD. Newborn sepsis and meningitis. In: Gleason CA, Juul SE, eds. *Avery's Diseases of the Newborn.* 10th ed. Philadelphia, PA: Elsevier Saunders; 2018:558-559.

17. (B) *S. aureus* is a Gram-positive, coccus-shaped organism that is coagulase positive. *Escherichia coli* is a Gram-negative rod. *Listeria monocytogenes* is typically a Gram-positive rod. *S. epidermidis* is coagulase negative.

Reference: Puopolo KM. Bacterial and fungal infections. In: Eichenwald EC, Hansen AR, Martin CR, Stark AR, eds. *Cloherty and Stark's Manual of Neonatal Care.* 8th ed. Philadelphia, PA: Lippincott Williams & Wilkins; 2017:861.

18. (D) Coagulase-negative staphylococci are the organisms that most commonly cause nosocomial infections in the NICU, accounting for approximately 50% of bloodstream infections. *Enterococcus*, Group B *Streptococcus* (GBS), and *S. aureus* are each responsible for fewer than 10% of nosocomial bloodstream infections.

Reference: Puopolo KM. Bacterial and fungal infections. In: Eichenwald EC, Hansen AR, Martin CR, Stark AR, eds. *Cloherty and Stark's Manual of Neonatal Care.* 8th ed. Philadelphia, PA: Lippincott Williams & Wilkins; 2017:860.

19. (A) Severe anemia is one of the most common side effects in infants receiving zidovudine (Retrovir). Retrovir may cause granulocytopenia; therefore neutropenia, rather than neutrophilia, is an adverse effect of its use. There are no common cardiovascular side effects related to Retrovir use. Electrolyte disturbances are not commonly reported with this drug.

Reference: Gomella T, Eyal F, Bany-Mohammed F. *Gomella's Neonatology: Management, Procedures, On-Call Problems, Diseases and Drugs.* 8th ed. New York: McGraw Hill; 2020:1316.

20. (A) A gestational age of less than 26 weeks, hyperglycemia, and postnatal steroid therapy are risk factors for invasive fungal dermatitis caused by microorganisms such as *Aspergillus* or *Candida* species in the first 2 weeks of life. The characteristic lesions typically appear on dependent surfaces such as the back or abdomen. Parvovirus B19 infections may be associated with an erythematous facial rash and a symmetric maculopapular, lacelike, and often pruritic rash on the trunk, arms, buttocks, and thighs. Clinical manifestations of infection with *E. coli* and *S. epidermidis* do not typically include erosive skin lesions.

References: Puopolo KM. Bacterial and fungal infections. In: Eichenwald EC, Hansen AR, Martin CR, Stark AR, eds. *Cloherty and Stark's Manual of Neonatal Care.* 8th ed. Philadelphia, PA: Lippincott Williams & Wilkins; 2017:872-873.

Rudd KM. Infectious diseases in the neonate. In: Verklan MT, Walden M, Forest S, eds. *Core Curriculum for Neonatal Intensive Care Nursing*. 6th ed. St. Louis, MO: Elsevier; 2021:601.

21. **(B)** Maternal history consisting of the follow risk factors indicates the need for intrapartum antibiotic prophylaxis: gestation less than 37 weeks, prolonged rupture of membranes (greater than 18 hours), maternal fever of 38°C (100.4°F) or higher, history of GBS bacteriuria during the current pregnancy, or a previous infant with GBS infection. An upper respiratory infection is not a contributing risk factor in this scenario. Although premature rupture of membranes is a concern, it is when the membranes have been ruptured for a prolonged period in which the risk of infection in the infant increases, thereby necessitating intrapartum antibiotic prophylaxis. Once the maternal temperature reaches 38°C (100.4°F), it is then considered a risk factor.

Reference: Pammi M, Brand C, Weisman L. Infection in the neonate. In: Gardner WL, Carter BS, Enzman-Hines M, Niermeyer S, eds. *Merenstein & Gardner's Handbook of Neonatal Intensive Care: An Interprofessional Approach*. 9th ed. St. Louis, MO: Elsevier; 2021:701-702.

22. **(D)** The mother is not exhibiting signs of infection or illness which would prohibit her from visiting her infant, continuing to provide milk, and providing direct contact. She should continue to perform good hand hygiene and ensure she is well enough to handle her infant. Infection Control notification is not indicated as the mother is not exhibiting any signs of communicable disease. Direct patient contact with standard precautions is acceptable; even if the mother is exhibiting fever in the postpartum period as long as she does not have a specific, communicable cause for her fever. Breastfeeding is rarely contraindicated in the case of maternal infection.

Reference: Kilpatrick SJ, Papile LA, eds. *Guidelines for Perinatal Care*. 8th ed. Elk Grove Village, IL: American Academy of Pediatrics; 2017:571.

23. **(D)** Treatment is always indicated in infants with proven or highly probable congenital syphilis. The preferred treatment, recommended by the Centers for Disease Control, is aqueous crystalline penicillin G 50,000 units/kg intravenously every 12 hours for the first 7 days and then every 8 hours thereafter, for a total of 10 days, even if the infant received empiric treatment ampicillin for possible sepsis. Intramuscular single dosing is only indicated when congenital syphilis is less likely in the instance the mother received adequate treatment during her pregnancy.

Reference: Gomella T, Eyal F, Bany-Mohammed F. *Gomella's Neonatology: Management, Procedures, On-Call Problems, Diseases and Drugs*. 8th ed. New York: McGraw Hill; 2020:1195.

24. **(B)** Although acyclovir (Zovirax) is generally well tolerated, it can be nephrotoxic and result in acute kidney injury/renal failure with elevations in the blood urea nitrogen and creatinine. Adequate hydration and administering the medication over at least 1 hour decreases the risk of renal injury. Hematologic dyscrasias such as neutropenia and neutrophilia, thrombocytopenia and thrombocytosis, anemia, and leucocytosis can be present as a result of acyclovir (Zovirax) administration. If neutropenia presents, the medication dose will need to be reduced. Acyclovir (Zovirax) has no effect on the respiratory system. Herpes simplex virus labs are obtained in the initial sepsis evaluation.

Reference: Gomella T, Eyal F, Bany-Mohammed F. *Gomella's Neonatology: Management, Procedures, On-Call Problems, Diseases and Drugs*. 8th ed. New York: McGraw Hill; 2020:1227.

25. **(B)** Current recommendations from the American Academy of Pediatrics (AAP) require infection control precautions until the infant tests negative in the first 72 hours of age. The timing/frequency of testing is dependent on each facility's protocols; however, the facility should follow the current AAP recommendations for ensuring a negative test in the first 72 hours of age. The AAP recommendations suggest the infant should be tested as the latest evidence of the risk of infection of the infant related to vertical transmission is 2.2%–5.6% and up to 13.6% in one registry, with the highest risk of infection occurring when a mother has onset of COVID-19 near the time of delivery.

Reference: American Academy of Pediatrics (AAP). *FAQs: Management of Infants Born to Mothers with Suspected or Confirmed COVID-19*. AAP. Available at: https://www.aap.org/en/pages/2019-novel-coronavirus-covid-19-infections/clinical-guidance/faqs-management-of-infants-born-to-covid-19-mothers/. Updated November 11, 2022; Accessed January 20, 2023.

26. **(C)** Stage II–III necrotizing enterocolitis (NEC) requires antibiotic therapy for 10–14 days and not routinely extended past 14 days unless other infectious problems present, which require more than 2 weeks of antibiotics. Infants presenting with clinical signs of medical NEC without diagnostic findings of pneumatosis on x-ray imaging (Stage I-suspected) will typically receive only 48 hours of antibiotics.

References: Gomella T, Eyal F, Bany-Mohammed F. *Gomella's Neonatology: Management, Procedures, On-Call Problems, Diseases and Drugs*. 8th ed. New York: McGraw Hill; 2020:995.

Weitkamp JH, Premjumar MH, Martin CR. Necrotizing enterocolitis. In: Eichenwald EC, Hansen AR, Martin CR, Stark AR, eds. *Cloherty and Stark's Manual of Neonatal Care*. 8th ed. Philadelphia, PA: Lippincott Williams & Wilkins; 2017:454-456.

Chapter 23

Dermatologic Disorders

1. Which statement is true when considering erythema toxicum?
   A. Erythema toxicum appears as yellow or pearly white papules on the brow, cheeks, and nose.
   B. Erythema toxicum has an erythematous base and can be transient, appearing on face, trunk, and limbs.
   C. Erythema toxicum appears as large white or yellow pustules in infants up to 3 months of age.
   D. Erythema toxicum is usually treated with antibiotic ointment.

2. The nurse is caring for an infant who is being treated for hypoxic ischemic encephalopathy with therapeutic hypothermia. Knowing that subcutaneous fat necrosis can be a complication of therapeutic hypothermia, the nurse monitors the infant for:
   A. abnormal serum calcium levels.
   B. abnormal complete blood count levels.
   C. soft, mobile, grey nodules in the subcutaneous tissue.
   D. scalp nodules presenting in a dermatomal pattern.

3. A 33-week African American infant born via a forceps-assisted vaginal delivery is admitted to the neonatal intensive care unit. The infant is comfortable on room air, and the physical exam is unremarkable except for a large blue–green patch over the lower back and buttocks. The father is concerned, after seeing the lower back and buttocks, that the infant may have suffered a birth injury from the forceps used at delivery. What is the nurse's best response to the father?
   A. "I will document presence of the bruise. It is likely not related to the use of forceps."
   B. "The bruise is from delivery and will fade with time. It is not painful to your infant."
   C. "These patches are consistent with Mongolian spots. They are common in African American and Hispanic infants. We will need to send blood tests to ensure your infant is not at risk for a bleeding disorder."
   D. "This patch of skin is consistent with hyperpigmented macules due to an increased number of melanocytes. They are a benign finding and will likely fade with time."

4. A newborn infant is diagnosed with cutis aplasia. The nurse knows this condition:
   A. is associated with trisomies 18 and 21.
   B. is infectious in origin.
   C. will heal slowly over several months, leaving hypertrophic or atrophic scar tissue.
   D. is associated with lateral abdominal wall defects.

5. A newborn infant presents with several vesicopustules on the scalp, lateral to the site of the fetal monitor electrode that was in place during labor and delivery. The nurse notifies the provider and expects the initial intervention to be:
   A. standard monitoring, because the nurse knows that seborrheic dermatitis is self-limiting.
   B. broad-spectrum antibiotics, such as vancomycin, because these findings are consistent with bacterial infection.
   C. an antiviral agent, such as acyclovir, because these findings are consistent with herpes infection.
   D. standard monitoring, because erythema toxicum does not require treatment.

6. The nurse has received the handover report on an infant diagnosed with Sturge-Weber syndrome. An expected finding on assessment is:
   A. port wine stain.
   B. multiple hemangiomas.
   C. more than six café au lait spots.
   D. hyperpigmented macules.

7. When planning care for an infant who has ichthyosis, the priority for treatment is:
   A. antibiotics as soon as possible due to risk of *Staphylococcus epidermidis* infection.
   B. moisturizing emollients to hydrate and lubricate the skin.
   C. NPO status to avoid associated gastrointestinal complication.
   D. skin biopsy to rule out malignancy.

8. A mother is concerned because her infant, who was born at 30 weeks' gestation, has multiple small infantile hemangiomas located on her chest and back. The mother says, "I've heard that they can grow so large, they can impede the functioning

of vital organs." What is the nurse's best response to the mother?
   A. "Hemangiomas always require treatment when the infant is older than 1 year. Laser therapy is the preferred method of treatment."
   B. "It is common for the hemangiomas to bleed and become ulcerated, but they won't interfere with organ functioning."
   C. "Hemangiomas are only a cosmetic concern and will not cause any physiologic problems for your baby."
   D. "Infantile hemangiomas will generally increase in size up to 6 months of age and then gradually get smaller. Most will go away without any treatment. They are treated if they interfere with vision or other organ functioning. They will be monitored closely to ensure there is no interference with any organ function."

ANSWERS AND RATIONALES

1. **(B)** Erythema toxicum, also known as *newborn rash*, is best characterized by small yellow or white pustules surrounded by an erythematous base seen in infants up to 3 months of age. The pustules can come and go on varying parts of the body but are never seen on the palms of the hands or the soles of the feet. Milia is better characterized by yellow or pearly white papules, approximately 1 mm in size, most commonly occurring on the brow, cheeks, and nose. Erythema toxicum does not require treatment.
Reference: Witt C. Neonatal dermatology. In: Verklan MT, Walden M, Forest S, eds. *Core Curriculum for Neonatal Intensive Care Nursing*. 6th ed. St. Louis, MO: Elsevier; 2021:678-690.

2. **(A)** Calcium levels should be monitored because both hypercalcemia and hypocalcemia may be noted in infants with subcutaneous fat necrosis. Subcutaneous fat necrosis does not alter complete blood count results. Nodules from subcutaneous fat necrosis are noted to be hard, circumscribed, and red or purple. Subcutaneous fat necrosis nodules appear on the trunk, extremities, or face, not on the scalp. A dermatome refers to an area of the skin that is supplied by a single spinal nerve. Since these subcutaneous fat nodules are from the subcutaneous tissue, they are not associated with the nervous system.
Reference: Witt C. Neonatal dermatology. In: Verklan MT, Walden MT, Forest S, eds. *Core Curriculum for Neonatal Intensive Care Nursing*. 6th ed. St. Louis, MO: Elsevier; 2021:678-690.

3. **(D)** The assessment is consistent with hyperpigmented macules, the most common pigmented lesion seen at birth, occurring in 80% of African American, Hispanic, and Asian infants and occasionally in lighter skinned infants. The areas can fade over time as surrounding skin gets darker. Hyperpigmented macules should not be referred to as Mongolian spots. Additionally, hyperpigmented macules do not indicate a bleeding disorder, therefore blood tests are not necessary. It is important to document the size and shape to avoid the question of nonaccidental trauma.
Reference: Witt C. Neonatal dermatology. In: Verklan MT, Walden M, Forest S, eds. *Core Curriculum for Neonatal Intensive Care Nursing*. 6th ed. St. Louis, MO: Elsevier; 2021:678-690.

4. **(D)** Cutis aplasia is a congenital disorder characterized by the absence of a portion of the skin. Lesions are most commonly seen midline on the scalp, but other areas of the body, including the extremities, may be affected. Generally, the lesions heal slowly over months, leaving scarring in the location of the defect. Large lesions, however, may require surgical excision or skin grafting. Cutis aplasia is associated with approximately 50% of infants with

trisomy 13. It is also associated with midline defects such as cleft lip and palate, heart disease, and tracheoesophageal fistula. Cutis aplasia is not infectious.

References: Narendram V. The skin of the neonate. In: Martin RJ, Fanaroff AA, Walsh MC, eds. *Fanaroff and Martin's Neonatal-Perinatal Medicine: Diseases of the Fetus and Infant.* 11th ed. Philadelphia, PA: Elsevier; 2020:1924.

Witt C. Neonatal dermatology. In: Verklan MT, Walden M, Forest S, eds. *Core Curriculum for Neonatal Intensive Care Nursing.* 6th ed. St. Louis, MO: Elsevier; 2019:678-690.

5. **(C)** Herpes rash appears as a vesicular or pustular rash. Treatment with an antiviral agent such as acyclovir should begin immediately after the rash is discovered or infection is suspected. Herpes can be transmitted during delivery and vesicopustules are often noted on the presenting body part. Seborrheic dermatitis is self-limiting, but it presents as plaques, rather than pustules, with a yellow waxy appearance. Vancomycin is used primarily to treat MRSA and late onset coagulase-negative staphylococci infections, the majority of which in the NICU are of late onset. Erythema toxicum presents with small white or yellow pustules with an erythematous base, usually on the face, trunk, and limbs.

References: Samies NL, James SH, Kimberlin DW. Neonatal herpes simplex virus disease. *Clin Perinatol.* 2021;48(2):263-274. doi:10.1016/j.clp.2021.03.003.

Witt C. Neonatal dermatology. In: Verklan MT, Walden M, Forest S, eds. *Core Curriculum for Neonatal Intensive Care Nursing.* 6th ed. St. Louis, MO: Elsevier; 2021:678-690.

6. **(A)** Port wine stain is a flat, vascular nevus that is present at birth, usually appearing pink, red or purple. It does not grow in size and is permanent, often getting darker and thicker with age. Sturge-Weber syndrome is characterized by port wine stains that are confined to a pattern similar to that of the trigeminal nerve. It is associated with atrophic changes in the cerebral cortex and calcium deposits in the walls of small vessels and areas of affected cortex. Infantile hemangiomas are not associated with Sturge-Weber syndrome. More than six café au lait spots can indicate neurofibromatosis. Neurofibromatosis causes tumors to form on the cutaneous nerves and along the thoracic, brachial, and lumbar nerve trunks. Hyperpigmented macules are the most common

pigmented lesion seen at birth, occurring in 80% of African American, Hispanic, and Asian infants and occasionally in lighter skinned infants. The areas can fade over time as surrounding skin gets darker.

References: Poliner A, Fernandez Faith E, Blieden L, Kelly KM, Metry D. Port-wine birthmarks: update on diagnosis, risk assessment for Sturge-Weber Syndrome, and management. *Pediatr Rev.* 2022;43(9):507-516. doi:10.1542/pir.2021-005437.

Witt C. Neonatal dermatology. In: Verklan MT, Walden M, Forest S, eds. *Core Curriculum for Neonatal Intensive Care Nursing.* 6th ed. St. Louis, MO: Elsevier; 2021:678-690.

7. **(B)** Ichthyosis is caused by excessive production of stratum corneum cells or faulty shedding of the stratum corneum. It is not infectious in origin and does not require prophylactic antibiotic treatment. Treatment for ichthyosis is limited to use of topical emollients to hydrate and lubricate the skin. Daily baths with water dispersible bath oil, with use of alpha hydroxyl acid ointments may be helpful. Prevention of infection of dry or cracked skin is important. Nutrition is vital to keep skin hydrated and intact. Skin biopsy is not recommended for ichthyosis.

Reference: Witt C. Neonatal dermatology. In: Verklan MT, Walden M, Forest S, eds. *Core Curriculum for Neonatal Intensive Care Nursing.* 6th ed. St. Louis, MO: Elsevier; 2021:678-690.

8. **(D)** Infantile hemangiomas will generally increase in size up to 6 months of age and then gradually spontaneously regress. Monitoring for bleeding or ulceration, interference with vision or other vital organ function, such as stridor, poor feeding, and difficulty swallowing is important to indicate if treatment is necessary. Treatment of choice is to allow the lesion to regress spontaneously. Intervention is considered if the hemangioma is bleeding or ulcerating, interfering with vision or other vital organ function, such as stridor, poor feeding, and difficulty swallowing. Bleeding and ulceration of infantile hemangiomas is not common and would require treatment.

Reference: Witt C. Neonatal dermatology. In: Verklan MT, Walden M, Forest S, eds. Core *Curriculum for Neonatal Intensive Care Nursing.* 6th ed. St. Louis, MO: Elsevier; 2021:678-690.

Chapter 24

Auditory and Ophthalmologic Disorders

1. Which of the following infants are at the greatest risk for developing retinopathy of prematurity?
   A. 26 weeks' gestation, female, weighing 990 g at birth, having never required supplemental oxygen
   B. 27 weeks' gestation, male, weighing 900 g at birth, having never required supplemental oxygen
   C. 29 weeks' gestation, female requiring mechanical ventilation and supplemental oxygen since birth
   D. 30 weeks' gestation male with extremely labile oxygen saturations, requiring supplemental oxygen, on phototherapy for hyperbilirubinemia with a symptomatic patent ductus arteriosus

2. An infant is to have an eye examination, and the nurse has just instilled a mydriatic agent into the infant's eyes. Which of the following is the most likely potential complication of the mydriatic agent?

   A. Tachycardia and restlessness
   B. Apnea and hypotension
   C. Periorbital edema and photophobia
   D. Lethargy and bradycardia

3. During evaluation of an infant's ears, the nurse notes a small pit anterior to the tragus. What is the best explanation for this finding?
   A. A normal variant that has no associated risks to the newborn
   B. A minor malformation that may communicate with the internal ear or brain and lead to infection
   C. A significant finding that is strongly associated with chromosomal anomalies
   D. A significant finding that is associated with hearing loss

4. The neonatal nurse is planning for the discharge of a full-term infant. What action is most appropriate when the nurse discovers the hearing screening has not yet been completed?
   A. Perform the hearing screening before the infant's discharge.
   B. Perform the hearing screening only if the infant received antibiotic therapy.
   C. Inform the parents that hearing screening is necessary only for preterm infants.
   D. If there is a family history of hearing loss, refer the infant for outpatient testing.

5. A full-term infant received ampicillin and gentamicin for suspected sepsis. Before discharge, the infant fails hearing screening in both ears. What information should the nurse provide to the parents at this time?
   A. Further evaluation of auditory function will be necessary.
   B. Immediate treatment for permanent hearing loss is required.
   C. Failing the hearing screening is a temporary side effect of antibiotic therapy.
   D. The hearing screening will be repeated until the infant passes the test in at least one ear.

6. After instillation of mydriatic eye drops, which of the following interventions should the nurse implement to reduce systemic absorption of the medication?
   A. Cover the eyes with eye shields.
   B. Turn head to the ipsilateral side.
   C. Apply a cool compress over eyes.
   D. Apply gentle pressure to the nasolacrimal duct for 1 minute.

7. When caring for a neonate with untreated peripartum exposure to *Neisseria gonorrhea*, the nurse expects which symptoms within how many days of age?
   A. Redness of conjunctivae and purulent discharge in 3–4 days
   B. Purulent discharge and intense edema of the eyelid in 5–7 days
   C. Purulent discharge causing matting of the eye in 5–14 days
   D. Redness and watering of the eye in 6–14 days

8. Which of these assessment findings would indicate a nasolacrimal obstruction in the premature neonate?
   A. Presence of conjunctival infection
   B. Minimal to excessive eye drainage at 4–5 weeks of life
   C. Purulent drainage from either punctum with pressure on nasolacrimal sac
   D. Occasional tearing when crying for the first 1–2 months of life

ANSWERS AND RATIONALES

1. **(A)** The incidence of retinopathy of prematurity (ROP) is inversely proportional to gestational age and birth weight. Therefore those infants at greatest risk for development of ROP are the smallest, most premature infants. The 26-week infant is therefore at greater risk than the 27-, 29-, and 30-week infants. Additionally, ROP occurs more often and with greater severity in male infants. Although supplemental oxygen, hypoxia, and hyperoxia are all proven risk factors for ROP, the single most important clinical factor is prematurity/low birth weight. The 27-week-gestational-age infant may weigh less than the 26-week infant, but the earlier gestation places the 26-week gestation infant at the greatest risk.

Reference: Fraser D, Diehl-Jones W. Ophthalmologic and auditory disorders. In: Verklan MT, Walden M, Forrest S, eds. *Core Curriculum for Neonatal Intensive Care Nursing.* 6th ed. St. Louis, MO: Elsevier; 2021:691-704.

2. **(A)** A mydriatic agent, an agent that dilates the pupil of the eye, is an anticholinergic, meaning it blocks acetylcholine in the central and peripheral nervous system. If systemic absorption occurs, other anticholinergic effects could be observed, including tachycardia and restlessness. Apnea can be a complication of mydriatic eye drops, but the nurse would expect hypertension, not hypotension, as a systemic effect of the anticholinergic eye drops. Photophobia is an expected finding after mydriasis, and the nurse should place protective eyewear on the infant after instillation of the eye drops. Periorbital edema is not pertinent to mydriatic agents.

Reference: Fraser D, Diehl-Jones W. Ophthalmologic and auditory disorders. In: Verklan MT, Walden M, Forest S, eds. *Core Curriculum for Neonatal Intensive Care Nursing.* 6th ed. St. Louis, MO: Elsevier; 2021:691-704.

3. **(B)** Preauricular skin pits are minor malformations that may be familial, congenital, or associated with other anomalies. The sinus may end in a blind pouch or communicate with the inner ear or brain and can lead to chronic infection, in which case the sinus tract would need to be removed. Preauricular skin pits are not associated with hearing loss.

References: Fraser D, Diehl-Jones W. Ophthalmologic and auditory disorders. In: Verklan MT, Walden M, Forest S, eds. *Core Curriculum for Neonatal Intensive Care Nursing.* 6th ed. St. Louis, MO: Elsevier; 2021:691-704.

Johnson PJ. Head, eyes, ears, nose, mouth, and neck assessment. In: Tappero EP, Honeyfield ME, eds. *Physical Assessment of the Newborn: A Comprehensive Approach to the Art of Physical Assessment.* 6th ed. New York: Springer Publishing Company, LLC; 2019:61-77.

4. **(A)** Hearing screening is recommended for all newborns. Failure on the hearing screening is an indication for referral for further evaluation.

References: Fraser D, Diehl-Jones W. Ophthalmologic and auditory disorders. In: Verklan MT, Walden M, Forest S, eds. *Core Curriculum for Neonatal Intensive Care Nursing.* 6th ed. St. Louis, MO: Elsevier; 2021:691-704.

The Joint Commission on Infant Hearing. Year 2019 position statement: principles and guidelines for early hearing detection and intervention programs. *J Early Hear Detect Int.* 2019;4(2):1-44. Available at: https://digitalcommons.usu.edu/cgi/viewcontent.cgi?article=1104&context=jehdi.

5. **(A)** Hearing screening aids in identifying infants at high risk for hearing loss. Infants who fail the screening should be referred for further evaluation. Failure on the hearing screening is not diagnostic of hearing loss. Gentamicin is a potentially ototoxic medication and can lead to permanent hearing loss. Repetition of the same screening test is not indicated. Infants who fail a hearing screening require further evaluation.

Reference: Fraser D, Diehl-Jones W. Ophthalmologic and auditory disorders. In: Verklan MT, Walden M, Forest S, eds. *Core Curriculum for Neonatal Intensive Care Nursing.* 6th ed. St. Louis, MO: Elsevier; 2021:691-704.

6. **(D)** Systemic absorption of mydriatic eye drops can lead to tachycardia and restlessness. Wiping away excess eye drops and applying gentle pressure over the nasolacrimal duct will minimize systemic absorption. Although covering the eyes after an eye examination protects them from bright light, it does not minimize systemic absorption of the medication. Turning the head to the ipsilateral side may result in excess eye drops on the face and subsequent systemic absorption through the skin. Applying a cool compress over the eyes may lead to hypothermia and does not minimize systemic absorption of the eye drops.

Reference: Fraser D, Diehl-Jones W. Ophthalmologic and auditory disorders. In: Verklan MT, Walden M, Forest S, eds. *Core Curriculum for Neonatal Intensive Care Nursing.* 6th ed. St. Louis, MO: Elsevier; 2021:691-704.

7. (A) *Neisseria gonorrhea* is transmitted through the peripartum environment and presents with symptoms of eyelid edema, purulent drainage, and redness of the conjunctivae typically within 3–4 days following birth, whereas *Chlamydia trachomatis* displays edema of eyelids and purulent discharge typically between days 5 and 7. Redness and matting of the eyes are common in *Staphylococcus aureus* infection typically noted between days 5–14. With herpes simplex infection redness, pain, and swelling is noted within 6–14 days and development of vesicles in the affected area is also noted in 50% of localized infections, appearing in 6–9 days of life.

References: Puopolo KM. Bacterial and fungal infections. In: Eichenwald EC, Hansen AR, Martin CR, Stark AR, eds. *Cloherty and Stark's Manual of Neonatal Care.* 8th ed. Philadelphia, PA: Wolters Kluwer; 2017:715-716.

Fraser D, Diehl-Jones W. Ophthalmologic and auditory disorders. In: Verklan MT, Walden M, Forest S, eds. *Core Curriculum for Neonatal Intensive Care Nursing.* 6th ed. St. Louis, MO: Elsevier; 2021:691-704.

8. (C) Purulent drainage noted from either punctum when pressure is applied to the nasolacrimal sac indicates obstruction, which is frequently caused by an imperforate membrane located at the distal end of the lacrimal duct. Care must be taken as firm digital pressure increases the hydrostatic pressure in the nasolacrimal sac potentially leading to rupture of the membranous obstruction. With massage, obstructed nasolacrimal ducts usually resolve within the first year of life. If drainage becomes mucopurulent, medicated eye drops or ointment are needed. Neonates with a nasolacrimal duct obstruction typically present within the first three weeks of life and do not present with infection. However, dacryocystitis, an inflamed, swollen lacrimal sac, may develop at a later time requiring treatment with antibiotic eye drops or antibiotic ointment. As a reflex to irritants in the environment, newborns, both term and preterm are capable of secreting tears due to these irritants, however neither population secrets emotional tears until 2–3 months of age.

Reference: Fraser D, Diehl-Jones W. Ophthalmologic and auditory disorders. In: Verklan MT, Walden M, Forest S, eds. *Core Curriculum for Neonatal Intensive Care Nursing.* 6th ed. St. Louis, MO: Elsevier; 2021:691-704.

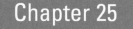

Chapter 25

Maternal–Fetal Complications

1. A 41-week neonate is delivered vaginally with vacuum extraction assistance. Within a few hours of birth, the neonate is noted to have increased work of breathing, pallor, and a head circumference measurement 2 cm larger than at birth. The nurse should anticipate this clinical presentation to be most consistent with:
   A. surfactant deficiency.
   B. subgaleal hemorrhage.
   C. neonatal encephalopathy.
   D. caput succedaneum.

2. A neonate is born to a 20-year-old primigravida mother with a history of cocaine use and daily cigarette smoking. Hypovolemia is noted on neonatal assessment after delivery. The nurse should anticipate this clinical presentation to be most consistent with which of the following maternal placental anomalies?
   A. Placenta previa
   B. Placenta accreta
   C. Placental abruption
   D. Circumvallate placenta

3. A 37-week neonate develops tachypnea and grunting at 6 hours of life. On chest radiograph the infant is found to have evidence of cardiomyopathy. What is the most likely maternal condition that results in neonatal cardiomyopathy?
   A. Diabetes
   B. Hypothyroidism
   C. Hemolysis, elevated liver enzymes, low platelet count syndrome
   D. Chronic hypertension

4. A 36-week neonate is born to a mother with known systemic lupus erythematosus. After delivery, the neonate is active and has the following vital signs: temperature 36.7°C (98°F), heart rate 64 bpm, respiratory rate 58, blood pressure 65/38 mm Hg, O_2 saturation 98%. Capillary refill is less than 2 seconds. What is the most appropriate response by the neonatal nurse?
   A. Provide positive pressure ventilation, anticipate intubation by the pediatric provider.
   B. Obtain order for chest radiograph.
   C. Obtain STAT electrocardiogram.
   D. Request provider place an emergent umbilical venous catheter and administer epinephrine.

5. During electronic fetal monitoring, the fetal heart rate slows with the initiation of a contraction, but returns to baseline as the contraction ends. Which of the following is the correct interpretation by the nurse of this tracing?
   A. Nonreassuring fetal heart rate
   B. Early deceleration
   C. Late deceleration
   D. Umbilical cord compression

6. A 40-week, 4.5-kg (10 lb, 2 oz) infant was born via vaginal delivery with forceps assistance. On examination, the infant has an internally rotated right arm with a pronated wrist and does not move the right arm. Moro reflex is absent on the right side of the neonate's upper extremity. The nurse should consider these findings most characteristic of:
   A. Klumpke paralysis.
   B. Erb-Duchenne paralysis.
   C. clavicle fracture.
   D. humerus fracture.

7. A set of monochorionic twins is admitted to the neonatal intensive care unit with a suspicion of twin-to-twin transfusion syndrome. The nurse should be aware that this syndrome is most commonly associated with which of the following findings?
   A. Recipient twin who presents with anemia
   B. Donor twin who presents with plethora
   C. Donor twin who is small for gestational age
   D. Recipient twin who is small for gestational age

8. A neonate is admitted following an emergent cesarean section. The obstetric team noted a cord prolapse on exam. Which of the following findings should the nurse anticipate given this delivery history?
   A. Apgar scores of 8 and 9 at 1 and 5 minutes, respectively
   B. Arterial pH 7.15 with base deficit –10
   C. Lactate level of 1.4 mmol/L
   D. Hemoglobin 15.8 g/dL and hematocrit 51%

9. A neonate is delivered to a mother with a history of oligohydramnios. The nurse recognizes an association of oligohydramnios with which of the following conditions?
   A. Renal agenesis
   B. Esophageal atresia
   C. Anencephaly
   D. Omphalocele

10. During intrapartum monitoring, a woman is noted to have the following vital signs: heart rate 110 beats per minute, respiratory rate 16 breaths per minute, oxygen saturation 99%, blood pressure 126/84, temperature 38.5°C (101.3°F), and reports uterine tenderness. The nurse should recognize this as indicative of which of the following?
    A. Placental abruption
    B. Placenta previa
    C. Umbilical cord prolapse
    D. Chorioamnionitis

11. On physical assessment, a 35-week-gestation neonate is noted to be small for gestational age (<3rd percentile) and microcephalic. Cataracts and a diffuse "blueberry muffin" rash are also noted. The nurse should suspect that the infant has which of the following conditions?
    A. Syphilis
    B. Herpes simplex virus
    C. Rubella
    D. Toxoplasmosis

12. At 28 weeks' gestation, a woman reports decreased fetal movement and measures large for gestational age. An ultrasound reveals fetal ascites and bilateral pleural effusions. The nurse should anticipate the infant is afflicted with which of the following conditions?
    A. Hydrops fetalis
    B. Trisomy 21
    C. Congenital diaphragmatic hernia
    D. Duodenal atresia

13. A 34-week-gestation neonate is found to have anemia (Hgb 8 g/dL) and hyperbilirubinemia (total bilirubin level 6 mg/dL) at 12 hours of life. The infant had a positive direct antiglobulin test. Which condition should the nurse consider as the most likely the etiology of these findings?
    A. Physiologic jaundice
    B. Vitamin K deficiency
    C. Cephalohematoma
    D. Rh isoimmunization

14. At 48 hours of life, a term neonate is noted to have jitteriness, irritability, sneezing, and elevated temperature. The maternal history is significant for sickle cell disease and chronic pain. The mother regularly takes prescribed opioids for pain management. Which of the following actions should the nurse take?
    A. Begin neonatal abstinence scoring.
    B. Discharge the infant with the parents.
    C. Administer intravenous fluids containing glucose.
    D. Draw blood cultures and place on antibiotics.

ANSWERS AND RATIONALES

1. **(B)** The traction associated with vacuum extraction can result in the rupture of blood vessels within the subgaleal space. This space can accommodate a large volume of blood which places at risk for ongoing blood loss and hypovolemic shock. Clinical symptoms include diffuse scalp swelling, a fluctuant mass, hypotonia, and pallor. Caput succedaneum is characterized by an area of self-limiting edema over the presenting part of the scalp and typically resolves within 48–72 hours. Neonatal encephalopathy can present with a decreased level of consciousness, hypotonia, abnormal reflexes, and seizures in the setting of a perinatal asphyxia. Surfactant deficiency related to prematurity can cause alveolar collapse and decreased lung compliance. A neonate with surfactant deficiency typically presents with tachypnea, grunting, retractions, and cyanosis.

References: Gomella TL, Eyal, FG, Bany Mohammed F. Chapter 83: Traumatic delivery. In: Gomella TL, Eyal FG, Bany Mohammed F, eds. *Gomella's Neonatology: Management, Procedures, On-Call Problems, Diseases, and Drugs*. 8th ed. New York: McGraw Hill; 2020.

Groenendaal F, de Vries LS. Hypoxic-ischemic encephalopathy. In: Martin RJ, Fanaroff AA, Walsh MC, eds. *Fanaroff and Martin's Neonatal-Perinatal Medicine*. 11th ed. Philadelphia, PA: Elsevier; 2020:989-1014.

AWHONN, Terese VM, Marlene W, Sharron F. *Core Curriculum for Neonatal Intensive Care Nursing*. 6th ed. St. Louis, MO: Elsevier Health Sciences (US); 2021.

2. **(C)** Placenta previa can present with bright, painless vaginal bleeding from cervical changes which may be associated with cigarette smoking and cocaine use, but occurs most frequently in multiparous and older women. Placenta accreta is an abnormal placental implantation and unless associated with placenta previa poses more risk for the mother than the newborn in terms of hemorrhage at delivery. Cocaine use and cigarette smoking are two risk factors commonly associated with placenta abruption due to a hypertensive state. Placental abruption can lead to acute blood loss at the time of delivery for mother and infant and reflect neonatal hypovolemia. Circumvallate placenta is an anomaly of the placental edges curling away from the uterine wall. It can be associated with recent or old hemorrhage and is noted on physical exam of the placenta after delivery.

Reference: Hurst HM. Antepartum-intrapartum complications. In: Verklan T, Walden M, Forest S, eds. *Core Curriculum for Neonatal Intensive Care Nursing*. 6th ed. Philadelphia, PA: Elsevier; 2021:20-37.

3. **(A)** Cardiomyopathy can present as thickened myocardium and/or septal hypertrophy in as many as 30% of infants of diabetic

mothers. Persistent maternal hyperglycemia results in increased fetal insulin production, resulting in a fetal hyperinsulinemic state. Increased circulating insulin promotes fetal growth, particularly in skeletal muscle and cardiac tissue. Neonates with cardiomyopathy may be asymptomatic, but may also present with respiratory distress or cardiac failure. Maternal hypertensive disorders result in fetal growth restriction and premature delivery. Hypothyroidism is not associated with cardiomyopathy.

References: Moore TR, Hauguel-De Mouzon S, Catalano P. Diabetes in pregnancy. In: Resnik R, Lockwood CJ, Moore TR, Greene MF, Copel JA, Silver RM, eds. *Creasy's & Resnik's Maternal-Fetal Medicine: Principles and Practice.* 8th ed. Philadelphia, PA: Elsevier; 2019:1067-1097.

Jeyabalan A. Hypertensive disorders of pregnancy. In: Martin RJ, Fanaroff AA, Walsh MC, eds. *Fanaroff and Martin's Neonatal-Perinatal Medicine.* 11th ed. Philadelphia, PA: Elsevier; 2020:288.

4. **(C)** Maternal systemic lupus erythematosus has been associated with neonatal congenital heart block. Infants with neonatal lupus should receive an electrocardiogram at birth. Neonates in complete heart block may require a permanent pacemaker to support systemic perfusion because the condition is irreversible. Positive pressure ventilation, intubation, and epinephrine are indicated per neonatal resuscitation protocol when there are signs of clinical decompensation, which the neonate did not exhibit.

Reference: Sammarito LR, Salmon Branch DW. Pregnancy and rheumatic diseases. In: Resnik R, Lockwood CJ, Moore TR, Greene MF, Copel JA, Silver RM, eds. *Creasy's & Resnik's Maternal-Fetal Medicine: Principles and Practice.* 8th ed. Philadelphia, PA: Elsevier; 2019:1192-1207.

5. **(B)** Early decelerations occur in conjunction with uterine contractions and have a uniform pattern with gradual deceleration and return to baseline. The increased intracranial pressure from the contraction causes vagal nerve stimulation resulting in transient fetal bradycardia. These are benign and not associated with fetal compromise. Late decelerations result from uteroplacental insufficiency and indicate a presence of fetal hypoxia. The nadir occurs after the contraction peaks, with the shape demonstrating a decrease and slow return to baseline. Variable decelerations are due to abrupt umbilical cord compression and exhibit a "V" or "W" nonuniform pattern. Variable decelerations typically have an abrupt onset and recovery and are often preceded by heart rate accelerations. A nonreassuring fetal heart rate (most often described as late or variable decelerations) is a heart rate nadir not achieved until after the contraction peaks and is followed by a slow return to baseline.

References: Gomella TL, Eyal FG, Bany Mohammed F. Chapter 1: Fetal assessment. In: Gomella TL, Eyal FG, Bany Mohammed F, eds. *Gomella's Neonatology: Management, Procedures, On-Call Problems, Diseases, and Drugs.* 8th ed. New York: McGraw Hill; 2020.

AWHONN, Terese VM, Marlene W, Sharron F. *Core Curriculum for Neonatal Intensive Care Nursing.* 6th ed. St. Louis, MO: Elsevier Health Sciences (US); 2021.

6. **(B)** Erb-Duchenne paralysis, Klumpke paralysis, and clavicle fractures may occur in difficult, prolonged deliveries. Erb-Duchenne and Klumpke paralyses result from excessive traction and stretching of the brachial plexus nerves. Neonates with Erb-Duchenne paralysis (upper arm) present with an internally rotated arm and a pronated, flexed wrist and typically have an absent Moro reflex. Klumpke paralysis is a lower arm and hand paralysis where the affected hand is flaccid with little control. Clavicle fractures are often asymptomatic, although crepitus may be palpated along the clavicle. The infant may exhibit decreased extremity movement on the side of the fracture. Humerus fractures can also be associated with decreased extremity movement and pain with manipulation, but it is a rare occurrence, even with a traumatic birth.

References: Gomella TL, Eyal FG, Bany-Mohammed F. Chapter 7: Newborn physical examination. In: Gomella TL, Eyal FG, Bany Mohammed F, eds.

Gomella's Neonatology: Management, Procedures, On-Call Problems, Diseases, and Drugs. 8th ed. New York: McGraw Hill; 2020.

AWHONN, Terese VM, Marlene W, Sharron F. *Core Curriculum for Neonatal Intensive Care Nursing.* 6th ed. St. Louis, MO: Elsevier Health Sciences (US); 2021.

7. **(C)** Twin–twin transfusion syndrome (TTTS) results from abnormal vascular connections within the placenta and allows for the exchange of volume and other substrates between the fetuses disproportionately. TTTS can be diagnosed in utero because there is discordance in amniotic fluid volume and growth parameters. The donor twin presents with oligohydramnios and smaller crown–rump length and abdominal circumference, whereas the recipient twin often presents with polyhydramnios and larger growth parameters. At birth, the donor twin is typically smaller and may present with anemia and hypovolemia, which can progress to congestive heart failure. The larger recipient twin is often polycythemic and may present with plethora and cardiomegaly.

Reference: Gomella TL, Eyal FG, Bany-Mohammed F. Chapter 107: Multiple gestation. In: Gomella TL, Eyal FG, Bany Mohammed F, eds. *Gomella's Neonatology: Management, Procedures, On-Call Problems, Diseases, and Drugs.* 8th ed. New York: McGraw Hill; 2020.

8. **(B)** This presentation is consistent with umbilical cord prolapse. These neonates can have prolonged bradycardia (from cord compression) as evidenced by severe variable decelerations and are at risk for fetal asphyxia. Umbilical cord prolapse and the subsequent compression of the cord can lead to respiratory acidosis and, if prolonged, anaerobic metabolism. The resulting blood gas is likely to demonstrate a mixed respiratory and metabolic acidosis. Immediate relief of cord compression (manually) and delivery are priorities for mother and neonate. Hemoglobin and hematocrit levels are not significantly affected with cord prolapse, given the absence of a hemorrhagic event. Lactate levels will be elevated in the case of a prolonged prolapse and asphyxia and 1.4 mg/dL would be normal. APGAR scores of 8 and 9 indicate an infant with successful transition to extrauterine life.

References: Ugwumadu A, Baskett TF. Cord prolapse. In: Arulkumaran S, Robson MS, eds. *Munro Kerr's Operative Obstetrics.* 13th ed. Philadelphia, PA: Elsevier; 2020:81-84.

Nageotte MP. Intrapartum fetal surveillance. In: Resnik R, Lockwood CJ, Moore TR, Greene MF, Copel JA, Silver RM, eds. *Creasy's & Resnik's Maternal-Fetal Medicine: Principles and Practice.* 8th ed. Philadelphia, PA: Elsevier; 2019:564-582.

9. **(A)** Fetal breathing, swallowing, and urine production and excretion regulate the amniotic fluid volume in utero. Amniotic fluid volume can be measured using ultrasonography and is reported as the amniotic fluid index, which is the summation of the measurement of the largest pocket of amniotic fluid in each quadrant. Oligohydramnios, low amniotic fluid volume, is associated with fetal anomalies, particularly of the renal and urinary system. Renal agenesis and urinary tract obstructions are commonly diagnosed if pregnancy is affected by oligohydramnios. Polyhydramnios, the overproduction of amniotic fluid, is often a result of impaired swallowing, gastrointestinal anomalies and obstructions, or neurologic anomalies. Anencephaly, a neural tube defect with absence of the fetal skull, is not commonly associated with oligohydramnios. Omphalocele, an abdominal wall defect, is not commonly associated with oligohydramnios.

References: Simmons PM, Magann EF. Amniotic fluid volume. In: Martin RJ, Fanaroff AA, Walsh MC, eds. *Fanaroff and Martin's Neonatal-Perinatal Medicine.* 11th ed. Philadelphia, PA: Elsevier; 2020:386-403.

AWHONN, Terese VM, Marlene W, Sharron F. *Core Curriculum for Neonatal Intensive Care Nursing.* 6th ed. St. Louis, MO: Elsevier Health Sciences (US); 2021.

10. **(D)** Pregnant women with chorioamnionitis present with fever >100.4°F, plus two other findings, including maternal (>100 bpm)

and fetal (>160 bpm) tachycardia, uterine tenderness, maternal leukocytosis, and foul-smelling/purulent amniotic fluid. Placental abruption can present with uterine tenderness, but vaginal bleeding is also a clinical finding. Placenta previa is defined when the placenta is covering the cervical opening. The woman may experience painless bleeding with previa in the absence of uterine tenderness. Umbilical cord prolapse occurs when the umbilical cord presents alongside or before the fetal presenting part. Umbilical cord prolapse is not associated with infection, rather fetal hypoxia and emergent need for delivery.

References: Polin R, Randis TM. Perinatal infections and chorioamnionitis. In: Martin RJ, Fanaroff AA, Walsh MC, eds. *Fanaroff and Martin's Neonatal-Perinatal Medicine*. 11th ed. Philadelphia, PA: Elsevier; 2020:404-414.

Hull AD, Resnik R, Silver RM. Placenta previa and accreta, vasa previa, sub-chorionic hemorrhage and abruptio placentae. In: Resnik R, Lockwood CJ, Moore TR, Greene MF, Copel JA, Silver RM, eds. *Creasy's & Resnik's Maternal-Fetal Medicine: Principles and Practice*. 8th ed. Philadelphia, PA: Elsevier; 2019.

Ugwumadu A, Baskett TF. Cord prolapse. In: Arulkumaran S, Robson MS, eds. *Munro Kerr's Operative Obstetrics*. 13th ed. Philadelphia, PA: Elsevier; 2020:81-84.

11. **(C)** Congenital rubella syndrome is a result of in utero transmission of the rubella virus with infected neonates exhibiting anomalies related to gestational age when the exposure occurred. Common clinical findings with congenital rubella syndrome can include a diffuse "blueberry muffin" rash, thrombocytopenia, growth restriction, hepatosplenomegaly, and jaundice. Microcephaly, cataracts, and sensorineural deafness are also commonly seen with congenital rubella syndrome. Infants with congenital herpes simplex virus can appear asymptomatic or present with localized skin lesions, such as vesicles and mucosal lesions, or more severely with diffuse central nervous system findings (seizures, temperature dysregulation, lethargy) and neurologic sequelae. Infants with congenital syphilis may not present with symptoms in the neonatal period. Affected infants often do not present with active disease until 3–8 weeks of life. Characteristic symptoms include intrauterine growth restriction, a maculopapular rash, nasal "snuffles," hepatosplenomegaly, generalized lymphadenopathy, and chorioretinitis. Congenital toxoplasmosis is rare and most likely results from in utero exposure toxoplasmosis protozoan host (cat feces) during the third trimester. Affected infants present with purpuric rash, hepatosplenomegaly, ventriculomegaly, and chorioretinitis. Diagnosis is often delayed until visual impairment, strabismus, or developmental delay is apparent.

References: Michaels MG, Williams JV. Infectious disease. In: Zitelli BJ, McIntire SC, Nowalk AJ, Garrison J, eds. *Zitelli and Davis' Atlas of Pediatric Physical Diagnosis*. 8th ed. Philadelphia, PA: Elsevier; 2023:459-510.

Polin R, Randis TM. Perinatal infections and chorioamnionitis. In: Martin RJ, Fanaroff AA, Walsh MC, eds. *Fanaroff and Martin's Neonatal-Perinatal Medicine*. 11th ed. Philadelphia, PA: Elsevier; 2020:404-414.

AWHONN, Terese VM, Marlene W, Sharron F. *Core Curriculum for Neonatal Intensive Care Nursing*. 6th ed. St. Louis, MO: Elsevier Health Sciences (US); 2021.

12. **(A)** Hydrops fetalis is characterized by excess fluid in two or more body cavities, defined as abdominal ascites, pleural or pericardial effusion, skin edema, polyhydramnios, or placentomegaly. Polyhydramnios and a fetus measuring large for gestational dates are often the first indicators of hydrops fetalis, with subsequent ultrasound findings confirming diagnosis. Hydrops fetalis is further defined as immune (around 10%) or nonimmune (around 90%) in the differential diagnosis. Immune hydrops fetalis is a combination of hydrops, fetal anemia, and jaundice that occurs when a Rh-negative mother is exposed to a Rh-positive fetal blood type. Antibodies produced by the mother transplacentally pass to the fetus, resulting in fetal hemolysis. Nonimmune hydrops fetalis encompasses many pathophysiologies resulting in excess fetal body fluid. Lymphatic malformations, liver failure, inborn errors

of metabolism, heart failure, and chromosomal abnormalities can be responsible for nonimmune hydrops fetalis and the condition often worsens until delivery, rarely resolving spontaneously. Ultrasonography findings commonly associated with trisomy 21 include increased nuchal translucency, absence of nasal bone, cardiac anomalies, specifically atrioventricular canal defect and shortened humerus and femur measurements. Congenital diaphragmatic hernia may be detected with a thoracic mass and visible peristalsis on the affected side of defect. The classic presentation of duodenal atresia on ultrasonography is the "double-bubble" sign which represents a dilated stomach and duodenum proximal to the atresia.

References: Simmons PM, Magann EF. Immune and nonimmune hydrops fetalis. In: Martin RJ, Fanaroff AA, Walsh MC, eds. *Fanaroff and Martin's Neonatal-Perinatal Medicine*. 11th ed. Philadelphia, PA: Elsevier; 2020:371-385.

Wapner RJ, Dugoff L. Prenatal diagnosis of congenital disorders. In: Resnik R, Lockwood CJ, Moore TR, Greene MF, Copel JA, Silver RM, eds. *Creasy's & Resnik's Maternal-Fetal Medicine: Principles and Practice*. 8th ed. Philadelphia, PA: Elsevier; 2019:493-538.

Wilkins I. Nonimmune hydrops. In: Resnik R, Lockwood CJ, Moore TR, Greene MF, Copel JA, Silver RM, eds. *Creasy's & Resnik's Maternal-Fetal Medicine: Principles and Practice*. 8th ed. Philadelphia, PA: Elsevier; 2019:645-653.

AWHONN, Terese VM, Marlene W, Sharron F. *Core Curriculum for Neonatal Intensive Care Nursing*. 6th ed. St. Louis, MO: Elsevier Health Sciences (US); 2021.

13. **(D)** Due to immature hepatic function, physiologic jaundice in preterm infants should be closely monitored. Physiologic jaundice in preterm neonates' peak between 10 and 12 mg/dL on the fifth day of life. There are a number of causes of pathologic unconjugated hyperbilirubinemia, with Rh isoimmunization being one of the more common causes. Rh isoimmunization results when fetal erythrocytes carry different antigens than maternal erythrocytes. The maternal immune system reacts against the foreign antigen and produces IgG antibodies, which bind to and then subsequently destroy the fetal erythrocyte. Infants with Rh incompatibility present with jaundice within a few hours of birth and pallor due to the destruction of fetal erythrocytes. Common laboratory findings with Rh isoimmunization include anemia, reticulocytosis, and a positive direct antiglobulin test. Infants have limited vitamin K stores at birth and are at high risk of bleeding because vitamin K plays a key role in the production of coagulation factors. Vitamin K deficiency often presents with abnormal bleeding, particularly from the gastrointestinal tract, the umbilical stump, or after circumcision. Cephalohematoma often develops slowly and does not extend across suture lines. The infant may develop anemia and hyperbilirubinemia if the hemorrhage is severe, but cephalohematoma typically resolves without any treatment.

References: Lee RH, Chung RT, Pringle P. Diseases of the liver, biliary system, and pancreas. In: Resnik R, Lockwood CJ, Moore TR, Greene MF, Copel JA, Silver RM, eds. *Creasy's & Resnik's Maternal-Fetal Medicine: Principles and Practice*. 8th ed. Philadelphia, PA: Elsevier; 2019:1173-1191.

Kaplan M, Wong RJ, Burgis JC, et al. Neonatal jaundice and liver diseases. In: Martin RJ, Fanaroff AA, Walsh MC, eds. *Fanaroff and Martin's Neonatal-Perinatal Medicine*. 11th ed. Philadelphia, PA: Elsevier; 2020:1788-1852.

Moise KJ, Queenan J. Hemolytic disease of the fetus and newborn. In: Resnik R, Lockwood CJ, Moore TR, Greene MF, Copel JA, Silver RM, eds. *Creasy's & Resnik's Maternal-Fetal Medicine: Principles and Practice*. 8th ed. Philadelphia, PA: Elsevier; 2019:632-644.

14. **(A)** Physiologic withdrawal symptoms can appear within the first 2–3 days of life, and nearly 60%–90% of exposed infants develop withdrawal symptoms. Women with chronic pain may be managed throughout a pregnancy with prescribed opioids. Symptoms of withdrawal can reflect gastrointestinal disturbances, such as emesis, loose stools, and poor feeding; central nervous system disturbances, such as irritability, hypertonicity, high-pitched cry, and exaggerated reflexes; and metabolic/

respiratory disturbances, such as sneezing, tachypnea, and fever. Infants with hypoglycemia that require intravenous glucose solutions may exhibit irritability, jitteriness, hypotonia, hypothermia, and seizures but will not exhibit sneezing as a symptom. Signs of early-onset sepsis typically manifest within 12–24 hours after birth. Infants with neonatal sepsis commonly present with neurologic changes (lethargy or irritability), apnea, respiratory distress, and temperature fluctuations with hypothermia more common than hyperthermia.

References: Gomella TL, Eyal FG, Bany-Mohammed F. Chapter 102: Infant of a mother with substance use disorder. In: Gomella TL, Eyal FG, Bany Mohammed F, eds. *Gomella's Neonatology: Management, Procedures, On-Call Problems, Diseases, and Drugs.* 8th ed. New York: McGraw Hill; 2020.

Ferrieri P, Wallen LD. Newborn sepsis and meningitis. In: Gleason CA, Juul SE, eds. *Avery's Diseases of the Newborn.* 10th ed. *Avery's Diseases of the Newborn.* 10th ed. Philadelphia, PA: Elsevier; 2018:553-565.

AWHONN, Terese VM, Marlene W, Sharron F. *Core Curriculum for Neonatal Intensive Care Nursing.* 6th ed. St. Louis, MO: Elsevier Health Sciences (US); 2021.

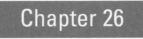

Pain Assessment and Management

1. The parent of a 4-day-old male infant born at 32 weeks' gestation does not want his infant to receive pain medication for a chest tube insertion for fear that his son will become addicted. Based on knowledge of opioids, the nurse:
   A. suggests subcutaneous lidocaine as an alternative intervention.
   B. respects the parent's decision and does not provide pain medication.
   C. explores the parent's beliefs about pain and pain medication.
   D. tells the parent that addiction is a psychologic dependence on a drug and preterm infants cannot become addicted.

2. A 6-week-old female infant with severe retinopathy of prematurity is scheduled for her third eye examination. The infant's mother indicates that the infant required reintubation after a prior examination. Which of the following is the best action?
   A. Provide 24% sucrose 2 minutes before the examination.
   B. Ask the mother to watch her daughter's response to the examination while the nurse assists the ophthalmologist.
   C. Instruct the mother to provide her daughter with containment while softly speaking to her during the procedure.
   D. Ask the mother if she knows what makes her daughter comfortable during painful procedures and explain that containment or offering a pacifier with or without sucrose may reduce pain.

3. A growing premature infant is preparing for discharge and scheduled to receive immunizations. His parents are unable to be present during the procedure. Nonnutritive sucking on a pacifier is recommended based on the knowledge that:
   A. nonnutritive sucking reduces pain transmission through opioid pathways.
   B. nonnutritive sucking effects are immediate.
   C. the pain-relieving properties of nonnutritive sucking increase with gestational age.
   D. the effects of nonnutritive sucking continue after the pacifier is removed.

4. In an emergency situation in which immediate pain relief is desired, the most appropriate medication to administer is intravenous (IV):
   A. fentanyl.
   B. morphine.

   C. midazolam (Versed).
   D. meperidine (Demerol).

5. When planning to perform a routine heel stick:
   A. cluster all other care procedures at the same time.
   B. ensure a rest period to follow.
   C. apply EMLA 1 hour before.
   D. play recorded lullaby music just before and during the procedure.

6. A growing premature infant requires intermittent heel sticks. The father has expressed an interest in soothing the infant with facilitated tuck for these procedures. The nurse instructs the father on the appropriate technique for holding gentle pressure as follows:
   A. Place one cupped hand on the top of the infant's head and the other on the bottom of the feet.
   B. Place one cupped hand on the back side of the infant's head and the other on the buttocks.
   C. Place both cupped hands on either side of the infant's shoulder/upper arm area.
   D. Hold the infant in a football hold.

7. A 37-week-old newborn weighing 2150 g has a complete repair of his gastroschisis and postoperatively is started on a fentanyl infusion at 2 mcg/kg/h and IV acetaminophen every 6 hours. An acute desaturation and increase in heart rate with an elevated pain score at 4 hours result in an as-needed fentanyl dose of 4 mcg. What additional intervention would be appropriate at this time?
   A. Oral sucrose
   B. Short-acting benzodiazepine
   C. Position with containment
   D. 0.1 mg morphine IV

8. A term infant had a complete surgical repair of a congenital diaphragmatic hernia 9 days ago. The infant was weaned off inhaled nitric oxide 2 days ago but remains on high-frequency oscillatory ventilation (HFOV). A morphine infusion has been continuous postoperatively and has been at 0.04 mg/kg/h for the last 3 days. Today, the plan is to wean HFOV. The nurse suggests the following approach to opiate management:

A. Wean in small increments and perform neonatal abstinence scoring.

B. Wean in small increments and perform serial sedation assessments.

C. Discontinue the infusion and perform neonatal abstinence scoring.

D. Discontinue the infusion and perform serial sedation assessments.

9. A nurse is caring for a 35-week-gestation newborn weighing 2.3 kg. The infant underwent a small bowel resection with an end-to-end anastomosis on day 1 of life. IV fentanyl 6 mcg is ordered as-needed every 4 hours for elevated pain scores. The initial postoperative assessment reveals a hypotonic infant without spontaneous respirations. Monitoring this infant for pain will require a focus on:

A. changes in vital signs.

B. changes in facial expression.

C. changes in behavioral signs.

D. changes in transcutaneous CO_2.

10. Subcutaneous lidocaine is an appropriate pain management strategy for what type of procedure?

A. Circumcision

B. Radial arterial puncture

C. Peripherally inserted central catheter

D. Lumbar puncture

11. Which of these actions is the most effective way to prevent pain?

A. Place the neonate in prone position in between assessments.

B. Reduce the number of procedures routinely performed in the neonatal intensive care unit.

C. Provide music therapy in between assessments.

D. Ensure IV access is available for emergent treatment of pain.

12. A neonatal nurse practitioner is planning to perform a suprapubic aspiration procedure on a former 26-week-gestation infant whose corrected age is 37 5/7 weeks. The nurse provides adequate pain management by:

A. providing nonnutritive sucking with sucrose administration and a topical anesthetic.

B. establishing IV access for morphine administration.

C. ensuring that the infant's mother can be present to provide skin-to-skin care.

D. providing bundling and repositioning.

13. Which pain assessment tool is used specifically to assess postoperative pain?

A. Premature Infant Pain Profile

B. Neonatal Infant Pain Scale

C. Échelle de Douleur et d'Inconfort du Nouveau-né

D. CRIES

14. The healthcare team is preparing for an insertion of a chest tube on a 3280 g infant. The provider orders fentanyl 16.4 mg IV. The nurse should:

A. administer the medication slowly.

B. administer the medication rapidly.

C. not administer the medication and suggest to the provider a lower dose.

D. not administer the medication and suggest a nonopioid be used instead.

15. Reduced brain microstructure and volumes, greater risk for diabetes mellitus and hypertension, and long-term stress-related psychosocial disabilities are all negative effects from:

A. necrotizing enterocolitis.

B. early life pain.

C. anemia of prematurity.

D. long-term use of mechanical ventilation.

ANSWERS AND RATIONALES

1. **(C)** Parents have many concerns and fears about their infant's pain and about the drugs used in the treatment of pain, thus the nurse should explore the father's concerns about pain medication. Suggesting subcutaneous lidocaine as an alternative intervention or telling the parent that addiction is a psychologic dependence on a drug does not address or explore the parent's concerns. If the nurse does not provide analgesia, then the nurse is not advocating for the infant.

References: Coughlin M. *Trauma Informed Care in the NICU: Evidence-Based Practice Guidelines for Neonatal Clinicians.* New York: Springer Publishing Company, LLC; 2017:123.

Walden M. Pain assessment and management. In: Verklan M, Walden M, Forest S, eds. *Core Curriculum for Neonatal Intensive Care Nursing.* 6th ed. St. Louis, MO: Elsevier; 2021:284.

2. **(D)** A key principle of family-centered neonatal care is that "parents and healthcare professionals must talk openly and honestly about acute and chronic pain associated with operative, diagnostic, and therapeutic procedures." Additionally, parents should be taught how to interpret their infant's pain cues. Providing 24% sucrose 2 minutes before the examination and asking the mother to watch her daughter's response to the examination while the nurse assists the ophthalmologist does not explore the mother's concerns nor does it facilitate family-centered care. Although it will be helpful to have the mother perform comfort measures, in the spirit of family-centered care, the nurse must first explore the mother's concerns and explain the benefits of the comfort measures.

Reference: Walden M. Pain assessment and management. In: Verklan M, Walden M, Forest S, eds. *Core Curriculum for Neonatal Intensive Care Nursing.* 6th ed. St. Louis, MO: Elsevier; 2021:284.

3. **(B)** The mechanism of action of nonnutritive sucking is thought to be related to its effect on nonopioid pathways. The effects of nonnutritive sucking are immediate and continue as long as the infant sucks on the pacifier. Once the pacifier is removed from the infant's mouth, the pain-relieving effects of nonnutritive sucking cease. The pain-relieving properties of sucking are not related to gestational age.

References: Walden M. Pain assessment and management. In: Verklan M, Walden M, Forest S, eds. *Core Curriculum for Neonatal Intensive Care Nursing.* 6th ed. St. Louis, MO: Elsevier; 2021:280.

Vu-Ngoc H, Minh Uyen NC, Thinh OP, et al. Analgesic effect of non-nutritive sucking in term neonates: a randomized controlled trial. *Pediatr Neonatol.* 2020;61(1):106-113.

4. **(A)** The onset of action for fentanyl is almost immediate, and it is the preferred analgesic when immediate pain relief is the goal. The onset of action for morphine is 5–15 minutes, thus morphine would not be the analgesic of choice in an emergency situation. Midazolam, a benzodiazepine, is a sedative without analgesic properties and should not be used for pain relief. Demerol is not recommended in preterm or term infants due to the accumulation of the active metabolite normeperidine. This accumulation may cause central nervous system stimulation and may lower the seizure threshold level.

References: Gardner SL, Enzman-Hines M, Agarwal R. Pain and pain relief. In: Gardner SL, Carter B, Enzman-Hines M, Niermeyer S, eds. *Merenstein & Gardner's Handbook of Neonatal Intensive Care: An Interprofessional Approach*. 9th ed. St. Louis, MO: Elsevier; 2021:306.

Donato J, Lewis T, Rao T. Pharmacology of common analgesic and sedative drugs used in the neonatal intensive care unit. *Clin Perinatol*. 2019;46(4): 673-692.

5. **(B)** After a painful procedure, the nociceptive pathways may remain active such that routine caregiving procedures that are ordinarily not painful may be perceived to be painful. Plan to give the infant time to recover from the painful procedure before resuming routine caregiving procedures. Clustering of care may not allow for sufficient time for the infant to rest between care intervals. EMLA is not effective for heel stick procedures. The use of music is not an evidence-based intervention for moderate pain associated with heel stick.

Reference: Walden M. Pain assessment and management. In: Verklan M, Walden M, Forest S, eds. *Core Curriculum for Neonatal Intensive Care Nursing*. 6th ed. St. Louis, MO: Elsevier; 2021:279.

6. **(B)** Facilitated tuck involves flexion of the neck and body which can be achieved by placing one cupped hand on the back side of the infant's head and the other on the buttocks. Pressure from the top of the head does not facilitate flexion. Bilateral containment limits the amount of flexion that can be supported. The football hold is an optional position used for breastfeeding, and the arms provide more support for the upper part of the infant's body rather than the lower part of the body.

References: Ranjbar A, Bernstein C, Shariat M, Ranjbar H. Comparison of facilitated tucking and oral dextrose in reducing the pain of heel stick in preterm infants: a randomized clinical trial. *BMC Pediatr*. 2020;20(1):162. doi:10.1186/s12887-020-2020-7.

Friedrichsdorf SJ, Eull D, Weidner C, Postier A. A hospital-wide initiative to eliminate or reduce needle pain in children using lean methodology. *Pain Rep*. 2018;3(1):e671. doi:10.1097/PR9.0000000000000671.

Pouraboli B, Mirlashari J, Fakhr AS, Ranjbar H, Ashtari S. The effect of facilitated tucking on the pain intensity induced by chest tube removal in infants. *Adv Neonatal Care*. 2022;22(5):467-472. doi:10.1097/ANC.0000000000000936.

Francisco ASPG, Montemezzo D, Ribeiro SNDS, et al. Positioning effects for procedural pain relief in NICU: systematic review. *Pain Manag Nurs*. 2021;22(2):121-132. doi:10.1016/j.pmn.2020.07.006.

7. **(C)** Nonpharmacologic interventions should accompany pharmacologic interventions to additionally support the infant's coping ability. Sucrose use in intubated babies has not been adequately studied, and the potential effect of sucrose administered orally in an infant with gastrointestinal dysfunction is unknown. Benzodiazepines should not be used to manage pain because they provide sedation, not analgesia. Fentanyl and morphine are both opioids; only one opioid should be used at a time.

Reference: Walden M. Pain assessment and management. In: Verklan M, Walden M, Forest S, eds. *Core Curriculum for Neonatal Intensive Care Nursing*. 6th ed. St. Louis, MO: Elsevier; 2021:273.

8. **(A)** Infants exposed to opioid therapy for several days are at risk for opioid withdrawal, therefore weaning rather than abrupt discontinuance of therapy is recommended. Abstinence scoring should be performed during weaning to monitor for withdrawal.

References: Walden M, Spruill CT. Pain assessment in the newborn. In: Honeyfield M, Tapparo E, eds. *Physical Assessment of the Newborn: A Comprehensive Approach to the Art of Physical Examination*. 6th ed. New York: Springer Publishing Company, LLC; 2019:239-254.

Walden M. Pain assessment and management. In: Verklan M, Walden M, Forest S, eds. *Core Curriculum for Neonatal Intensive Care Nursing*. 6th ed. St. Louis, MO: Elsevier; 2021:282.

9. **(A)** Behavioral indicators of pain, including facial expression, may be suppressed in this infant due to the effects of anesthesia. Thus vital sign changes such as an elevated heart rate and/or blood pressure may indicate the need for additional pain medication. No measure of CO_2 has been identified as an indicator of pain in a unidimensional or multidimensional pain assessment tool.

References: Campbell-Yeo M, Eriksson M, Benoit B. Assessment and management of pain in preterm infants: a practice update. *Children (Basel, Switzerland)*. 2022;9(2):1-18. doi:10.3390/children9020244.

Perry M, Tan Z, Chen J, Weidig T, Xu W. Neonatal pain: perceptions and current practice. *Crit Care Nurs Clin North Am*. 2018;30(4):549-561. doi:10.1016/j.cnc.2018.07.013.

10. **(D)** Subcutaneous lidocaine should be considered for lumbar puncture and chest tube insertion. A dorsal penile nerve block or other regional block or a topical anesthetic would be appropriate for a circumcision. A topical anesthetic would be appropriate for a radial arterial stick or peripherally inserted central catheter.

Reference: Bailey TB, Maltsberger HL. Common invasive procedures. In: Verklan M, Walden M, Forest S, eds. *Core Curriculum for Neonatal Intensive Care Nursing*. 6th ed. St. Louis, MO: Elsevier; 2021:266.

11. **(B)** Reducing the number of procedures routinely performed in the neonatal intensive care unit is the most effective way to prevent pain in the neonate. Neonates should always be placed supine in between assessments, unless a different position is ordered by the physician. Music therapy may be used to treat short-term pain and stress relief however, it is not the most effective treatment for pain relief. Further study is needed on the use of music therapy. Ensuring intravenous access for a neonate that is not requiring treatment with medication or intravenous fluid is an unnecessary painful and stressful procedure.

References: Arnon S, Maitre N. Music Therapy for neonatal stress and pain—music to our ears. *J Perinatol*. 2020;(40):1734-1735.

Coughlin M. *Trauma Informed Care in the NICU: Evidence-Based Practice Guidelines for Neonatal Clinicians*. New York: Springer Publishing Company, LLC; 2017:101-136.

12. **(A)** Providing nonpharmacologic interventions such as nonnutritive sucking with sucrose administration and a topical anesthetic is an appropriate intervention to prevent pain associated with a bladder aspiration. Morphine is not indicated for this procedure. The procedure requires the infant's abdomen to be exposed, therefore skin-to-skin care and bundling are not appropriate.

References: Peters A, Medina-Blasini Y. Suprapubic aspiration. In: *StatPearls*. Treasure Island, FL: StatPearls Publishing; 2022. Available at: https://www.ncbi.nlm.nih.gov/books/NBK557545/.

13. **(D)** The CRIES Neonatal Postoperative Pain Assessment Score is used to assess postoperative pain in infants between 32 and 60 weeks' gestation. The premature infant pain profile is used to assess procedural pain in infants between 28 and 40 weeks' gestation. The Neonatal Infant Pain Scale is used to assess procedural pain in infants between 26 and 47 weeks' gestation. The Échelle de Douleur et d'Inconfort du Nouveau-né (EDIN) Pain Scale is used to assess pain in infants between 25 and 36 weeks' gestation who are experiencing prolonged pain.

Reference: Walden M. Pain assessment and management. In: Verklan M, Walden M, Forest S, eds. *Core Curriculum for Neonatal Intensive Care Nursing*. 6th ed. St. Louis, MO: Elsevier; 2021:274-279.

14. **(C)** An opioid is an appropriate option to prevent procedural pain associated with a chest tube insertion. The recommended dose of fentanyl for intermittent pain is 0.5–3 mcg/kg, given slowly to prevent chest wall rigidity. For this infant, the correct dose would be 1.64–9.84 mcg. Since the provider ordered too high of a dose, the nurse should not administer the medication and suggest a lower dose be used.

Reference: Walden M. Pain assessment and management. In: Verklan M, Walden M, Forest S, eds. *Core Curriculum for Neonatal Intensive Care Nursing.* 6th ed. St. Louis, MO: Elsevier; 2021:281.

15. **(B)** Reduced brain microstructure and volumes, greater risk for diabetes mellitus and hypertension, and long-term stress related psychosocial disabilities are all negative effects from early life pain. Complications of necrotizing enterocolitis include failure to thrive, short bowel syndrome, neurodevelopmental delay, gastrointestinal issues, adhesions, and/or strictures. Symptoms of anemia of prematurity includes tachycardia, poor feeding, diminished activity and weight gain. Long-term effects of mechanical ventilation include bronchopulmonary dysplasia.

References: Walden M. Pain assessment and management. In: Verklan M, Walden M, Forest S, eds. *Core Curriculum for Neonatal Intensive Care Nursing.* 6th ed. St. Louis MO: Elsevier; 2021:576.

Williams MD, Lascelles B. Early neonatal pain – a review of clinical and experimental implications on painful conditions later in life. *Front Pediatr.* 2020;8:30. doi:10.3389/fped.2020.00030.

Chapter 27

Perinatal Substance Abuse

1. An infant is admitted to the neonatal intensive care unit (NICU) and is displaying severe signs of neonatal abstinence syndrome. What nonpharmacologic supportive measure does the nurse take to help reduce the symptoms and offer support to the infant?
   A. Rock the infant after feedings.
   B. Swaddle the infant.
   C. Encourage the mother to stroke and talk with infant while visiting.
   D. Offer infant larger feeding volumes to decrease hunger feelings initiated by neonatal abstinence syndrome.

2. A newborn in the NICU is receiving morphine in the correct prescribed dose for sedation while on mechanical ventilation. After several days the mechanical ventilation and the morphine are discontinued, and the newborn becomes restless and agitated. The nurse suspects:
   A. sepsis.
   B. hypoxia.
   C. iatrogenic neonatal abstinence syndrome.
   D. overstimulation from the neonatal intensive care environment.

3. The provider orders urine toxicology on an infant whose mother is suspected of substance abuse. The nurse knows that:
   A. urine toxicology should be performed 48 hours after birth.
   B. urine toxicology will not detect marijuana.
   C. urine toxicology can detect drug metabolites from 20 weeks' gestational age.
   D. urine toxicology is associated with a high false-negative rate.

4. A preceptor and orientee are caring for a 36-week-gestation premature infant born to a mother with an opioid use disorder. While discussing neonatal opioid withdrawal syndrome (NOWS), the preceptor explains which of the following?
   A. Signs and symptoms of withdrawal are exacerbated in premature infants.
   B. The plan of care for infants with NOWS should include nonpharmacologic interventions once pharmacologic treatment has started.
   C. Signs and symptoms of NOWS primarily reflect central nervous system irritability, excessive autonomic activity, and gastrointestinal dysfunction.

   D. Onset of withdrawal symptoms from opioids typically begins within 2 hours of birth.

5. When developing the plan of care for an infant born to a mother prescribed buprenorphine during pregnancy, the nurse includes which of the following interventions?
   A. Encourage mother to breastfeed.
   B. Limit maternal visitation.
   C. Assess for facial dysmorphology.
   D. Offer nonnutritive sucking with oral sucrose if signs of withdrawal occur.

6. A 38-week-gestation infant is admitted to the NICU for meconium aspiration syndrome. Maternal history is notable for no prenatal care and heroin use. The infant was intubated at 1 hour of life and remained on mechanical ventilation for 24 hours. At 36 hours of life, the infant is on oxygen via nasal cannula and has begun feeding. Assessment reveals respiratory rate of 60 breaths per minute, oxygen saturation 96%, tremors, irritability, vomiting, and temperature instability. A priority action is to:
   A. start oral morphine to treat opioid withdrawal.
   B. obtain laboratory tests to assess for glucose and electrolyte disturbances.
   C. obtain meconium for drug screening.
   D. begin antibiotics to treat sepsis.

7. An infant's care team has decided to begin pharmacologic treatment for an infant with severe signs of NOWS. The mother has a history of polysubstance abuse during pregnancy, is in a substance use treatment program, and is taking buprenorphine as prescribed in her program. The nurse expects which of the following medications to be ordered for the infant?
   A. Paregoric
   B. Phenobarbital
   C. Clonidine
   D. Morphine

8. Compared to mothers using methadone during pregnancy, use of buprenorphine has been found to be associated with:
   A. a shorter hospital length of stay for the infant.
   B. higher neonatal abstinence scores.

C. a higher incidence of seizures in infants.

D. a later onset of withdrawal symptoms in the infant.

9. Meconium drug screening (MDS) is the gold standard for testing neonates with perinatal drug exposure. An advantage of MDS over urine toxicology is that MDS testing can identify a neonate who has been exposed to drugs during which of the following time periods?

A. The second and third trimesters of the pregnancy.

B. The last 30 days of the pregnancy.

C. The entire pregnancy.

D. The last 48 hours prior to delivery.

10. If the mother's prenatal history is positive for cocaine abuse, what should the nurse most likely suspect?

A. The newborn to show signs and symptoms of neonatal abstinence syndrome within 4 hours of birth.

B. The newborn to have a low birth weight and length.

C. The newborn to have facial dysmorphology.

D. The newborn to display decreased tone and activity.

11. A term infant with a maternal history of substance use, including heroin, is being cared for in the NICU. When developing the plan of care for this infant, the nurse includes which of the following interventions?

A. Provide nutrition to meet 100 cal/kg/day.

B. Minimal handling while sleeping.

C. Begin using the Finnegan abstinence scoring tool once signs and symptoms of withdrawal appear.

D. Maintain bright lighting to observe for signs and symptoms of withdrawal.

12. A NICU nurse is a team member for a quality improvement project aimed at improving outcomes of infants with neonatal abstinence syndrome. The nurse recommends which of the following strategies?

A. Establishing set times for maternal visitation

B. Observation of opioid exposed infants for 3 days

C. Admission to the NICU for all infants with neonatal abstinence syndrome

D. A standardized assessment approach by using a commonly used tool to measure presence and severity of withdrawal symptoms

13. What is the minimum duration of observation time for an infant born to a mother receiving buprenorphine for opioid use disorder before the asymptomatic infant can be discharged home?

A. 1 day

B. 3 days

C. 4 days

D. 10 days

14. Regarding pregnancy and lactation, the American College of Obstetricians and Gynecologist discourages:

A. the use of any marijuana while pregnant or breastfeeding.

B. the use of marijuana unless prescribed for medical reasons.

C. the use of marijuana while pregnant.

D. the use of marijuana while breastfeeding.

15. Which of the following statements made by a mother of an infant diagnosed with NOWS indicates further teaching is needed?

A. "I should watch for signs of withdrawal for 6 months."

B. "My baby sucks her fists all the time, I think I need to feed her more often."

C. "I will pay close attention to my baby's diaper area and keep it clean because she is at risk for skin breakdown."

D. "When I lay my baby down to go to sleep, I will put her on her back."

16. Infants exposed to opioids in utero should be seen by a pediatrician within 48 hours of discharge to assess for:

A. the potential need for an ophthalmologic evaluation.

B. nystagmus, strabismus, or other refractive errors.

C. neonatal abstinence symptoms, adequate weight gain, or potential feeding problems.

D. neurodevelopmental issues.

ANSWERS AND RATIONALES

1. **(B)** Swaddling the infant is a measure that can be used to support symptoms such as hypertonia, tremors, and inability to sleep. Minimal stimulation offers the best support for infants with neonatal abstinence syndrome. Noises, talking, and lighting should be reduced to offer environmental support. Rocking an infant with neonatal abstinence syndrome is overstimulating and may exacerbate withdrawal symptoms. Slow, rhythmic swaying is the preferred motion as opposed to rocking. Providing support to the mother is an essential foundation of care in the opioid exposed infant. Coaching caregivers in supportive nonpharmacologic care promotes bonding. To provide supportive care, the nurse can encourage the mother to provide firm soft touch without stroking the infant. Infants should be offered small frequent or on demand feedings. The display of agitation and fist sucking seen in neonatal abstinence syndrome is related to drug withdrawal and not hunger.

References: Jackson J, Knappen B, Olsen S. Drug withdrawal in the neonate. In: Gardner SL, Carter BS, Enzman-Hines M, Niermeyer S, eds. *Merenstein and Gardner's Handbook of Neonatal Intensive Care: An Interprofessional Approach.* 9th ed. St. Louis, MO: Elsevier; 2021:264-265.

Patrick S. Maternal drug use, infant exposure, and neonatal abstinence syndrome. In: Eichenwald EC, Hansen AR, Martin CR, Stark AR, eds. *Cloherty and Stark's Manual of Neonatal Care.* 8th ed. Philadelphia, PA: Wolters Kluwer; 2017:141-157.

Patrick SW, Barfield WD, Poindexter BB, Committee on Fetus and Newborn, Committee on Substance Use and Prevention. Neonatal opioid withdrawal syndrome. *Pediatrics.* 2020;146(5):e2020029074. doi:10.1542/peds.2020-029074.

2. **(C)** Prolonged use of opioids can result in physical dependence, a state in which continued use of the drug is needed to prevent withdrawal. The withdrawal symptoms are similar to symptoms seen in infants born to mothers with an opioid use disorder (OUD) and are more likely occur in infants receiving fentanyl versus morphine and higher total doses or of longer duration. The newborn with neonatal sepsis is most likely to present with decreased tone, activity and lethargy. Hypoxia in the newborn would be best indicated by a decrease in oxygen saturation, tachypnea, and increased work of breathing. Overstimulation from the neonatal intensive care environment can lead to stress signs such as tremors and frequent squirming in the infant. However, overstimulation is not likely the cause for the infant's agitation in this scenario.

References: Gardner SL, Enzman-Hines M, Agarwal R. Pain and pain relief. In: Gardner S, Carter B, Enzman-Hines M, Niermeyer S, eds. *Merenstein and Gardner's Handbook of Neonatal Intensive Care: An Interprofessional Approach.* 9th ed. St. Louis, MO: Elsevier; 2021:319-320.

Hudak M. Infants of substance-using mothers. In: Martin R, Fanaroff A, Walsh M, eds. *Fanaroff and Martin's Neonatal-Perinatal Medicine: Diseases of the Fetus and Infant.* 11th ed. Philadelphia, PA: Elsevier; 2020:735-750.

Jackson J, Knappen B, Olsen S. Drug withdrawal in the neonate. In: Gardner SL, Carter BS, Enzman-Hines M, Niermeyer S, eds. *Merenstein and Gardner's Handbook of Neonatal Intensive Care: An Interprofessional Approach.* 9th ed. St. Louis, MO: Elsevier; 2021:252.

Walden M. Pain assessment and management. In: Verklan MT, Walden M, Forest S, eds. *Core Curriculum for Neonatal Intensive Care Nursing.* 6th ed. St. Louis, MO: Elsevier; 2021:283.

3. **(D)** A limitation of urine testing is that many drugs are metabolized and excreted rapidly. Only infants who had a recent exposure will screen positive. This is also the reason that urine testing should be performed as soon as possible after birth. Urine toxicology can detect numerous substances, including marijuana, opioids, amphetamines, benzodiazepines, cocaine, and barbiturates. Drug metabolites are found in meconium, not urine, from 20 weeks gestational age.

References: D'Apolito K. Perinatal substance abuse. In: Verklan MT, Walden M, Forest S, eds. *Core Curriculum for Neonatal Intensive Care Nursing.* 6th ed. St. Louis MO: Elsevier; 2021:40.

Patrick SW, Barfield WD, Poindexter BB, Committee on Fetus and Newborn, Committee on Substance Use and Prevention. Neonatal opioid withdrawal syndrome. *Pediatrics.* 2020;146(5):e2020029074. doi:10.1542/peds.2020-029074.

4. **(C)** Because opioid receptors are concentrated in the central nervous system and gastrointestinal tract, the predominant signs of opioid withdrawal primarily reflect central nervous system irritability, excessive autonomic activity, and gastrointestinal tract dysfunction. Signs of withdrawal are less evident in premature infants. This decreased severity of signs may be related to their immature central nervous system, lower fat depots of drug, and differences in total drug exposure rather than a protective mechanism against withdrawal. Additionally, the tools developed to assess for withdrawal were primarily developed for term or late preterm infants and may not be sensitive enough to identify withdrawal in premature infants. Nonpharmacologic interventions are recommended for all infants beginning at birth with opioid exposure, regardless of the need for pharmacologic treatment. Nonpharmacologic interventions should include providing support to the mother and creating a supportive environment for the infant. Although withdrawal symptoms may appear shortly after birth, timing of withdrawal depends on the opioid(s) used. Withdrawal from opioids with a short half-life, such as heroin, often begins within 24 hours of birth. Withdrawal from opioids with a longer half-life, such as methadone, usually begins around 24–72 hours of age.

References: D'Apolito K. Perinatal substance abuse. In: Verklan MT, Walden M, Forest S, eds. *Core Curriculum for Neonatal Intensive Care Nursing.* 6th ed. St. Louis, MO: Elsevier; 2021:46.

Hudak M. Infants of substance-using mothers. In: Martin R, Fanaroff A, Walsh M, eds. *Fanaroff and Martin's Neonatal-Perinatal Medicine: Diseases of the Fetus and Infant.' Diseases of the Fetus and Infant.* 11th ed. Philadelphia PA: Elsevier; 2020:740.

Patrick SW, Barfield WD, Poindexter BB, Committee on Fetus and Newborn, Committee on Substance Use and Prevention. Neonatal opioid withdrawal syndrome. *Pediatrics.* 2020;146(5):e2020029074. doi:10.1542/peds.2020-029074.

5. **(A)** Buprenorphine is a partial μ-opioid receptor agonist and partial κ-opioid antagonist used to treat OUD. The American Academy of Pediatrics recommends that breastfeeding be supported for infants born to mothers in treatment of OUD with buprenorphine or methadone who have not had a relapse for 90 days or more. Breast milk contains a small amount of buprenorphine and no short-term effects have been reported. Keeping the mother–infant dyad together during observation and treatment may promote bonding and facilitate breastfeeding. Rooming-in has been associated with less use of pharmacotherapy for withdrawal and shorter

lengths of hospital stay. The preferred model of care for infants born to substance using mothers is rooming-in, even in the neonatal intensive care unit (NICU). Facial dysmorphology in newborns is associated with exposure to alcohol during gestation. Because infants exposed to opioids in utero have poorly functioning endogenous opioid systems, oral sucrose is not effective in calming infants displaying symptoms of opioid withdrawal.

References: D'Apolito K. Perinatal substance abuse. In: Verklan MT, Walden M, Forest S, eds. *Core Curriculum for Neonatal Intensive Care Nursing.* 6th ed. St. Louis MO: Elsevier; 2021:40, 48.

Patrick SW, Barfield WD, Poindexter BB, Committee on Fetus and Newborn, Committee on Substance Use and Prevention. Neonatal opioid withdrawal syndrome. *Pediatrics.* 2020;146(5):e2020029074. doi:10.1542/peds.2020-029074.

6. **(B)** Metabolic derangements such as hypoglycemia, hypocalcemia, and hypomagnesemia can produce symptoms similar to neonatal abstinence syndrome. Because neonatal abstinence syndrome mimics these and other conditions such as hyperthyroidism, intracranial hemorrhage, hypoxic–ischemic encephalopathy, and polycythemia/hyperviscosity, a diagnosis of neonatal abstinence syndrome should be made and treatment begun only after other potential causes of the infant's symptoms have been ruled out. With a history of opioid use, drug testing should be performed soon after birth. If testing has not been done, it is reasonable to do so, however other potential causes of the infant's symptoms should be pursued first. Although sepsis can produce symptoms similar to neonatal abstinence syndrome, blood cultures should be obtained prior to initiating antibiotics.

References: Jackson J, Knappen B, Olsen S. Drug withdrawal in the neonate. In: Gardner SL, Carter BS, Enzman-Hines M, Niermeyer S, eds. *Merenstein and Gardner's Handbook of Neonatal Intensive Care: An Interprofessional Approach.* 9th ed. St. Louis, MO: Elsevier; 2021:261.

Patrick SW, Barfield WD, Poindexter BB, Committee on Fetus and Newborn, Committee on Substance Use and Prevention. Neonatal opioid withdrawal syndrome. *Pediatrics.* 2020;146(5):e2020029074. doi:10.1542/peds.2020-029074.

7. **(D)** Opioids are recommended as the first-line pharmacologic treatment for neonatal opioid withdrawal syndrome (NOWS). Morphine is the most commonly used opioid. Recommended pharmacological treatment for NOWS includes morphine, methadone, and buprenorphine. Paregoric (tincture of opium) contains anise oil, benzoic acid, camphor, and glycerin in an alcohol base. Some of the effects of these additives are unknown and the alcohol base is irritating to the gastrointestinal tract. The American Academy of Pediatrics recommends against the use of paregoric for NOWS. Clonidine, an α-2 adrenergic receptor agonist, and phenobarbital, a barbiturate, are used as adjunct therapy if an opioid alone does not control symptoms.

References: Jackson J, Knappen B, Olsen S. Drug withdrawal in the neonate. In: Gardner S, Carter B, Enzman-Hines M, Niermeyer S, eds. *Merenstein and Gardner's Handbook of Neonatal Intensive Care: An Interprofessional Approach.* 9th ed. St. Louis, MO: Elsevier; 2021:263-267.

Patrick SW, Barfield WD, Poindexter BB, Committee on Fetus and Newborn, Committee on Substance Use and Prevention. Neonatal opioid withdrawal syndrome. *Pediatrics.* 2020;146(5):e2020029074. doi:10.1542/peds.2020-029074.

8. **(A)** Buprenorphine is a partial μ-opioid receptor agonist and partial κ-opioid antagonist used to treat OUD. Use of buprenorphine in pregnant women has been found to be associated with less total amount of morphine needed to treat neonatal opioid withdrawal symptoms and a shorter hospital stay. Studies have not found a difference in peak neonatal abstinence scores or incidence of seizures in infants born to mothers receiving buprenorphine versus methadone. Buprenorphine has a shorter half-life than methadone, thus withdrawal typically begins between 4 and 7 days compared to 5 and 7 days for methadone.

References: Jackson J, Knappen B, Olsen S. Drug withdrawal in the neonate. In: Gardner SL, Carter BS, Enzman-Hines M, Niermeyer S, eds. *Merenstein* *and Gardner's Handbook of Neonatal Intensive Care: An Interprofessional Approach.* 9th ed. St. Louis, MO: Elsevier; 2021:254.

Patrick SW, Barfield WD, Poindexter BB, Committee on Fetus and Newborn, Committee on Substance Use and Prevention. Neonatal opioid withdrawal syndrome. *Pediatrics.* 2020;146(5):e2020029074. doi:10.1542/peds.2020-029074.

9. **(A)** Meconium drug screening is the most popular test for detecting perinatal drug exposure because it provides a more extensive drug exposure history than urine and it reports drug exposure as far back as 20 weeks gestation. A limitation to this advantage is that meconium analysis may not reflect periods of abstinence close to delivery. Urine toxicology reflects only recent exposure to most substances and may not detect previous, more remote exposure. Both meconium and urine toxicology can identify exposure to substances in the 48 hours prior to delivery.

References: Hudak M. Infants of substance-using mothers. In: Martin R, Fanaroff A, Walsh M, eds. *Fanaroff and Martin's Neonatal-Perinatal Medicine: Diseases of the Fetus and Infant. Diseases of the Fetus and Infant.* 11th ed. Philadelphia, PA: Elsevier; 2020:740.

Patrick SW, Barfield WD, Poindexter BB, Committee on Fetus and Newborn, Committee on Substance Use and Prevention. Neonatal opioid withdrawal syndrome. *Pediatrics.* 2020;146(5):e2020029074. doi:10.1542/peds.2020-029074.

10. **(B)** Newborns exposed to cocaine prenatally are born with lower birth weights and birth lengths. Cocaine has vasoconstriction properties which decreases blood flow to the placenta and fetus, contributing to fetal growth restriction. Symptoms such as irritability, hyperactivity, tremors, high-pitched cry, excessive sucking, and poor alertness and orientation are frequently seen in infants exposed to cocaine most commonly on day 2 or 3 of life. However, these abnormalities more likely reflect drug effect rather than withdrawal. Unlike opioids, cocaine does not have a clearly defined abstinence syndrome. Facial dysmorphology such as a smooth philtrum, thin upper lip, and short palpebral fissure, is associated with in utero exposure to alcohol.

References: Hudak M. Infants of substance-using mothers. In: Martin R, Fanaroff A, Walsh M, eds. *Fanaroff and Martin's Neonatal-Perinatal Medicine: Diseases of the Fetus and Infant.* 11th ed. Philadelphia, PA: Elsevier; 2020:745-746.

Jackson J, Knappen B, Olsen S. Drug withdrawal in the neonate. In: Gardner SL, Carter BS, Enzman-Hines M, Niermeyer S, eds. *Merenstein and Gardner's Handbook of Neonatal Intensive Care: An Interprofessional Approach.* 9th ed. St. Louis, MO: Elsevier; 2021:256.

11. **(B)** Nonpharmacologic interventions are recommended for all infants with opioid exposure beginning at birth, regardless of the need for pharmacologic treatment. Interventions include minimal handling while sleeping, dim room lighting, quiet environment, swaddling, rooming-in, and responding quickly to distress cues. Term infants require 100–120 cal/kg/day. Infants with neonatal abstinence syndrome may require up to 150–250 cal/kg/day because of increased energy expenditure. The onset and presentation of withdrawal is dependent on several factors, including the drug, timing of most recent exposure, maternal use of other substances such as cigarettes and benzodiazepines, genetic predisposition, gestational age, and infant metabolism and excretion. Infants exposed to opioids in utero may display signs of withdrawal shortly after birth. The initial assessment for neonatal abstinence syndrome should be done within 2–4 hours of admission to the nursery. This score reflects all infant behaviors from admission until the infant is scored.

References: D'Apolito K. Perinatal substance abuse. In: Verklan MT, Walden M, Forest S, eds. *Core Curriculum for Neonatal Intensive Care Nursing.* 6th ed. St. Louis, MO: Elsevier; 2021:42.

Hudak M. Infants of substance-using mothers. In: Martin R, Fanaroff A, Walsh M, eds. *Fanaroff and Martin's Neonatal-Perinatal Medicine: Diseases of the Fetus and Infant.* 11th ed. Philadelphia, PA: Elsevier; 2020:740.

Patrick SW, Barfield WD, Poindexter BB, Committee on Fetus and Newborn, Committee on Substance Use and Prevention. Neonatal opioid withdrawal syndrome. *Pediatrics.* 2020;146(5):e2020029074. doi:10.1542/peds.2020-029074.

Parker LA. Nutritional management. In: Verklan MT, Walden M, Forest S, eds. *Core Curriculum for Neonatal Intensive Care Nursing.* 6th ed. St. Louis, MO: Elsevier; 2021:155.

12. **(D)** Several scoring systems are available to assess for the presence and severity of withdrawal symptoms. Current guidelines do not endorse one tool over another, but rather recommend that each hospital establish a consistent approach and adherence to assessment. Keeping the mother–infant dyad together during observation and treatment may promote bonding and facilitate breastfeeding. Rooming-in has been associated with less use of pharmacotherapy for withdrawal and shorter lengths of hospital stay. The preferred model of care for infants born to substance using mothers is rooming-in, even in the NICU. The observation period for opioid exposed infants is based on the opioid(s) used during pregnancy. The 2020 American Academy of Pediatrics clinical report on NOWS recommends the following approach: immediate-release opioids (e.g., hydrocodone): 3 days; buprenorphine and sustained-release opioids: 4–7 days; methadone: 5–7 days. In the absence of other conditions requiring intensive care, infants with neonatal abstinence syndrome can be safely observed and treated in non-NICU settings.

References: Jackson J, Knappen B, Olsen S. Drug withdrawal in the neonate. In: Gardner S, Carter B, Enzman-Hines M, Niermeyer S, eds. *Merenstein and Gardner's Handbook of Neonatal Intensive Care: An Interprofessional Approach.* 9th ed. St. Louis, MO: Elsevier; 2021:259-263.

Patrick SW, Barfield WD, Poindexter BB, Committee on Fetus and Newborn, Committee on Substance Use and Prevention. Neonatal opioid withdrawal syndrome. *Pediatrics.* 2020;146(5):e2020029074. doi:10.1542/peds.2020-029074.

13. **(C)** The observation period for opioid exposed infants is based on the opioid(s) to which the infant was exposed. The 2020 American Academy of *Pediatrics* clinical report on NOWS recommends the following approach: immediate-release opioids (e.g., hydrocodone): 3 days; buprenorphine and sustained-release opioids: 4–7 days; and methadone: 5–7 days.

References: D'Apolito K. Perinatal substance abuse. In: Verklan MT, Walden M, Forest S, eds. *Core Curriculum for Neonatal Intensive Care Nursing.* 6th ed. St. Louis, MO: Elsevier; 2021:45.

Patrick SW, Barfield WD, Poindexter BB, Committee on Fetus and Newborn, Committee on Substance Use and Prevention. Neonatal opioid withdrawal syndrome. *Pediatrics.* 2020;146(5):e2020029074. doi:10.1542/peds.2020-029074.

14. **(A)** There are concerns about neurodevelopment impairment with fetal exposure to marijuana, therefore women who are pregnant or contemplating pregnancy should be screened for marijuana use and discouraged from using any marijuana during pregnancy. There is insufficient data to support the effects of any marijuana use on infants during breastfeeding, therefore use of marijuana during breastfeeding should be discouraged.

References: D'Apolito K. Perinatal substance abuse. In: Verklan MT, Walden M, Forest S, eds. *Core Curriculum for Neonatal Intensive Care Nursing.* 6th ed. St. Louis, MO: Elsevier; 2021:40.

Committee Opinion No. 722: marijuana use during pregnancy and lactation. *Obstet Gynecol.* 2017;130:e205-e209.

15. **(B)** Constant sucking of the fists is a sign of withdrawal, not hunger, and may lead to overfeeding if misinterpreted. The mother requires further teaching on the signs of withdrawal and appropriate management. Withdrawal symptoms may persist for 2–6 months. The mother has demonstrated understanding of the duration of time she should observe for withdrawal symptoms. Loose stools are a sign of withdrawal, and the mother has demonstrated understanding of this issue and how to care for her infant. Some evidence suggests that infants with substance exposure are at an increased risk for sleep-related deaths. The mother has demonstrated understanding of a safe sleep position for her infant.

References: Jackson J, Knappen B, Olsen S. Drug withdrawal in the neonate. In: Gardner S, Carter B, Enzman-Hines M, Niermeyer S, eds. *Merenstein and Gardner's Handbook of Neonatal Intensive Care: An Interprofessional Approach.* 9th ed. St. Louis, MO: Elsevier; 2021:268-269.

Patrick SW, Barfield WD, Poindexter BB, Committee on Fetus and Newborn, Committee on Substance Use and Prevention. Neonatal opioid withdrawal syndrome. *Pediatrics.* 2020;146(5):e2020029074. doi:10.1542/peds.2020-029074.

16. **(C)** Early pediatrician follow-up within 48 hours of hospital discharge should be arranged prior to hospital discharge to assess the infant for withdrawal symptoms, adequate weight gain, and any potential feeding problems. Pediatric providers should be aware infants with neonatal abstinence syndrome do have the potential need for ophthalmologic evaluation for nystagmus, strabismus, or other refractive errors. However, these conditions do not occur immediately after birth. Neurodevelopmental issues can be related to neonatal abstinence syndrome but are rarely noted soon after birth.

References: Kanukollu VM, Sood G. Strabismus. In: *StatPearls.* Treasure Island, FL: StatPearls Publishing. Available at: https://www.ncbi.nlm.nih.gov/books/NBK560782/. Updated 08.08.22.

Patrick SW, Barfield WD, Poindexter BB, Committee on Fetus and Newborn, Committee on Substance Use and Prevention. Neonatal opioid withdrawal syndrome. *Pediatrics.* 2020;146(5):e2020029074. doi:10.1542/peds.2020-029074.

PSYCHOSOCIAL AND BEHAVIORAL ADJUSTMENTS

Chapter 28

Family Integration and Culturally Sensitive Care

1. Which of the following is true about family and infant bonding?
   A. Bonding is unaffected by birth of a premature infant or infant born ill.
   B. Bonding occurs on the same timetable for mothers and fathers.
   C. Bonding is displayed by parents identifying negative characteristics of their infant.
   D. Bonding is gradual and occurs over time and is reciprocal between both infant and parent.

2. Which of the following interventions can nurses integrate into their practice in order to encourage parent–infant bonding?
   A. Encourage parents to participate in providing care for their infant.
   B. Limit holding of their infant.
   C. Remind parents of visiting hours.
   D. Communicate with parents only when they are at the bedside.

3. When providing culturally sensitive care, what should the nurse consider or have knowledge of?
   A. To address disparities in healthcare, staff must be trained in every culture.
   B. The incorporation of cultural competence into health care practice has not been shown to decrease overall medical care expenditures.
   C. Cultural competence has not been shown to impact the incidence of breastfeeding.
   D. Cultural sensitivity is demonstrated when nurses focus on being learners and approaching patients with humility.

4. An infant is born at 28 weeks' gestation and needs to be transferred to a children's hospital 100 miles away. Which is the most appropriate action the transport nurse should take initially after physiologic stabilization?
   A. Have the mother's nurse tell the parents they will be called when the team and infant arrive at the receiving hospital.
   B. Bring the infant to the parents in the delivery room/recovery area and encourage them to touch and see their infant.
   C. Take a picture and e-mail it to the parents when the transport team arrives at the children's hospital.
   D. Tell the parents they can come see the baby after the mother is discharged from the delivery hospital.

5. An infant is brought to the special care nursery to be treated for sepsis. The infant's mother is single and a victim of domestic violence. The nurses have noticed that the mother visits infrequently and stays only a short time. She avoids feeding times and rarely wants to hold the baby. This mother's behavior is consistent with:
   A. adaptation.
   B. normal parenting.
   C. inadequate bonding.
   D. positive attachment behavior.

6. To foster family-centered care the nurse will:
   A. welcome parents during change of shift report, rounds, and admissions.
   B. individualize the infant's plan of care based on what the nurse thinks is best for the infant.
   C. offer parents to participate in care once their infant has stabilized.
   D. ask parents to leave the bedside when IVs are to be started on their infant.

7. What should a nurse know about a father's experience that will help support early father–infant attachment?
   A. Both mother and father have the same starting points of attachment.
   B. When fathers are more engaged in caring for their babies, they experience stronger hormonal and neurological changes than when not engaged.
   C. Mothers and fathers feel powerless and distant.
   D. The mother's and father's support needs are similar.

8. A preterm infant is diagnosed with a significant intraventricular hemorrhage. The physicians have explained the damage to the brain and are discussing treatment options with the adolescent parents. The maternal grandmother insists on telling the mother the best treatment plan for the infant. The mother and father do not want the grandmother telling them what to do. The parents' reactions are not unusual, because as adolescents they:
   A. feel like the staff will not accept their decision.
   B. are able to think abstractly and anticipate future problems.

C. have realistic expectations of their role as parents.

D. may be trying to take on adult responsibilities and feel they are being treated like children.

9. An infant was diagnosed prenatally with congenital anomalies and is now born. The family has increased levels of anxiety and fear. What attachment behaviors would the nurse assess/observe that would be of concern in evaluating mother–infant bonding?

A. The mother has named the infant.

B. The mother is demonstrating increasing skill in holding the baby/caregiving.

C. The mother does not hold her infant close to her body but rather at a distance.

D. The mother makes positive comments about the baby.

10. What can the neonatal intensive care unit (NICU) nurse do to support sibling participation?

A. Encourage visitation with siblings that are age 10 and older.

B. Suggest the parents spend more time at home with the siblings.

C. Have parents give the siblings a picture of their baby sister or brother to hang in their room at home.

D. Encourage sibling visitation and activities such as drawing pictures to hang at the sick sibling's bedside.

11. How is parent adaptation and coping with the birth of a premature infant evidenced?

A. Mother and father visit infrequently and separately.

B. Parents are ready to learn discharge needs of the infant upon admission.

C. Father has returned to work and mother has been eating and sleeping well.

D. Parents are not participating in care.

12. A new mother who has held her premature infant but never provided kangaroo care is very anxious. She shares that she may not hold her baby correctly and he might not do well. The nurse can alleviate these fears best by:

A. sharing that every mother feels this way.

B. encouraging the mother to do it despite her fear.

C. reassuring mother that she will sit with the mother the entire time.

D. providing positive reinforcement about when she held her baby previous times.

13. Which of the following interventions could be improved upon to provide positive family support?

A. Allowing parent participation in daily rounds every other day

B. Offering education programs to facilitate communication between parents and staff

C. Purposeful development of the NICU physical environment allowing overnight accommodations near their infant

D. Encouraging parents to learn their infant's developmental cues

14. A 17-year-old Pakistani father is not visiting his female premature infant as regularly as does the teen mother. Which of the following is the most appropriate initial action?

A. Consider that cultural differences may be at play.

B. Report to the NICU team that the infant is at risk for poor bonding.

C. Include in the care plan as a goal for the father to provide skin-to-skin care.

D. Consider grief counseling only for the teen mother.

ANSWERS AND RATIONALES

1. **(D)** Bonding is a gradual and reciprocal process that occurs over time and differently for both parents. Bonding begins with acquaintance. It is a unique and specific relationship between two people and endures across time. Disruptions in early attachment between the infant and parent, such as premature delivery or delivery of a sick newborn, increase the parents' vulnerability and ability for them to establish a nurturing relationship. Alteration in the parental role related to the infant's sickness and hospitalization might lead to diminished parental attachment to the infant and decreased parental confidence in their own abilities to give care to and keep their infant safe. Bonding occurs on a different timetable for mothers than fathers. A mother's attachment is thought to take a rise around the fifth month of pregnancy and grows, whereas a father's attachment grows slowly during the pregnancy and becomes strong after the birth of the infant. Positive bonding and attachment behaviors include the parent visits frequently, has named the infant, makes positive comments when talking to or about the infant, demonstrates increasing skill in caregiving/holding the infant, and displays increasing eye and body contact (e.g., kissing, fondling, stroking, and nuzzling). Negative comments about their infant are behaviors of concern when evaluating parent–infant bonding.

References: Fegran L, Fageermoenm MS, Helseth S. A comparison of mothers' and fathers' experiences of the attachment process in a neonatal intensive care unit. *J Clin Nurs.* 2008;17:810-816.

Kenner C, Boykova M. Intrafacility and interfacility neonatal transport. In: Verklan MT, Walden M, Forest S, eds. *Core Curriculum for Neonatal Intensive Care Nursing.* 6th ed. St. Louis, MO: Elsevier; 2021:288-289, 292.

2. **(A)** Caregiving is the final step in the attachment process and is important for bonding. Encouraging the parents to participate in providing care for their infant as soon as possible helps begin this process. Developing skills in caregiving of an infant in the neonatal intensive care unit (NICU) is expected to occur over time. Early touch aids in establishing that the infant is real; therefore, encouraging the parents to hold their infant as soon as possible helps begin infant attachment. Parents should be welcomed as partners in care and not "visitors." Therefore the concept of visiting hours for parents should be eliminated in the NICU. Encouraging "parenting" is vital to bonding. Parents are not always able to be in the NICU, so limiting communication to when they are at the bedside also limits nurses' ability to partner with families in the manner most useful for them.

References: Kenner C, Boykova M. Families in crisis. In: Verklan MT, Walden M, Forest S, eds. *Core Curriculum for Neonatal Intensive Care Nursing.* 6th ed. St. Louis, MO: Elsevier; 2021:292-293.

Gardner SL, Voos K. Families in crisis: theoretical and practical considerations. In: Gardner SL, Carter BS, Enzman-Hines M, Niermeyer S, eds. *Merenstein & Gardner's Handbook of Neonatal Intensive Care: An Interprofessional Approach.* 9th ed. St. Louis, MO: Elsevier; 2021:1041-1046.

3. **(D)** Cultural sensitivity, an affective construct, includes values, attitudes, and beliefs. Attitude about self and others, as well as openness to new experiences, affects cultural sensitivity. Sensitivity is demonstrated when nurses focus on being learners and approaching patients with humility. When nurses approach patients with cultural humility, they display cultural sensitivity by treating

patients as they wish to be treated. Patients presenting with one or more of the following factors: racial or ethnic background, religion, age, sexual orientation, socioeconomic status, gender identity, or other characteristics historically linked to discrimination or exclusion are more likely to become victims of health disparity. One solution to address disparity is to adopt Culturally Congruent Care. Culturally Congruent Care does not require that every staff member be trained in every culture, but rather that the staff be trained on how to adopt an attitude of curiosity and investigation as to what cultural norms are important and what adaptations the staff can make to be more inclusive to the family. The incorporation of cultural competence into health care practice has been shown to have numerous benefits, including greater health equality, increased patient satisfaction, enhanced communication, better pain control, greater medication adherence, and increased seeking and sharing of information during health care visits. Cultural competence may also decrease overall medical care expenditures. Cultural competence also affects the health behaviors of women related to pre- and postnatal care. For example, cultural competence has been reported to increase the incidence of breastfeeding.

References: Heitzler ET. Cultural competence of obstetric and neonatal nurses. *J Obstetr Gynecol Neonatal Nurs.* 2017;46:423-433.

Torr C. Culturally competent care in the neonatal intensive care unit, strategies to address outcome disparities. *J Perinatol.* 2022;42(10):1424-1427. doi:10.1038/s41372-022-01360-2.

4. **(B)** The NICU team should make every attempt for the parents to see and touch their infant before being separated. Allowing the parents to see and touch their infant provides assurance that the infant is real. Although letting the parents know that the NICU team will call once at the receiving facility supports open communication, it does not replace seeing and touching the infant to begin the attachment process. Parents are partners in care and should be encouraged to see and hold the infant as the infant's condition allows. Providing families with pictures, telephone numbers, and information about the NICU is helpful, but also does not replace seeing and touching to begin attachment. Encouraging families to call anytime creates open communication and helps parents understand their infant's care and status. Letting the parents know they can visit their infant is helpful and can be done before the transport team leaves the referring hospital. Although the mother may not be able to visit until after she is discharged, the father should be encouraged to visit at any time.

Reference: Bowen SL. Intrafacility and interfacility neonatal transport. In: Verklan MT, Walden M, Forest S, eds. *Core Curriculum for Neonatal Intensive Care Nursing.* 6th ed. St. Louis, MO: Elsevier; 2021:368-369.

5. **(C)** An abnormal visiting pattern is a sign of inadequate bonding. Positive bonding and attachment behaviors include the parent changes his/her schedule to accommodate the care schedule of the infant, visits frequently, has named the infant, makes positive comments when talking to or about the infant, demonstrates increasing skill in caregiving/holding the infant, and displays increasing eye and body contact (e.g., kissing, fondling, stroking, and nuzzling). Normal parenting would be characterized by a more consistent visitation pattern and longer visits. If parents are not visiting frequently, be careful to determine the reasons (e.g., home environment/dynamics/relationships/support, cultural practices after childbirth, conflicting obligations between work and family roles, or lack of transportation to the hospital) before assuming that the parents are unconcerned or that parenting difficulties exist.

Reference: Kenner C, Boykova M. Families in crisis. In: Verklan MT, Walden M, Forest S, eds. *Core Curriculum for Neonatal Intensive Care Nursing.* 6th ed. St. Louis, MO: Elsevier; 2021:292.

6. **(A)** Family-centered care requires that parents have full access to their infant. Evidence is growing regarding the benefits of parent participation on rounds, including improved parent satisfaction regarding communication and knowledge gained, reduced anxiety, increased confidence in the healthcare team, and a high level of participation by parents. Additionally, the nurse should offer the parent access to their infant during simple procedures and whether the parent participates becomes their decision. Family-centered care also requires that parents are seen as partners in care. Involving parents in developing the infant's plan of care supports principles of family-centered care in the NICU. Before offering the parents to participate in care, the nurse needs to first assess the parent's readiness to participate in care after the initial stress of the NICU admission. There are a number of important assessments and treatments for NICU infants that parents can safely and effectively perform *only* after parents receive training and support from skilled healthcare providers.

References: Gardner SL, Voos K. Families in crisis: theoretical and practical considerations. In: Gardner SL, Carter BS, Enzman-Hines M, Niermeyer S, eds. *Merenstein & Gardner's Handbook of Neonatal Intensive Care: An Interprofessional Approach.* 9th ed. St. Louis, MO: Elsevier; 2021:1046-1050.

Franck LS, O'Brien K. The evolution of family-centered care: from supporting parent-delivered interventions to a model of family integrated care. *Birth Defect Res.* 2019;111(15):1044-1059.

7. **(B)** Oxytocin increases in fathers as in mothers through physical contact such as skin-to-skin and decreases less quickly than it does in mothers post-skin-to-skin. Testosterone decreases in men when a baby is born. If the father is more involved in caring, the testosterone decreases further. Fathers with lower testosterone are more affectionate and sensitive towards their babies. Skin-to-skin care is associated with a drop in cortisol in fathers, as in mothers, with the effect being longer lasting in fathers post-skin-to-skin. Prolactin is associated with breastfeeding, but it increases in new fathers as well. Prolactin levels are highest when babies are most needy and vulnerable. These changes are, in turn, associated with short and longer-term benefits for the baby. Neuroscience has identified two areas of the brain associated with caregiving and both can be activated in fathers like mothers, the more so when the father cares for his baby. The "emotional empathy" brain network enables an automatic understanding of the baby's mental state, allowing the parent to "feel" and experience in herself/himself the physical pain or emotional distress of the baby. The "sociocognitive" brain network is associated with mentalizing, cognitive empathy, and social understanding. It enables a parent to infer the baby's mental state from behavior, predict the baby's needs, and plan future caregiving activities. The active engagement of fathers in neonatal units triggers these biological and neurobiological processes. This new science helps to explain the feelings of love expressed by fathers holding their babies.

Mothers and fathers have different starting points of attachment. Bonding occurs on a different timetable for mothers than fathers. A mother's attachment is thought to take a rise around the fifth month of pregnancy and grows, whereas a father's attachment grows slowly during the pregnancy and becomes strong after the birth of the infant. Mothers feel they have lost a relationship with their child built during the pregnancy, whereas fathers feel it is the beginning of a relationship. After delivery, mothers feel powerless and distant, and fathers feel "shocked" and are concerned for both their spouse and infant and look to the health care team to gauge the acuteness of the situation. While mothers of NICU infants tend to be the primary focus of support by the nursing staff, fathers have unique support needs that are frequently not met. Fathers of NICU infants describe feelings of inequality as a parent, lack of NICU staff communication, difficulty with work constraints and visiting the NICU, and an overall lack of situational control. In addition, these fathers struggle with role transitions, work–life–home imbalances, emotional stress, and their concern for the well-being of both the mother and the infant. When NICU fathers perceive a lack of support during their infant's hospitalization, they experience an increase in self-doubt and distress, with the potential to have negative long-term effects on the cognitive, social, and emotional growth and development of their infants. Conversely, NICU fathers who perceive adequate support during their infant's hospitalization report meaningful father–infant bonding, increased parental functioning confidence, and increased engagement in caregiving activities, even after discharge.

References: Kenner C, Boykova M. Families in crisis. In: Verklan MT, Walden M, Forest S, eds. *Core Curriculum for Neonatal Intensive Care Nursing.* 6th ed. St. Louis, MO: Elsevier; 2021:288.

LeDuff III, LD, Carter BM, Cunningham DA, Braun LA, Gallaher KJ. NICU fathers. *Adv Neonatal Care.* 2020;21(5):387-398.

Fisher D, Khashu M, Adama EA, et al. Fathers in neonatal units: improving infant health by supporting the baby-father bond and mother-father coparenting. *J Neonatal Nurs.* 2018;24(6):306-312. doi:10.1016/j.jnn.2018.08.007.

Stefana A, Biban P, Padovani EM, Lavelli M. Fathers' experiences of supporting their partners during their preterm infant's stay in the neonatal intensive care unit: a multi-method study. *J Perinatol.* 2022;42(6):714-722. doi:10.1038/s41372-021-01195-3.

8. **(D)** Parents who are adolescents have some unique needs. Adolescence is a turning point that moves a child from childhood toward the maturation of the adult. Some developmental tasks of this period are independence from adults and role identification which can cause conflict with the family. Adolescent parents may be trying to take on adult responsibilities while feeling that they are being treated like children. Nevertheless, as parents, they do have legal rights to decision-making for their infant. The NICU staff knows, and the adolescent parents should be made aware, that once a teenage girl delivers a baby, she is considered an emancipated minor who can make independent decisions for herself and her child. Teenagers have difficulty anticipating the long-term implications of their decision. Developmentally the teen mother may feel ready to take on critical health care decisions about her infant. The reality is that adolescent parents need to be assessed for their knowledge, level of crisis, and available support. It has been shown that adolescents often underestimate the severity of their infant's illness and require increased levels of informational, and esteem/appraisal supports. Teenage parents often have unrealistic expectations of their role as parents and lack parenting skills.

Reference: Kenner C, Boykova M. Families in crisis. In: Verklan MT, Walden M, Forest S, eds. *Core Curriculum for Neonatal Intensive Care Nursing.* 6th ed. St. Louis, MO: Elsevier; 2021:290-291.

9. **(C)** Holding the infant at distance would be cause for concern. Predictors of positive bonding and attachment behaviors include the parent naming the infant, displaying increasing eye and body contact (e.g., kissing, fondling, stroking, and nuzzling), increasing skill in caregiving/holding, and making positive comments about the infant.

Reference: Kenner C, Boykova M. Families in crisis. In: Verklan MT, Walden M, Forest S, eds. *Core Curriculum for Neonatal Intensive Care Nursing.* 6th ed. St. Louis, MO: Elsevier; 2021:291-292.

10. **(D)** All siblings are affected by the delivery of a premature or sick sibling. Activities that encourage sibling attachment are drawing pictures and placing them at the bedside, creating tape recordings, and/or visiting the infant in the NICU according to visitation guidelines. Many children, even those younger than 10 years, benefit from visiting their brother or sister in the NICU. A qualified child life specialist is a helpful resource that can help prepare siblings for what they will see and hear in the NICU. While it is

important for parents to maintain their relationship with the infant's siblings, just spending time with the siblings does not develop attachment behaviors. Although giving a picture of the infant to siblings may be helpful for older children, sibling attachment is more effectively promoted by having the siblings draw pictures or create tape recordings for the infant.

References: Kenner C, Boykova M. Families in crisis. In: Verklan MT, Walden M, Forest S, eds. *Core Curriculum for Neonatal Intensive Care Nursing.* 6th ed. St. Louis, MO: Elsevier; 2021:294-295.

Gardner SL, Voos K. Families in crisis: theoretical and practical considerations. In: Gardner SL, Carter B, Enzman-Hines M, Niermeyer S, eds. *Merenstein & Gardner's Handbook of Neonatal Intensive Care: An Interprofessional Approach.* 9th ed. St. Louis, MO: Elsevier; 2021:1081-1083.

11. **(C)** Adaptation and coping with premature birth may be evidenced by the resumption of activities of daily living, such as personal grooming, eating, appropriate clothing. Parents should be assessed as to whether they can maintain the lifestyle they led before the crisis; for instance, if they are returning to work, able to do housekeeping activities, care for any other children in the household, or have financial issues. Frequent parent visits are positive behaviors. If parents are not visiting frequently or are not visiting together, it is important to determine the reasons (e.g., cultural practices after childbirth, conflicting obligations between work and family roles, or lack of transportation to the hospital) before assuming that the parents are unconcerned or that parenting difficulties exist. The birth of a premature or sick infant is an unexpected life event; such events are referred to as *situational or accidental stressors* for which a person or family is often psychologically unprepared. There are several psychological tasks and phases that the mother/father must accomplish to cope with the crisis of a premature birth or the birth of a sick infant. Preparing for taking the infant home is not a psychological task that occurs on admission. Preparing to go home is a psychologic task parents need to accomplish after adaptation has been established. In addition, parents must come to understand the special needs and characteristics of the premature or sick infant and the precautions that must be taken. Positive attachment behaviors include participating in caregiving activities such as feeding, bathing, and clothing the infant. To feel more comfortable with their infant, parents need to understand what they contribute as parents to the care of their infant. If there is no participation, their parental role may be compromised.

Reference: Kenner C, Boykova M. Families in crisis. In: Verklan MT, Walden M, Forest S, eds. *Core Curriculum for Neonatal Intensive Care Nursing.* 6th ed. St. Louis, MO: Elsevier; 2021:288-289, 292.

12. **(D)** Giving positive reinforcement to parents as they interact with their infant helps parents to recognize positive changes in the infant in response to their caregiving. Assisting parents to recognize positive changes in the infant in response to their caregiving has a strong impact on the parents and increases their feelings of success. Negating a parent's feelings of fear or pushing a parent to participate in care beyond his or her desire and comfort is not supportive. Knowledge, caregiving skills, and competency develop over time. Simply sitting with the mother would not be as effective as listening to her fears and providing positive reinforcement.

Reference: Kenner C, Boykova M. Families in crisis. In: Verklan MT, Walden M, Forest S, eds. *Core Curriculum for Neonatal Intensive Care Nursing.* 6th ed. St. Louis, MO: Elsevier; 2021:294, 297.

13. **(A)** Interventions that focus on the parent–NICU team communication and relationship are relatively new and include parent participation on daily, rather than every other day, clinical rounds. Evidence is growing regarding the benefits of parent participation on rounds, including improved parent satisfaction regarding communication and knowledge gained, reduced anxiety, increased confidence in the healthcare team, high level of participation by

parents, and almost unanimous support by parents. Interventions that focus on the parent–NICU team communication also include specific education programs to facilitate the communication between staff and parents. The physical environment of the hospital and NICU has also been shown to impact parent involvement in their infant's care. Families who are provided with purposely built overnight accommodations near their ill infant or child report a better hospital experience and feel more involved in their child's care. An approach that supports family-centered care involves encouraging parents to learn their infant's developmental cues (e.g., assessment of feeding readiness, signs of stress, or readiness for social interaction). Parents can provide the infant with positive stimuli through smell, positioning or holding, skin-to-skin contact, feeding, or other sensitive and appropriate developmental stimulation.

Reference: Franck LS, O'Brien K. The evolution of family-centered care: from supporting parent-delivered interventions to a model of family integrated care. *Birth Defects Res*. 2019;111:1044-1059.

14. **(A)** Parent–infant bonding and attachment concerns must be considered within the context of the culture of the parents. In some cultures, the adolescent mother will have full rights to determine the future for her child without consultation with the father or other family members. But in other cultures, the father must make the decisions about the family—no matter what the marital status may be. Different cultures approach parenthood and parent–infant interaction in different ways. Before reporting that the infant is at risk for poor bonding, the nurse should explore the reasons, including cultural, for why the father is not visiting as often as the mother. An individualized care plan would involve plans to assess the father's desire to participate in care and those assessments and preferences should be clearly written into the care plan. The extent to which both parents are experiencing grief must be determined. The grief responses do not necessarily occur in the same sequence for all people. Grief reactions are mediated by cultural beliefs and values as well as the parents' developmental stage. In some cases, it may not be acceptable for parents to express grief or worries to outsiders.

Reference: Kenner C, Boykova M. Families in crisis. In: Verklan MT, Walden M, Forest S, eds. *Core Curriculum for Neonatal Intensive Care Nursing*. 6th ed. St. Louis, MO: Elsevier; 2021:291-292.

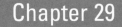

Chapter 29

Discharge Planning and Transition to Home

1. The nurse should consider which of the following as the most important component of discharge planning?
   A. Successful rooming-in by the parents
   B. Plan completed 1–2 weeks before discharge
   C. Involvement of family and members of interdisciplinary discharge planning/transition to home team
   D. Compliance with hospital policy and protocols

2. An infant born at 30 weeks' gestation, currently 38 weeks post conceptual age, is being discharged home. The nurse should consider the infant ready for discharge when which of the following criteria are met?
   A. Parents complete rooming-in and cardiopulmonary resuscitation training.
   B. Infant demonstrates physiologic stability consistent weight gain, tolerance of enteral feedings, and maintenance of body temperature in open crib.
   C. Parents have secured necessary supplies for home care, including car seat.
   D. Infant approaches original estimated date of confinement.

3. An infant born at 26 weeks' gestation is now medically ready for discharge. On the day of discharge the nurse notices that the mother is unusually anxious despite ongoing involvement. Which of the following should the nurse consider as the basis for the mothers' behavior?
   A. Guilt about delivering her infant prematurely
   B. Regret about the pediatrician they selected
   C. Concern for not effectively bonding with their infant
   D. Fear about leaving the security of the intensive care nursery

4. Parent education should be targeted for which of the following reading levels?

A. 6th grade
B. 8th grade
C. 10th grade
D. 12th grade

5. A former 30-week-gestation infant is scheduled for neonatal intensive care unit (NICU) discharge within 36 hours. The parents have brought to the hospital the car seat they are planning to use for testing. The nurse should be aware that the period of observation recommended by the American Academy of Pediatrics for infants born at less than 37 weeks' gestation is:
   A. 15–30 minutes
   B. 45–60 minutes
   C. 90–120 minutes
   D. 3–4 hours

6. An infant born at 28 weeks' gestation, currently 40 weeks post conceptual age, is being discharged in the month of January. Which of the following prophylactic medications should be given by the nurse immediately before discharge?
   A. Influenza vaccine
   B. Palivizumab (Synagis)
   C. Diphtheria, tetanus toxoids/acellular pertussis vaccine
   D. *Haemophilus influenzae* vaccine

7. Parents of a former 24-week infant question the nurse about the need for developmental follow-up after discharge. Which of the following statements by the nurse most accurately describes the purpose of the clinic?
   A. Allows for early identification of developmental disability.
   B. Minimizes the need for home therapy services.
   C. Serves to reinforce medication teaching after discharge.
   D. Substitutes for primary pediatric care.

8. A former 33-week infant, currently 2 months old, presents with lethargy a few days after being left with another caregiver. The caregiver verbalized to the parents that the infant "likes to be bounced around a lot." Which of the following should the nurse consider as the likely cause of the lethargy?
   A. Shaken baby syndrome
   B. Acute infection
   C. Metabolic disorder
   D. Anemia of prematurity

9. The nurse should instruct the parents of a former 25-week-gestation infant that proper sleeping position after NICU discharge is:
   A. side-lying.
   B. prone.
   C. supine.
   D. head of bed elevated 45 degrees.

10. Parents of a term infant diagnosed with trisomy 13 and complex cardiac disease want to keep the infant in the room with them following delivery if a live birth occurs. Which of the following is the most appropriate conversation to have with the parents?
    A. Counsel the parents that it is best to not see the infant due to the poor prognosis.
    B. Discuss a wait-and-see approach once their infant is born versus having a delivery plan.
    C. Discuss with the parents that once their infant is born, palliative care will be instituted with a progression to hospice care if needed.
    D. Inform the parents that policy dictates the infant must be immediately admitted to the nursery.

11. A set of former 34-week twins are being prepared for discharge. The parents show the nurse a picture of their nursery with one crib, decorated with fluffy linens, pillows, blankets, and stuffed animals. Upon seeing this picture and congratulating them on nursery preparation, which is the most appropriate discussion for the nurse to have with the parents?
    A. Inform them that their twins will enjoy cobedding every night with all the pillows and stuffed animals in the crib.
    B. Inform them that it is highly recommended that each infant has their own crib with a firm mattress; with no pillows, crib bumpers, or stuffed animals; and be in the parents' room until 6 months of age.
    C. Share with the parents that when their daughters are older, they can share the same crib, but until then they need to each have their own separate sleeping space.
    D. Suggest that they should also add cameras to the room as an additional safety measure.

ANSWERS AND RATIONALES

1. **(C)** Discharge planning begins on admission and incorporates a family-centered multidisciplinary team consisting of physicians, nurse practitioners, nurses, respiratory therapists, occupational/physical/speech therapists, pharmacists, dietitians, social workers, and the family. Integration of these family-centered principles will help facilitate better parental adaptation to the transition to home. Successful rooming-in and compliance with hospital protocols does not fulfill all of the elements to achieve a safe discharge and does not address medical readiness of the infant.
Reference: Hummel P. Discharge planning and transition to home care. In: Verklan MT, Walden M, eds. *Core Curriculum for Neonatal Intensive Care Nursing*. 6th ed. St. Louis, MO: Saunders; 2021:329-330.

2. **(B)** The American Academy of Pediatrics (AAP); Committee on Fetus and Newborn has published specific guideline criteria for hospital discharge of the high-risk neonate. Infants ready for discharge must be medically and physiologically stable and have completed all well-child care screening requirements. The infant's original estimated date of confinement is used only as a guide for a potential discharge time frame in an uncomplicated hospitalization. Medical readiness for the infant is not contingent on whether parents' room-in, complete cardiopulmonary resuscitation, or have secured all infant care supplies.
Reference: Hummel P. Discharge planning and transition to home care. In: Verklan MT, Walden M, eds. *Core Curriculum for Neonatal Intensive Care Nursing*. 6th ed. St. Louis, MO: Saunders; 2021:331-332.

3. **(D)** Feelings of fear are not uncommon because the intensive care nursery has been a place of safety and support. Regret about the pediatrician selection is not likely the source because that choice is determined before discharge. A feeling of not effectively bonding with her infant is unlikely because she has been an ongoing active participant in her infant's care. Guilt is commonly an emotion expressed immediately following delivery but unlikely to be a primary emotion at the time of discharge.
Reference: Hummel P. Discharge planning and transition to home care. In: Verklan MT, Walden M, eds. *Core Curriculum for Neonatal Intensive Care Nursing*. 6th ed. St. Louis, MO: Saunders; 2021:331-332.

4. **(A)** A sixth-grade reading level or lower will meet the cognitive baseline of the lay public and allow health care providers to assure that the materials are targeted to meet specific learning needs.
Reference: Rooney MK, Santiago G, Perni S, et al. Readability of patient education materials from high-impact medical journals: a 20-year analysis. *J Patient Exp*. 2021. doi:10.1177/2374373521998847.

5. **(C)** The AAP indicates a period of observation in a car seat for a minimum of 90–120 minutes is needed to determine the potential for desaturation events and/or episodes of apnea and bradycardia. The recommendation includes infants born at less than 37 weeks' gestation.
Reference: Hummel P. Discharge planning and transition to home care. In: Verklan MT, Walden M, eds. *Core Curriculum for Neonatal Intensive Care Nursing*. 6th ed. St. Louis, MO: Saunders; 2021:335.

6. **(B)** Infants born at less than 29 weeks' gestation and discharged during respiratory syncytial virus (RSV) season (November through March) should receive palivizumab (Synagis) prophylaxis at discharge and then monthly during RSV season up to a maximum of five doses, according to the AAP, along with other scheduled immunizations. The influenza vaccine is given when infants are older than 6 months of age. The diphtheria, tetanus toxoids/acellular pertussis vaccine and *Haemophilus influenzae* vaccine are part of the routine immunization schedule and would have been given when the infant was 2 months old and given again at 4 months of age.
Reference: Hummel P. Discharge planning and transition to home care. In: Verklan MT, Walden M, eds. *Core Curriculum for Neonatal Intensive Care Nursing*. 6th ed. St. Louis, MO: Saunders; 2021:335.

7. **(A)** The developmental clinic works collaboratively with the infant's pediatrician to ensure that all of the medical needs are addressed and is not intended to be used in lieu of a pediatrician.

Referrals by developmental clinics to early intervention programs are essential components of follow-up care and facilitate and maximize home-based services. Medication teaching should be fully accomplished before discharge to minimize any potential for error.

Reference: Hummel P. Discharge planning and transition to home care. In: Verklan MT, Walden M, eds. *Core Curriculum for Neonatal Intensive Care Nursing*. 6th ed. St. Louis, MO: Saunders; 2021:332.

8. **(A)** When an infant is vigorously shaken, the head moves back and forth in a confined space, causing a whiplash motion that can lead to intracranial bleeding or retinal hemorrhages. Infection is an unlikely cause of the lethargy given the caregiver description. A metabolic disorder is generally identified through routine screening processes after birth. Although anemia can cause lethargy in addition to pallor and tachycardia, the onset of lethargy would be gradual.

Reference: Hummel P. Discharge planning and transition to home care. In: Verklan MT, Walden M, eds. *Core Curriculum for Neonatal Intensive Care Nursing*. 6th ed. St. Louis, MO: Saunders; 2021:335-336.

9. **(C)** Infants who sleep prone and side-lying have a much higher rate of sudden infant death syndrome than infants who sleep supine whether the head of bed is elevated or not. The supine sleep position is recommended by the AAP and does not increase the risk of choking and aspiration, even those with gastroesophageal reflux due to protective airway mechanisms.

Reference: American Academy of Pediatrics, Task Force on Sudden Infant Death Syndrome. SIDS and other sleep-related infant deaths: expansion of recommendations for a safe infant sleeping environment. *Pediatrics*. 2011; 128(5):1030-1039.

10. **(C)** Palliative care can be instituted prior to delivery and transitioned to hospice care as circumstances dictate after delivery or during hospitalization. The goal is to maximize quality of life for infants with life limiting conditions and their families. A plan formulated by care givers and the family will provide comfort and dignity to all involved and may include parental desire to see and hold the infant, if nursery admission is necessary or any other plans for care.

Reference: Hummel P. Discharge planning and transition to home care. In: Verklan MT, Walden M, eds. *Core Curriculum for Neonatal Intensive Care Nursing*. 6th ed. St. Louis, MO: Saunders; 2021:342.

11. **(B)** Safe sleep includes placing the infant supine in a crib on a firm mattress without pillows, blankets, bumper pads, or stuffed animals. Infants should not sleep with other children and adults when at home or away. The crib should be kept in the parents' room until the infant has reached 6 months of age and can roll from side to side. Cameras may be used but are not a substitute for safe sleep practices.

Reference: Hummel P. Discharge planning and transition to home care. In: Verklan MT, Walden M, eds. *Core Curriculum for Neonatal Intensive Care Nursing*. 6th ed. St. Louis, MO: Saunders; 2021:334.

Chapter 30

Grieving Process

1. A neonate is admitted to the neonatal intensive care unit (NICU) with a diagnosis of trisomy 13 and is receiving palliative care. The mother expresses concern about the ability to deal with her emotions from the birth of a less than perfect baby with a short life expectancy. What is this an example of?
   A. Anticipatory grieving
   B. Pathologic grief
   C. Chronic sorrow
   D. Incongruent grieving

2. The initial stage of grief is characterized by:
   A. emotional numbness.
   B. anger.
   C. depression.
   D. bargaining.

3. An infant is withdrawn from life support while being held in the mother's arms. The father is also at the bedside. The mother cries softly for 2 hours at the bedside. The father grows impatient with the mother and verbalizes, "It's over, there's no use in crying anymore." What is this an example of?
   A. Incongruent grieving
   B. Parental disassociation
   C. Guilt
   D. Apathy

4. A child is diagnosed with trisomy 21 and is being followed in a NICU developmental clinic. During the interview, the mother expresses a daily sadness regarding nonachievable developmental milestones. What is this an example of?
   A. Chronic sorrow
   B. Maladaptation
   C. Pathologic grief
   D. Incongruent grief

5. A 10-year-old child experiences the loss of a 23-week sibling at 1 week of life. The mother questions the nurse regarding the impact of the death on her 10-year-old child. The nurse should explain that the sibling:
   A. will consider the death as temporary.
   B. may have regressive behaviors.
   C. will express philosophic reasoning about the death.
   D. may demonstrate a death phobia.

6. A mother expresses psychosomatic complaints 2 years after losing her infant son. What is this an example of?
   A. Chronic sorrow
   B. Delayed grief
   C. Pathologic grief
   D. Guilt

7. An infant is unexpectedly born with multiple congenital anomalies that are incompatible with life. The mother had chosen to breastfeed prior to delivery. Which course of action by the nurse is most appropriate for lactation suppression?
   A. Assist mother to apply breast binder.
   B. Encourage continual breast pumping every 3 hours.
   C. Offer donation of any pumped milk to a local milk bank.
   D. Instruct mother to completely empty breasts with each pumping session.

ANSWERS AND RATIONALES

1. **(A)** Anticipatory grieving prepares an individual to process the loss of an imperfect baby and ultimate death. It is the most applicable for this clinical situation. This is not a long-term grief response so would not be demonstrative of pathologic grief or chronic sorrow. Incongruent grieving is not applicable given that only the mother is expressing her concerns rather than both parents.

Reference: Gardner S, Carter B. Grief and perinatal loss. In: Gardner SL, Carter BS, Enzman-Hines M, Niermeyer S, eds. *Merenstein & Gardner's Handbook of Neonatal Intensive Care.* 9th ed. St. Louis, MO: Elsevier; 2021:1100.

2. **(A)** Emotional numbness is the initial stage of grief and is characterized by overwhelming feelings of being stunned and surprised. It is a defense mechanism used to help the individual adapt slowly to the crisis. Anger will often follow the initial emotional numbness, then bargaining and depression as the grief is processed by the affected individual to the final stage of acceptance.

Reference: Gardner S, Carter B. Grief and perinatal loss. In: Gardner SL, Carter BS, Enzman-Hines M, Niermeyer S, eds. *Merenstein & Gardner's Handbook of Neonatal Intensive Care.* 9th ed. St. Louis, MO: Elsevier; 2021:1102-1103.

3. **(A)** There is a lag in physiologic reality and lag of investment of the father versus the mother, indicating incongruent grieving. Failure to share grief leads to isolation and alienation in the relationship and may result in parental disassociation in the long term. Although guilt and apathy may be emotions expressed by both parents, they affect the mother more often than the father.

Reference: Gardner S, Carter B. Grief and perinatal loss. In: Gardner SL, Carter BS, Enzman-Hines M, Niermeyer S, eds. *Merenstein & Gardner's Handbook of Neonatal Intensive Care.* 9th ed. St. Louis, MO: Elsevier; 2021:1104-1106.

4. **(A)** Sorrow and grief may last a lifetime for families of children with lifelong and incurable conditions. Parents have a constant reminder of what is not and what the child will never be and can never do. Chronic sorrow is grieving on a daily basis. This is not considered a maladaptive behavior given the child's diagnosis. The grief is appropriate for the situation and not pathologic. Given the mother's verbalization of the grief, it is unclear if incongruent grief exists between the parents.

Reference: Gardner S, Carter B. Grief and perinatal loss. In: Gardner SL, Carter BS, Enzman-Hines M, Niemeyer S, eds. *Merenstein & Gardner's Handbook of Neonatal Intensive Care.* 9th ed. St. Louis, MO: Elsevier; 2021:1103, 1107.

5. **(B)** Attempts to protect children from feelings of grief and mourning due to perinatal loss isolate the child. Age-based, developmentally appropriate explanations should include the child in the family loss experience. Regressive behaviors such as enuresis are common in the school-age child (6–12 years) upon the death of a sibling. Eight-year-olds demonstrate a death phobia and have thoughts of their own possible death. Preschoolers view death as a temporary state and expect the dead to return. Adolescents are able to have philosophic reasoning about the death.

Reference: Gardner S, Carter B. Grief and perinatal loss. In: Gardner SL, Carter BS, Enzman-Hines M, Niermeyer S, eds. *Merenstein & Gardner's Handbook of Neonatal Intensive Care.* 9th ed. St. Louis, MO: Elsevier; 2021:1131.

6. **(C)** A maladaptive response to perinatal loss includes complaints of psychosomatic conditions and is an indication for the need to refer to specialized care because the grief has become pathologic. Chronic sorrow afflicts families with disabled children, not children who have died. Guilt is a stage of grief, but the guilt will begin to dissipate within the first few months after the death. Delayed grief may be evident for a period when an immediate grief reaction would be expected and appropriate. It is a conscious, intentional decision to postpone or dismiss the grief to meet the needs of others.

Reference: Gardner S, Carter B. Grief and perinatal loss. In: Gardner SL, Carter BS, Enzman-Hines M, Niermeyer S, eds. *Merenstein & Gardner's Handbook of Neonatal Intensive Care.* 9th ed. St. Louis, MO: Elsevier; 2021:1118, 1132-1133.

7. **(C)** The wearing of a well-fitted and supportive bra will cause the mother less pain and discomfort during lactation suppression than a breast binder. If the mother pumps until she is comfortable, prolonging the intervals between pumping will gradually suppress lactation. An incomplete emptying of the breasts versus a complete emptying will result in a gradual decrease in milk production. Mothers who have pumped and stored breast milk can donate as an act of altruism.

Reference: Gardner S, Carter B. Grief and perinatal loss. In: Gardner SL, Carter BS, Enzman-Hines M, Niermeyer S, eds. *Merenstein & Gardner's Handbook of Neonatal Intensive Care.* 9th ed. St. Louis, MO: Elsevier; 2021: 1110, 1121.

PROFESSIONAL PRACTICE

Chapter 31

Quality Improvement

1. Which improvement strategy supports a culture of safety awareness among neonatal nursing staff through information sharing throughout the day/week?
   A. Safety briefings
   B. Forcing functions
   C. Time-outs
   D. Read-backs

2. Which one of the following quality improvement models provides the opportunity for rapid cycle testing?
   A. Root-cause analysis
   B. Failure mode effect analysis
   C. Plan, do, study, act
   D. Six Sigma modeling

3. What term represents a standard of performance or best practice for a particular process or outcome?
   A. Outcome measure
   B. Benchmarking
   C. Qualitative research
   D. Quantitative research

4. Quality improvement and creating a culture of safety represent a focus in organizations to improve patient outcomes. Each leader within the organization has a specific responsibility, and senior leaders must engage key stakeholders in creating a culture of safety. Which of the following people represent key stakeholders in the neonatal intensive care unit (NICU)?
   A. Neonatologists, NICU nurses, respiratory therapists, nonfamily visitors, unit secretary
   B. Lactation consultants, electricians, laboratory technicians, nonfamily visitors
   C. Neonatal nurse practitioners, family members, NICU nurses, neonatologist, respiratory therapist
   D. Neonatologists, pharmacists, physical therapists, nonfamily visitors, family members, social workers

5. Which of the following is essential to conducting quality improvement work?
   A. Involving leadership only in the initial stages of quality improvement work
   B. Fostering and sustaining a culture of change and safety
   C. Hypothesizing a problem that will be addressed
   D. Committing to applying only one quality improvement tool

6. Standardized reporting guidelines were developed to support transparency, value, and accuracy in conducting and disseminating outcomes of quality improvement. Among the recommendations with use of the Standards for Quality Improvement Reporting Excellence (SQUIRE) guidelines for reporting quality improvement is:
   A. generating new empirical evidence and reporting it accurately.
   B. indicating clear evidence of institutional review board approval as human subject research.
   C. ensuring that the methodology used supports generalizability of findings across settings.
   D. applying a theoretical rationale for the planning, implementation, and/or evaluation of the quality improvement initiative.

7. When considering practice change in an organization, it is important to distinguish between research, evidence-based practice, and quality improvement. Which of the following statements is true?
   A. Results of research, evidence-based practice, and quality improvement are all generalizable across practice settings.
   B. Quality improvement integrates existing knowledge into process/practice improvement while research generates new discipline knowledge.
   C. Research and evidence-based practice aim to generate new empirical evidence that will inform and evaluate practice.
   D. Research typically integrates critical appraisal of existing evidence while quality improvement aims to generate new knowledge about nursing practice or health systems.

8. Which of the following is true about the quality improvement process?
   A. Quality improvement utilizes validated tools to contrast findings against benchmarks, determines a root cause that can be targeted, and tests a change that can be generalized across multiple settings.
   B. Quality improvement is a systematic approach to quality, safety, or efficiency changes that aims to standardize processes that are measurable and sustainable.
   C. Quality improvement begins with a focus of clinical inquiry and results in generation of new research evidence that can impact care.
   D. Quality improvement typically contrasts and tests two different strategies, protocols, or processes.

9. Which quality improvement schema provides a visual representation for root-cause analysis, using organizing categories to guide understanding of the "5 whys" involved with a problem?
   A. Fishbone cause-and-effect diagram
   B. Iowa model
   C. Stetler model
   D. Advancing research and clinical practice through close collaboration (ARCC) model

ANSWERS AND RATIONALES

1. **(A)** A safety briefing is a safety awareness model that supports staff sharing of patient safety information with other staff. It encourages an environment for staff to feel safe in speaking up as part of the daily unit routine. Forcing functions are interventions that prevent errors by enforcing a correct, safe action. An example is designing oral syringes in a way that they cannot be inadvertently connected to an intravenous port or removing concentrated medication from the medication cart. Time-outs refer to planned periods of quiet or stoppage, to allow discussion of key procedural details. An example of this is a surgical procedure time-out to allow the opportunity for staff to double-check key procedural elements before proceeding with a planned procedure. Read-backs are components of closed-loop communication. A read-back allows the receiver of the information to repeat back what is heard and allows the transmitter of the information to confirm that what is transmitted is correctly heard and interpreted.

Reference: Smith JR, Donze A. Patient safety. In: Verklan M, Walden M, Forest S, eds. *Core Curriculum for Neonatal Intensive Care Nursing*. 6th ed. St. Louis, MO: Elsevier; 2021:301-328.

2. **(C)** The plan–do–study–act or plan–do–check–act process is a four-stage quality improvement model that incorporates rapid-cycles and focuses on the relationship between changes in processes and outcomes. The stages include: **planning** and observation; **doing** the change on a small scale; **studying** the result of the change to determine what was learned and next steps; and **acting** to refine the change. The small tests of change continually build knowledge and allow for advancing the change on a broader scale. Root-cause analysis focuses on a specific event to reveal the underlying cause(s) and circumstance(s) that contributed to an outcome such as a medical error. It involves an analysis of the event and proposes a specific action plan to remedy the problem such as procedure changes or additional education. A failure mode effect analysis identifies and analyses potential failures within a system and predicts the probability and consequences of the failure. Six sigma is an approach used when there is a need for a large-scale change within an organization. Methodologies to define, measure, analyze, design, improve, and sustain occur over multiple months to years, and result in outcomes that align with organizations goals. Used in conjunction with *Lean*, this approach can reduce waste, improve errors and positively impact processes, care and patient satisfaction.

References: Fineout-Overholt E, Stevens KR. Critically appraising knowledge for clinical decision making. In: Melnyk BM, Fineout-Overholt E, eds. *Evidence-Based Practice in Nursing and Healthcare: A Guide to Best Practice*. 4th ed. Philadelphia, PA: Wolters Kluwer; 2019:109-123.

Giardino ER. Evaluation in quality improvement. In: Hickey JV, Giardino ER, eds. *Evaluation of Quality in Healthcare for DNPs*. 3rd ed. New York: Springer Publishing Co; 2021:215-246.

Johnson J. Quality improvement. In: Sherwood G, Barnsteiner J, eds. *Quality and Safety in Nursing. A Competency Approach to Improving Outcomes*. 3rd ed. Hoboken, NJ: John Wiley & Sons; 2022:155-184.

Langabeer JR. Glossary of key terms. In: Langabeer JR, ed. *Performance Improvement in Hospitals and Health Systems: Managing Analytics and Quality in Healthcare*. 2nd ed. Boca Raton, FL: Taylor and Francis Group; 2018: 213-224.

3. **(B)** Benchmarking is a standard of performance or best practice for a particular process or outcome. It is a process of measuring and comparing the results of key work processes with those of other leading organizations. An outcome measure indicates the result of the performance or nonperformance of a function or process. Outcomes are often expressed as a metric for the success or failure of a project or process. Qualitative research refers to investigation of phenomena and generation of narrative data that explain and inform that data. It is an iterative design that continually examines and interprets data and generates themes that build a rich examination of the phenomenon of interest. Sampling is guided by the data until the point of saturation is achieved. Quantitative research investigates phenomena using precise mathematical measurement and applies rigorous design and statistical analysis. It is a scientific, multiphase process that conceptualizes, designs, plans, collects, and analyzes data to form conclusions.

References: Langabeer JR. Glossary of key terms. In: Langabeer JR, ed. *Performance Improvement in Hospitals and Health Systems: Managing Analytics & Quality in Healthcare*. 2nd ed. Boca Raton, FL: Taylor and Francis Group; 2018: 213-224.

Polit D, Beck C. Glossary. In: Polit D, Beck C, eds. *Essentials of Nursing Research*. 10th ed. Philadelphia, PA: Wolters Kluwer; 2020:375-404.

4. **(C)** Key neonatal intensive care unit (NICU) stakeholders must be actively and credibly involved in discussions of safety culture and planning for any needed change. Neonatologists, NICU nurses, respiratory therapists, lactation consultants, laboratory technicians, neonatal nurse practitioners, pharmacists, physical therapists, social workers, and the unit secretary are all key stakeholders that provide either direct or indirect patient care. Family members are considered key stakeholders in their infant's care. Nonfamily visitors and electricians are not key stakeholders because the sharing of patient information is protected.

Reference: Ravi D, Tawfik DS, Sexton JB, Profit J. Changing safety culture. *J Perinatol*. 2021;41(10):1-9. doi:10.1038/s41372-020-00839-0.

5. **(B)** It has been suggested that quality improvement requires five essential elements for success: fostering and sustaining a culture of change and safety; clarifying an understanding of the problem; involving key stakeholders; testing change strategies; and continuous monitoring of performance and reporting of findings to sustain the change. Involving all key stakeholders, including leadership, nurses, providers, and family members, throughout the process is an important component of quality improvement. A key element of quality improvement is identifying and addressing an existing problem that is amenable to change. It differs from research in that it does not begin with generating of a hypothesis that will be rigorously tested. Quality improvement is a dynamic, rapid-cycle process that often employs more than one quality improvement tool.

Reference: Giardino ER. Evaluation in quality improvement. In: Hickey JV, Giardino ER, eds. *Evaluation of Quality in Healthcare for DNPs*. 3rd ed. New York: Springer Publishing Co; 2021:215-246.

6. **(D)** A recommendation of the Standards for Quality Improvement Reporting Excellence (SQUIRE) guidelines is to indicate the informal or formal theories or frameworks that were used as rationale for the project. This was intended to align the measures and assumptions of quality improvement more clearly with the expected outcomes and support its inclusion in scholarly literature. Quality improvement is not focused on generating new evidence and there is no expectation of generalizability with the findings beyond a specific setting. Quality improvement protocols do not typically create risks for patients and are typically eligible for

expedited review or exempt status. Individual organizational rules apply regarding the level of approval expected with quality improvement, however quality improvement is not considered human subject research.

References: Giardino ER. Evaluation in quality improvement. In: Hickey JV, Giardino ER, eds. *Evaluation of Quality in Healthcare for DNPs.* 3rd ed. New York: Springer Publishing Co; 2021:215-246.

Hu ZJ, Fusch G, Hu C, et al. Completeness of reporting of quality improvement studies in neonatology is inadequate. A systematic literature survey. *BMJ Open Quality.* 2021;10(2):1-8.

Ogrinc G, Armstrong GE, Dolansky MA, Singh MK, Davies L. SQUIRE-EDU (Standards for Quality Improvement Reporting Excellence in Education): Publication guidelines for educational improvement. *Acad Med.* 2019; 94(10):1461-1470.

7. (B) Quality improvement is setting specific and benefits the specific organization by uncovering actionable processes that can be improved. It is not meant to be generalizable beyond the individual setting nor is its aim to generate new practice knowledge. Research applies the scientific process to hypotheses and generates new knowledge and evidence that can be translated into practice and generalized. Evidence-based practice translates research and other evidence into practice, but does not generate new empirical evidence.

Reference: Melnyk BM, Fineout-Overholt E. Making the case for evidence-based practice and cultivating a spirit of inquiry. In: Melnyk BM, Fineout-Overholt E, eds. *Evidence-Based Practice in Nursing and Healthcare: A Guide to Best Practice.* 4th ed. Philadelphia: Wolters Kluwer; 2019:7-32.

8. (B) Quality improvement systematically applies metrics to determine performance against benchmarks, with a goal of organization-specific standardized and sustainable benefits. Quality improvement applies strategies that can improve benchmark indicators and identify process or practice issues that can be targeted for improvement. It does not aim to make findings generalizable beyond a specific setting. Quality improvement identifies and addresses current issues but does not aim to generate research evidence. Research evidence is generated through a rigorous, scientific approach that is beyond the scope of setting-specific quality improvement processes. Quality improvement directly impacts and benefits a process, system, or outcome at a specific setting. This contrasts with research that may compare different approaches to care and the impact on outcomes.

Reference: Giardino ER. Evaluation in quality improvement. In: Hickey JV, Giardino ER, eds. *Evaluation of Quality in Healthcare for DNPs.* 3rd ed. New York: Springer Publishing Co; 2021:215-246.

9. (A) Quality improvement is a systematic process that assesses progress toward identified goals. Work is mapped to established practice benchmarks and continually evaluated to improve practice. Organizing schema can help with identifying areas or processes to address, such as people, equipment, environment, materials or management. Developed in the 1960s, the Fishbone cause-and-effect diagram has been used by teams to brainstorm ideas and intensively target one to two areas for action. The Iowa, Stetler, and advancing research and clinical practice through close collaboration (ARCC) models are all evidence-based practice models used to translate research findings into practice. According to a recent US survey, over 90% of nursing leaders indicate use of an evidence-based practice model, and the Iowa, Stetler, and ARCC models were the most commonly used for evidence-based practice.

References: Johnson J. Quality improvement. In: Sherwood G, Barnsteiner J, eds. *Quality and Safety in Nursing. A Competency Approach to Improving Outcomes.* 3rd ed. Hoboken, NJ: John Wiley & Sons; 2022:155-184.

Langabeer JR. Glossary of terms. In: Langabeer JR, ed. *Performance Improvement in Hospitals and Health Systems: Managing Analytics and Quality in Healthcare.* 2nd ed. Boca Raton, FL: Taylor and Francis Group; 2018:213-224.

Speroni KG, McLaughlin MK, Friesen MA. Use of evidence-based practice models and research findings in Magnet-designated hospitals across the United States. National survey results. *Worldviews Evid Based Nurs.* 2020;17(2):98-107.

Chapter 32

Patient Safety

1. Of the following interventions implemented to reduce medication errors, which has been most effective?
   A. Pediatric-trained pharmacists on rounds
   B. Bar code–assisted medication administration
   C. Smart pump technology
   D. Double-checking of medications

2. The neonatal intensive care unit (NICU) that has a "culture of safety" is focused on which of the following?
   A. Promoting a no-blame approach to error reporting
   B. Focusing on individual performance with each error event
   C. Sharing error reports as a method of learning and improving
   D. Measuring the effectiveness of safety efforts by a reduction in the number of errors reported

3. A nonpunitive approach to patient safety errors means that health care providers:
   A. are human and mistakes happen.
   B. are the focus of patient safety efforts.
   C. are accountable for safety procedures.
   D. will not receive disciplinary action for an error regardless of the circumstances.

4. Distractions during medication administration:
   A. can be easily reduced.
   B. are not a major contributing factor in errors.
   C. are a major contributing factor in errors.
   D. are caused mostly by patients and their families.

5. Most patient safety events in the NICU are:
   A. harmless.
   B. preventable.
   C. voluntarily reported.
   D. the result of human error.

6. Syringe pumps are used commonly in the NICU for medication administration and use of these pumps is associated with:
   A. specialized intravenous tubing increasing dead space and inaccurate medication delivery.
   B. accurate drug delivery in all conditions.
   C. rapid detection of occlusions.
   D. variable infusion flow including delayed drug delivery, overdosing, and underdosing.

7. Patients in the NICU are at an increased risk of wrong patient errors when compared to other hospitalized patients primarily due to:
   A. frequently moving a patient to a different NICU bed space during a shift.
   B. arm/leg band commonly removed during routine care and not replaced.
   C. lack of identification photo in the electronic medical record.
   D. lack of nondistinctive naming conventions.

8. Transparency and full disclosure when unexpected events occur in the NICU may be associated with:
   A. increased malpractice claims.
   B. reduced patient safety climate.
   C. reduced reporting of patient safety events.
   D. reduced liability and malpractice claims.

9. Standardized hand-offs that are integrated within the electronic health record are associated with:
   A. reduced patient safety due to increased workload and poor usability.
   B. reduced distractions during hand-off and increased accuracy of information.
   C. reduced provider efficiency, as hand-off processes take longer to complete.
   D. increased patient safety errors, as computers are a distraction.

10. In the patient safety literature, the term "high-reliability" organization describes a NICU in which:
    A. a comprehensive education program is provided as a method of retraining.
    B. a systems approach is used with adverse events including analysis of trends, a focus on near misses to improve error-prone processes, and a multipronged approach to patient safety.
    C. adverse event reporting is focused on improving individual performances.
    D. leaders are the expert and drive unit changes.

11. A NICU with staff that rate teamwork as high is associated with:
    A. reduced healthcare-associated infections.
    B. individual staff characteristics of isolation and burnout.
    C. poor interdepartmental teamwork.
    D. daily bedside clinical rounds.

ANSWERS AND RATIONALES

1. **(A)** Pediatric pharmacists on rounds have been shown to significantly reduce medication errors primarily in the prescribing phase of medication use. Widely adopted barcode-assisted medication administration research results demonstrate a reduction in medication administration error; however, limited research has been conducted or reported for patients in the neonatal intensive care unit (NICU). While smart pump technology has the potential to reduce medication errors in the NICU, more research is needed to confirm its overall effectiveness. Because there may be a mismatch between the capabilities of a smart pump and demands of care, workarounds in their use have been identified. Independent double-checks may not be performed with every medication administration and must be performed independently to be effective. *Independent* means that each registered nurse compares the medication with the order and the medication label, checking the important components (minimally, the "five rights") separately.

References: Hermanspann T, Schoberer M, Robel-Tillig E, et al. Incidence and severity of prescribing errors in parenteral nutrition for pediatric inpatients at a neonatal and pediatric intensive care unit. *Front Pediatr.* 2017;5:149. doi: 10.3389/fped.2017.00149.

Institute for Safe Medication Practices. *ISMP Medication Safety Alert! The Virtues of Independent Double Checks—They Really Are Worth Your Time!* 2003;8(5):1. Available at: http://www.ismp.org/Newsletters/acutecare/articles/20030306.asp.

Brennan-Bourdon LM, Vazquez-Alvarez AO, Gallegos-Llamas J, Koninckx-Canada M, Marco-Garbayo JL, Huerta-Olvera SG. A study of medication errors during the prescription stage in pediatric critical care services of a secondary-tertiary level public hospital. *BMC Pediatr.* 2020;20(1):549. doi:10.1186/s12887-020-02442-w.

Melton KR, Timmons K, Walsh KE, Meinzen-Derr JK, Kirkendall E. Smart pumps improve medication safety but increase alert burden in neonatal care. *BMC Med Inform Decis Mak.* 2019;19:213. doi:10.1186/s12911-019-0945-2.

2. **(C)** A safety culture is one that is focused on reducing safety problems by using a nonpunitive approach to errors, transparently sharing error reports as a method for learning and improving and focusing on systems issues rather than individual performance. An atmosphere of mutual trust is established in which all staff members can talk freely about safety problems and how to solve them without fear of retribution. Often, when a safety culture is present, error reporting increases as staff feel confident about reporting issues. A no-blame approach reduces the accountability of health care professionals for following established safety procedures.

References: Aydon L, Hauck Y, Zimmer M, Murdoch J. Factors influencing a nurse's decision to question medication administration in a neonatal clinical care unit. *J Clin Nurs.* 2016;25(17-18):2468-2477. doi:10.1111/jocn.13277.

Rogers E, Griffin E, Carnie W, Melucci J, Weber RJ. A just culture approach to managing medication errors. *Hosp Pharm.* 2017;52(4):308-315. doi:10.1310/hpj5204-308.

3. **(C)** A nonpunitive approach to patient safety errors includes achieving a balance between understanding human error and holding health care professionals accountable for following established safety procedures. A no-blame approach reduces the accountability of health care professionals for adhering to established safety procedures whereas a nonpunitive approach does not disregard reckless behavior of an employee who knowingly violates a rule. When a nonpunitive approach is followed, the focus of patient safety efforts is on systems issues.

Reference: Alsabri M, Castill F, Wiredu S, et al. Assessment of patient safety culture in a pediatric department. *Cureus.* 2021;13(4):e14646. doi:10.7759/cureus.14646.

4. **(C)** Distraction is a major contributing factor to medication errors in health care. Reducing distractions in the health care environment is a challenge and requires a combination of interventions, including behavioral changes in health care providers, workflow modifications, and use of new technology. Although there are multiple sources of distractions, one study demonstrated that other staff members are the most common source.

References: Melton K, Ni Y, Tubbs-Cooley H, Walsh K. Using health information technology to improve safety in neonatal care: A systematic review of the literature. *Clin Perinatol.* 2017;44(3):583-616. doi:10.1016/j.clp.2017.04.003.

Esque Ruiz MT. Medication errors in a neonatal unit: one of the main adverse events. *An Pediatr (Barc).* 2016;84(4):211-217.

5. **(B)** Most patient safety events in the NICU are preventable. Most patient safety events are not reported via a voluntary reporting system, but rather are identified via a "trigger" tool that is used concurrently or retrospectively. Trigger methods have been shown to be superior to other identification strategies such as voluntary reporting, nontriggered chart review, and administrative databases in the identification of adverse events in the NICU. Most patient safety events identified using a trigger tool result in harm to the patient. System issues and communication problems are the most common causes of errors.

Reference: Alghamdi AA, Keers RN, Sutherland A, Ashcroft DM. Prevalence and nature of medication errors and preventable adverse drug events in paediatric and neonatal intensive care settings: a systematic review. *Drug Saf.* 2019;42(12):1423-1436. doi:10.1007/s40264-019-00856-9.

6. **(D)** Syringe pump use in the NICU is high as the device delivers small volume infusions with a strong degree of accuracy. However, the FDA issued a safety communication highlighting the risks associated with syringe pump use including variable flow delivery that can result in under-/overdosing problems. Syringe pumps require low-volume tubing which reduces dead space and improves accuracy of delivery. Syringe pumps may not deliver accurately in all conditions, especially when syringe pumps are positioned above or below the level of the patient's heart. Timely detection of occlusions that occur along the fluid pathway may be delayed due to syringe pump piston delivery system.

References: FDA. Syringe pump problems fluid flow continuity at low infusion rates can result in serious clinical consequences: FDA safety communication. Issued August 25, 2016; retrieved April 19, 2021.

Institute for Safe Medication Practices (ISMP). *ISMP Guidelines for Optimizing Safe Implementation and Use of Smart Infusion Pumps.* 2020. Available at: https://www.ismp.org/node/972.

7. **(D)** The Joint Commission in 2019 issued new requirements for distinct newborn naming conventions as an evidenced-based intervention to reduce wrong patient errors. Recent published research and quality reports have determined that nondistinctive naming conventions, common among newly delivered newborns significantly increases the risk of wrong-patient errors in this population. Although moving NICU patients to different bed spaces in the NICU may be common as compared to other patients in the hospital, this practice has not been well-studied as contributing factor in wrong-patient errors. Difficulties in both maintaining and utilizing NICU patient identification bands consistently prior to interventions has been cited as a barrier to safe practice in the NICU. Identification bands may be removed during routine care and may not be replaced leading to nonuse prior to medication administration, laboratory blood draws, and other diagnostic tests. However, lack of ID band wearing in the NICU has not been further explored as a patient safety issue since the widespread use of medication administration using barcode technology. Use of photo identification integrated into the electronic health record (EHR) has recently been explored as method to reduce wrong patient safety events. However, this has not be specifically studied in the NICU population and may not have significant impact in reducing wrong patient errors.

References: Adelman J, Applebaum J, Southern W, et al. Risk of wrong-patient orders among multiple vs singleton births in the neonatal intensive care units of 2 integrated health care systems. *JAMA Pediatr.* 2019;173(10):979-985. doi:10.1001/jamapediatrics.2019.2733.

The Joint Commission. *R3 Report Issue 17: Distinct Newborn Identification Requirement.* 2018. Available at: https://www.jointcommission.org/standards/r3-report/r3-report-issue-17-distinct-newborn-identification-requirement/#.Y1Qe7HZlCUk. Accessed October 22, 2022.

8. **(D)** Health care providers are both ethically and morally required to discuss with patients and their families when unexpected outcomes or events have occurred. Additionally, transparency and full disclosure with families regarding events is associated with reduced malpractice claims, reduced liability, and increased settling of claims. There are no data suggesting that full disclosure policies or practices are associated with reduced reporting of neither safety events nor a reduced patient safety climate.

Reference: Kaldjian L. Communication about medical errors. *Patient Educ Couns.* 2021;104:989-993.

9. **(B)** Integrating a standardized hand-off within the EHR has demonstrated improvement in the accuracy of information exchanged, reduces preparation time for the provider, and reduces distractions. Utilization of an integrated hand-off improves efficiency and accuracy as information within the EHR autopopulates necessary and vital hand-off components. New technology can introduce unexpected safety events such as distractions; however, an integrated hand-off has not been associated with an increase in safety events.

References: Melton K, Ni Y, Tubbs-Cooley H, Walsh K. Using health information technology to improve safety in neonatal care: a systematic review of the literature. *Clin Perinatol.* 2017;44(3):583-616.

Nikel N, Amin D, Shakeel F, Germain A, Machry J. Handoff standardization in the neonatal intensive care unit with an EMR-based handoff tool. *J Perinatol.* 2020;41:634-640.

10. **(B)** High-reliability organizations (HROs) are described as environments that are preoccupied with providing safe, quality care; for example, HROs promote reporting of safety events in the spirit of analyzing core processes that contribute to the safety events, use expertise to find solutions, and test and retest to assure processes are correct. Retraining individuals will not address the system failures that contribute to the safety event, and thus the same safety event is likely to reoccur. Leaders in HROs value and defer to experts who inform and guide the organization. Focusing on efforts to improve individual performances alone does not address the system failures that contribute to the safety event, and thus the same safety event is likely to reoccur.

References: Gupta M, Soll R, Suresh G. The relationship between patient safety and quality improvement in neonatology. *Sem Perinatol.* 2019;43(8):1-11.

Tawfik D, Sexton JB, Adair K, Kaplan H, Profit J. Context in quality of care: improving teamwork and resilience. *Clin Perinatol.* 2017;44(3):541-552.

11. **(A)** The presence or absence of teamwork in an NICU is independently and significantly associated with hospital-acquired infection (HAI) rates. With every 10% increase in the reporting by NICU staff of good teamwork, HAI decreased by 18%; high-quality teamwork is also associated with higher-quality newborn resuscitation. Burnout and individual isolation are associated with reduced teamwork scores. Although daily bedside team rounding is preferred, this methodology does not necessarily incur high teamwork scores.

Reference: Profit J, Sharek PJ, Kan P, et al. Teamwork in the NICU setting and its association with health care associated infections in very low–birth-weight infants. *Am J Perinatol.* 2017;34:1032-1040.

Chapter 33

Research

1. A study of preterm infants examined how feedings of expressed breast milk affected the incidence of necrotizing enterocolitis (NEC). In this study, NEC is the:
   A. dependent variable.
   B. extraneous variable.
   C. antecedent variable.
   D. independent variable.

2. The extent to which the findings of a research study can be applied to populations beyond the study's sample is referred to as the study's:
   A. validity.
   B. reliability.
   C. testability.
   D. generalizability.

3. An investigation into the effect of co-bedding on weight gain in preterm infants used a process in which each baby had an equal chance of being assigned to either an experimental group or a control group. This process is referred to as:
   A. blinding.
   B. control.
   C. anonymity.
   D. randomization.

4. To achieve improved patient outcomes, evidence-based practice integrates the best research evidence, clinical expertise, and which of these additional elements?
   A. Corporate directives
   B. Clinician preferences
   C. Patient–family values
   D. Quality improvement principles

5. A study determined that tympanic membrane temperature recordings provide consistent temperature readings in stable, term newborns. This study demonstrated that the instrument used to record tympanic membrane temperatures has which of these attributes?
   A. Validity
   B. Accuracy
   C. Precision
   D. Reliability

6. When considering the use of evidence to inform nursing practice, which of these represent the highest level of evidence?
   A. Descriptive studies
   B. Meta-analyses
   C. Reports from expert committees
   D. Case–control studies

7. When considering the application of a quantitative research study's findings to evidence-based practice, the nurse determines that the study's statistically significant findings indicate that:

A. findings of the study should be used in clinical practice.
B. the relationship between the study's variables did not occur by chance.
C. there are no significant limitations described in the study.
D. the study's demographic variables are heterogeneous.

8. The aim of a descriptive research study is to:
   A. deepen knowledge about a target population.
   B. understand the lived experience of the study's participants.
   C. determine relationships among the study variables.
   D. establish a cause-and-effect relationship.

   Evolve Rationale:
   A. A descriptive study aims to increase the understanding of a population or phenomenon.
   B. Qualitative studies examine the lived experience of the study's participants.
   C. A correlational study seeks to determine the relationships among the variables in the study.
   D. Experimental and quasi-experimental studies aim to identify cause-and-effect relationships.

9. The nurse is collecting data for a qualitative research study, and notices redundancy in the data. This phenomenon refers to:
   A. confirmability.
   B. saturation.
   C. trustworthiness.
   D. triangulation.

10. The nurse researcher asks nurses to voluntarily complete a survey about their satisfaction with a new staffing protocol. Which of these sampling techniques is the nurse researcher using?
    A. Cluster sampling
    B. Purposive sampling
    C. Convenience sampling
    D. Snowball sampling

ANSWERS AND RATIONALES

1. **(A)** A dependent variable represents the outcome variable or result of interest in a study. An extraneous variable is one that is outside the variables of interest and may obscure the relationship between the dependent and independent variables. An antecedent variable is a type of independent variable that occurs before the main independent variable and has the potential to explain the relationship between the dependent and independent variables. An independent variable is the phenomenon that has a presumed effect on the dependent variable.

Reference: Haber J. Appraising Research questions, hypotheses, and clinical questions. In: LoBiondo-Wood G, Haber J, eds. *Nursing Research: Methods and Critical Appraisal for Evidence-Based Practice*. 10th ed. St. Louis, MO: Elsevier; 2022:24-46 [chapter 2].

2. **(D)** The generalizability of a study allows the study results to be applied to a similar phenomenon in a wider population. Validity refers to the ability of an instrument used to collect data to measure the attribute that it is intended to measure. Reliability refers to the ability of an instrument used to collect data to consistently measure the attribute of interest. Testability refers to the degree to which a variable lends itself to being measured, observed, and analyzed.

Reference: McEwen M. Theoretical frameworks for research. In: LoBiondo-Wood G, Haber J, eds. *Nursing Research: Methods and Critical Appraisal for Evidence-Based Practice.* 10th ed. St. Louis, MO: Elsevier; 2022:71-77 [chapter 4].

3. **(D)** Randomization refers to the random assignment of study subjects to either control or treatment groups for the purposes of an experimental study. Blinding refers to the withholding of information from the study subjects, the researchers implementing the study, or both. Control involves several strategies to hold study conditions constant so true relationships between variables can be understood. Anonymity refers to a study participant's right to privacy and the expectation that the data a participant provides cannot be linked to that study participant.

Reference: Sullivan-Bolyai S, Bova C. Appraising experimental and quasi-experimental designs. In: LoBiondo-Wood G, Haber J, eds. *Nursing Research: Methods and Critical Appraisal for Evidence-Based Practice.* 10th ed. St. Louis, MO: Elsevier; 2022:174-188 [chapter 9].

4. **(C)** Evidence-based practice is the result of integrating research, clinical expertise, and patient-family values into patient care. Although corporate directives can provide guidance when implementing evidence-based practice, they are not an essential component of evidence-based practice. Clinician preferences are not considered a component of evidence-based practice and should be incorporated only when they are in line with current research and patient–family values and expectations. Quality improvement is an essential component of an optimal health care system; however, it is not an essential component of evidence-based practice.

Reference: Titler M. Developing an evidence-based practice. In: LoBiondo-Wood G, Haber J, eds. *Nursing Research: Methods and Critical Appraisal for Evidence-Based Practice.* 10th ed. St. Louis, MO: Elsevier; 2022:338-415 [chapter 20].

5. **(D)** Reliability refers to the ability of an instrument to consistently measure the attribute of interest. Validity refers to the ability of an instrument to measure the attribute that it is intended to measure. Accuracy indicates the degree to which the value obtained for an attribute is congruent with its true value. Precision denotes the exactness with which an attribute is measured.

Reference: Lo-Biondo-Wood G, Haber J. Appraising reliability and validity. In: LoBiondo-Wood G, Haber J, eds. *Nursing Research: Methods and Critical Appraisal for Evidence-Based Practice.* 10th ed. St. Louis, MO: Elsevier; 2022: 275-292 [chapter 15].

6. **(B)** Metaanalyses provide the highest level of evidence on which to base nursing practice, because they are based on a comprehensive literature review, using a rigorous set of specific criteria. Descriptive studies are observational studies that give an overview of a particular phenomenon. Although reports from expert committees can provide useful information to guide practice, they are not always backed by research, so they represent the lowest level of evidence on which to base nursing practice. Case–control studies are retrospective investigations that compare a group that has a particular outcome of interest with a group that does not.

References: American Association of Critical-Care Nurses. *AACN Levels of Evidence.* Available at: https://www.aacn.org/clinical-resources/practice-alerts/aacn-levels-of-evidence. Accessed January 19, 2022.

Lo-Biondo-Wood G, Haber J. Appraising reliability and validity. In: LoBiondo-Wood G, Haber J, eds. *Nursing Research: Methods and Critical Appraisal for Evidence-Based Practice.* 10th ed. St. Louis, MO: Elsevier; 2022:275-292 [chapter 15].

7. **(B)** The statistical significance tells the nurse if there is a true relationship between the study's variables, or if the relationship is due to chance; however, statistical significance does not indicate whether the research findings are of practical value to clinical nursing practice. A study's limitations are weaknesses or shortcomings in methodology that could limit its generalizability or usefulness in clinical nursing practice. If the demographic variables, which are the characteristics of the study's participants, are heterogenous, this means there is a wide range of values within the sample, which increases its generalizability.

Reference: McEwen M. Appraising theoretical frameworks for research. In: LoBiondo-Wood G, Haber J, eds. *Nursing Research: Methods and Critical Appraisal for Evidence-Based Practice.* 10th ed. St. Louis, MO: Elsevier; 2022:71-77 [chapter 4].

8. **(A)** A descriptive study aims to increase the understanding of a population or phenomenon. Qualitative studies examine the lived experience of the study's participants. A correlational study seeks to determine the relationships among the variables in the study. Experimental and quasi-experimental studies aim to identify cause-and-effect relationships.

References: Flores DD, Barroso J. Qualitative approaches to research. In: LoBiondo-Wood G, Haber J, eds. *Nursing Research: Methods and Critical Appraisal for Evidence-Based Practice.* 10th ed. St. Louis, MO: Elsevier; 2022:109-128 [chapter 6].

LoBiondo-Wood G. Introduction to quantitative research. In: LoBiondo-Wood G, Haber J, eds. *Nursing Research: Methods and Critical Appraisal for Evidence-Based Practice.* 10th ed. St. Louis, MO: Elsevier; 2022:159-173 [chapter 8].

9. **(B)** Saturation refers to redundancy in the data, and that adequate data has been collected. Confirmability in a qualitative study is an indication of neutrality and freedom from bias. Trustworthiness refers to the credibility of data and the strength of a qualitative study's findings. Triangulation is a method where multiple sources of data, data analysis, theories, and methods are used in a single qualitative study to mitigate bias and other weaknesses to converge on the truth about a phenomenon.

Reference: Carpenter DR. Appraising qualitative research. In: LoBiondo-Wood G, Haber J, eds. *Nursing Research: Methods and Critical Appraisal for Evidence-Based Practice.* 10th ed. St. Louis, MO: Elsevier; 2022:129-154 [chapter 7].

10. **(C)** Convenience sampling, also called accidental sampling, is when available subjects are surveyed. A researcher uses cluster sampling by dividing populations into groups, and then randomly selecting subjects from each group. When purposive sampling is used, the researcher uses personal knowledge of a population to handpick a study sample that is deemed typical of the population of interest. Snowball sampling, sometimes called network sampling, is used when study subjects are asked to identify additional individuals to participate in the study.

Reference: Haber J. Sampling. In: LoBiondo-Wood G, Haber J, eds. *Nursing Research: Methods and Critical Appraisal for Evidence-Based Practice.* 10th ed. St. Louis, MO: Elsevier; 2022:223-242 [chapter 12].

Chapter 34

Legal Issues

1. A nurse makes a medication error by giving twice the ordered dose of ampicillin. This is discovered after the first dose, and the infant ultimately recovers from the infection without any adverse outcome. Which of the following statements is true?
   A. The nurse could be sued for negligence in this case.
   B. The physician could be sued for providing an unclear order.
   C. The nurse could not be sued because there was no injury related to the error.
   D. The nurse should document the correct dose because there was no injury.

2. A patient's critical value laboratory result is reported to the nurse by the laboratory. This is reported to the primary care provider who does nothing in response to this laboratory value. The best way to document this is:
   A. "Physician notified of laboratory result."
   B. "Dr. Jones notified of laboratory result without response."
   C. "Dr. Jones notified of (specific laboratory result). No orders at this time."
   D. "Physician notified of (specific laboratory result). Requested no action even though this was a critical value."

3. Fundamental criteria must be met to establish negligence in a medical malpractice case. Which of the following best describes these criteria?
   A. Duty to patient, a defective product, injury results.
   B. Duty to patient established, breach of duty, causal connection, injury results.
   C. Injury to a person through an error that occurred even though not assigned to that nurse.
   D. Error is made by the nurse assigned to the patient and injury occurs with or without causal connection.

4. In the case of legal action, the registered nurse's practice is judged by:
   A. policies and procedures in place when the event occurred.
   B. the state's nurse practice act in which the nurse is now licensed.
   C. the nurse's level of basic education (associates, baccalaureate, or diploma).
   D. standards from The Joint Commission in place when the event occurred.

5. A neonatal nurse is working at a hospital where there is a policy in place to double-check specific medications with another registered nurse. He is asked to cosign that he double-checked a medication that is already drawn up and unlabeled. After viewing the syringe and having the nurse tell him what she drew up, he agrees to cosign. Which of the following is true about this case?
   A. As a cosigner, he carries liability in case of an error.
   B. This activity reflects correct practice for double-checking of medications.

C. There is only liability for his cosignature because there is a policy in place.
   D. If this particular medication is not on the list of medications requiring a double check, the cosigner does not carry any liability for an error.

6. The nurse is aware that informed consent has not been obtained for a procedure to be done on an infant. Which of the following is the best action?
   A. Call the parents and inform them of the procedure.
   B. Do nothing—this is the responsibility of the primary care provider.
   C. Stop the procedure until informed consent can be obtained.
   D. Remind the physician that informed consent is not present in the medical record.

7. An infant of 23 weeks' gestation is now 7 days old. A head ultrasound shows a grade 4 intraventricular hemorrhage, and the infant is now showing signs of necrotizing enterocolitis. Parents have been informed of the infant's grave condition and voice that they want every measure possible taken to prolong their infant's life. The nurse is uncomfortable with the parent's decision. Which of the following describes the best action on the nurses' part?
   A. Tell the charge nurse he/she can no longer care for the infant.
   B. Continue caring for the infant and suggest to the healthcare team to reevaluate the plan of care to avoid painful procedures that no longer benefit the infant.
   C. Consult the hospital ethics committee as soon as possible.
   D. Remind parents when they visit how much the infant is suffering so that they understand the futility of care.

8. The nurse is working with an unlicensed assistive person (UAP). The nurse will be delegating duties to this person. The nurse's responsibilities regarding this process are best described as:
   A. the nurse must provide all of the direct patient care to the infants. The UAP can perform only nonclinical duties.
   B. the nurse must evaluate the UAP's abilities before delegating routine tasks to him/her and still maintain supervision while retaining accountability.
   C. the nurse may transfer responsibility and accountability for performance of tasks to the UAP.
   D. if the UAP is experienced, the nurse need not supervise his/her work and is not accountable for the outcome of what he/she does.

9. Standards of care in a specific clinical situation under legal review are determined by:
   A. federal regulations only, as they do not vary by location.
   B. policies and procedures in place when the lawsuit is filed.
   C. the testimony of a physician familiar with nursing care.
   D. the expected actions of a reasonable and prudent nurse in a similar situation.

ANSWERS AND RATIONALES

1. **(C)** Every case of negligence must meet four criteria. These are duty, breach, proximate cause, and injury. In the instance of a medication error that does not result in harm to the client, injury has not occurred, and therefore all necessary elements for a lawsuit have not been met. Therefore, the nurse could not be sued even though he or she made an error. There is insufficient information to determine whether the physician's order was indeed unclear. Even if the order was unclear, the nurse has a duty to clarify the order, and no injury occurred. Documentation should include the facts of care provided, whether injury occurred, and whether or not orders were followed.

References: Cypher RL. Demystifying the 4 elements of negligence. *J Perinat Neonatal Nurs.* 2020;34(2):108-109. doi:10.1097/JPN.0000000000000479.

Verklan MT. Legal issues. In: Verklan MT, Walden M, Forest S, eds. *Core Curriculum for Neonatal Intensive Care Nursing.* 6th ed. St. Louis, MO: Elsevier; 2021:720-733.

2. **(C)** Although there are few absolute rules about documentation, it should include information relayed as this serves as a record in the future if it should be needed. Documentation should remain neutral and nonjudgmental in the medical record. "Physician notified of laboratory result" is an incomplete description of what occurred because it does not indicate any acknowledgment of the information and does not indicate the specific laboratory result communicated, nor the specific physician notified when often more than one physician may be involved. "Dr. Jones notified of laboratory result without response" does not accurately describe the exchange because the physician did respond that there were no new orders. "Physician notified of (specific laboratory result). Requested no action even though this was a critical value" does not indicate the specific physician notified. In addition, this information would imply that "no action" was not appropriate because it was a critical value, making this documentation judgmental of the physician response.

Reference: Verklan MT. Legal issues. In: Verklan MT, Walden M, Forest S, eds. *Core Curriculum for Neonatal Intensive Care Nursing.* 6th ed. St. Louis, MO: Elsevier; 2021:720-733.

3. **(B)** Establishing negligence in a medical malpractice case requires that four criteria are met. These include that a duty to the patient has been established, that duty was not met (breach of duty) and injury resulted that can be shown to be related to the breach of duty (causal connection). Defective products are rarely involved in negligence cases and certainly are not a required element to establish negligence. Negligence may be established even though the nurse is not assigned to the patient if there is duty established such as the nurse is present during the event and had some responsibility to the patient. But a breach of duty and causal connection would also need to be established.

Reference: Cypher RL. Demystifying the 4 elements of negligence. *J Perinat Neonatal Nurs.* 2020;34(2):108-109. doi:10.1097/JPN.0000000000000479.

4. **(A)** Policies and procedures in place when the event occurred are the most useful in establishing an expected standard of practice amongst the responses provided. These also must reflect national, state, and Joint Commission standards of care. This is further communicated by an expert witness who is a nurse. The nurse practice act in the state where the event occurred would be considered primarily in scope of practice issues. The nurse's basic level of education does not change the standard of practice. This only changes from basic nursing practice to advanced-level practice.

Reference: Verklan MT. Legal issues. In: Verklan MT, Walden M, Forest S, eds. *Core Curriculum for Neonatal Intensive Care Nursing.* 6th ed. St. Louis, MO: Elsevier; 2021:720-733.

5. **(A)** The responsibilities of the cosigner are the same as those of the administrator of the medication. By cosigning the medication administration record, he is accepting joint responsibility (liability) for the care provided, in this case, the medication being administered. Since this medication was already drawn up and unlabeled, the cosigner is unable to double-check the medication itself and the dose. Whether or not a policy is in place to double-check the specific medication, cosigning indicates all rights of medication administration have been met.

Reference: Verklan MT. Legal issues. In: Verklan MT, Walden M, Forest S, eds. *Core Curriculum for Neonatal Intensive Care Nursing.* 6th ed. St. Louis, MO: Elsevier; 2021:720-733.

6. **(D)** To meet both ethical and legal standards, the nurse must notify the provider and encourage the patient to discuss the details of the procedure and ask questions regarding the core components of informed consent: risks, benefits, alternatives, and implications for the future. The nurse has no legal responsibility to obtain informed consent, in fact, this responsibility rests with the ordering provider. Doing nothing would not be legally wrong but does not rise to the level of ethical standards. Because the nurse has no legal responsibility for informed consent, there is no need to stop the procedure due to a lack of informed consent. Although calling the parents to inform them of the procedure may be done in some circumstances, it is not the best response to this scenario. There may be an urgency to the procedure when consent cannot be obtained quickly enough.

Reference: Verklan MT. Legal issues. In: Verklan MT, Walden M, Forest S, eds. *Core Curriculum for Neonatal Intensive Care Nursing.* 6th ed. St. Louis, MO: Elsevier; 2021:720-733.

7. **(B)** In situations where parents are in disagreement with the healthcare team, and the nurse feels the care is causing harm or suffering, the nurse has the right to conscientious objection. In doing so, the nurse should discuss their point of view with the healthcare team. As a whole, the team should adopt the "dual track method," in which the infant continues to receive curative care, but efforts are directed toward comfort and pain avoidance. The nurse may request relief from the assignment but cannot legally abandon the patient. A referral to the ethics committee is not likely to help the outcome. The ethics committee provides recommendations for care trajectory rather than a decision or mandate that must be accepted by all parties. It is likely that the parents will come to appreciate the futility of care over time. Parents should be supported through the process while the healthcare team provides pain relief and pain avoidance as much as possible.

Reference: Sudia T, Catlin A. Ethical issues. In: Verklan MT, Walden M, Forest S, eds. *Core Curriculum for Neonatal Intensive Care Nursing.* 6th ed. St. Louis, MO: Elsevier; 2021:714-719.

8. **(B)** Nurses are often in a position to delegate tasks to others. State nurse practice acts provide guidance on delegation which is allowed when certain conditions/circumstances apply. Nursing delegation has three components. The registered nurse holds authority for care delivery, may transfer responsibility for performance of a task but retains accountability for a safe outcome of that task. The nurse must have knowledge of the person's capabilities before transferring responsibility and retains accountability for the outcome of the tasks assigned. This holds true regardless of level of experience of the delegatee.

References: Delegation: legal issues for clinicians. *J Perinat Neonatal Nurs.* 2018;32(2):104-106. doi:10.1097/JPN.0000000000000327.

ANA. *National Guidelines for Nursing Delegation.* Available at: https://www.ncsbn.org/public-files/NGND-PosPaper_06.pdf. Effective April 29, 2019; Accessed January 20, 2023.

9. **(D)** The policies and procedures in place at the time of the event, the state or federal regulations, and the testimony of expert witnesses all go to establish the expected actions of a reasonable

and prudent nurse in the same or similar situation, which is what is used to judge the actions of a nurse in a specific situation. Federal regulations are generally quite broad and allow for flexibility in state practice acts. Standards of care do not vary by location and are not specified by federal regulations. Policies and procedures are important to establish the expected standard of care in a specific case. However, these are based on policies and procedures in place at the time of the event, not when the lawsuit is filed which may be months or years after the event. While physician testimony may be required to establish causality in a negligence case, the standard of care for nursing is provided by a nurse expert witness familiar with the expected level of performance of a nurse.

Reference: Verklan MT. Legal issues. In: Verklan MT, Walden M, Forest S, eds. *Core Curriculum for Neonatal Intensive Care Nursing.* 6th ed. St. Louis, MO: Elsevier; 2021:720-733.

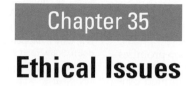

Chapter 35

Ethical Issues

1. To achieve true informed consent, what principle must be present?
   A. Beneficence
   B. Justice
   C. Fidelity
   D. Nonmaleficence

2. An infant is born with a life-limiting disease, and an order is written to give morphine as needed for pain. The nurse administers the dose, and the infant becomes apneic and has bradycardia. This is known as a(an):
   A. adverse drug reaction.
   B. double effect.
   C. overdose.
   D. intended effect.

3. A term infant is born after a placental abruption and is taken to the neonatal intensive care unit (NICU) for whole-body cooling. The infant is having seizures at birth that continue throughout cooling, then worsen when rewarming occurs. The magnetic resonance image after rewarming is consistent with hypoxic ischemic encephalopathy. The infant is nonresponsive, and the electroencephalogram is flat. The medical team approaches the family to discuss a redirection of care to comfort care based on the poor prognosis. Who can make the decision to redirect care?
   A. Nurse
   B. Chaplain
   C. Parents or legal guardian
   D. Ethics committee

4. What are the four major principles of biomedical ethics?
   A. Fidelity, truth telling, confidentiality, privacy
   B. Veracity, confidentiality, privacy, fidelity
   C. Do no harm, do good, be truthful, be respectful
   D. Autonomy, beneficence, nonmaleficence, justice

5. The nurse is caring for an infant who has a metabolic disorder and is slowly dying. The family visits infrequently and does not want to redirect care to comfort care. The parents want to be notified of the infant's death even if it happens at night. The nurse feels the parents are causing the infant to suffer, but he continues to provide care. What is this an example of?
   A. Ethical dilemma
   B. Poor parenting
   C. Moral distress
   D. Professional dilemma

6. An infant is being admitted to the NICU. A nurse from the medical surgical floor calls to see how the infant is because the mother is her neighbor. The infant's nurse gives the medical surgical nurse an update of the infant's diagnosis. What is this an example of?
   A. Breach of confidentiality
   B. Fidelity
   C. Beneficence
   D. Information sharing

   Rationale:
   A. Breach of confidentiality is the disclosure of information originally disclosed within a confidential relationship.
   B. Fidelity is evidenced when promises are kept.
   C. Beneficence means acting to benefit others.
   D. Information sharing is health care practitioners communicating and sharing complete and unbiased information with patients and families in ways that are affirming and useful. Patients and families receive timely, complete, and accurate information in order to effectively participate in care and decision making.

7. The bedside nurse does not agree with the treatment plan because she believes the care is futile. She discusses it with the doctor, and the conflict escalates. With whom should the nurse discuss the conflict to enable resolution?
   A. Nurse colleagues in the lounge
   B. Staff meeting
   C. Parents
   D. Ethics committee

8. An extremely low-birth-weight infant has been diagnosed with periventricular leukomalacia. The family has decided to redirect care to comfort care. They have decided to withhold fluids and nutrition. The nurse taking care of the infant does not agree with the plan and asks not to take care of the infant. The nurse is expressing:
   A. justice.
   B. respect for autonomy.
   C. conscientious objection.
   D. nonmaleficence.

9. The nurse is caring for an infant who is going into multiorgan system failure. The nurse advocates for a family conference with all the specialists. The family says they still want everything done despite the poor prognosis. This is an example of:
   A. nonmaleficence.
   B. justice.
   C. autonomy.
   D. selfishness.

ANSWERS AND RATIONALES

1. **(C)** Fidelity means promise keeping, the duty to keep promises to promote the greatest good and is a key principle in informed consent. Beneficence can be discussed during the informed consent discussion but is not a primary principle that must be present during informed consent. Justice means fairness. Justice is an important part of informed consent but not the primary principle that must be present. Nonmaleficence means doing no harm. Informed consent can promote nonmaleficence, the latter is not the primary principle that must be present.

Reference: Beauchamp T, Childress J. *Principles of Biomedical Ethics.* 8th ed. New York: Oxford University Press; 2019:118-119.

2. **(B)** Double effect means an action may be good if the intent of the action is a positive value, even if the secondary effects of the action might be considered harmful if undertaken as the primary goal; further, the effect should be commensurate with the harm. Adverse drug reaction is an effect of a drug that may not be wanted and may be harmful. Overdose occurs when a lethal or toxic dose is given. Intended effect is the medicine doing what it is prescribed to do. In this scenario, the intent of giving morphine was to relieve suffering.

Reference: Beauchamp T, Childress J. *Principles of Biomedical Ethics.* 8th ed. New York: Oxford University Press; 2019:167-171.

3. **(C)** The parents or legal guardian are the legal decision-makers and bear the consequences of their decisions. The nurse provides medical information but does not make medical treatment decisions. The chaplain provides spiritual support to the family. The ethics committee provides guidance and helps improve communication among the team.

Reference: Beauchamp T, Childress J. *Principles of Biomedical Ethics.* 8th ed. New York: Oxford University Press; 2019:167-171.

4. **(D)** The four major principles of biomedical ethics are autonomy, beneficence, justice, and nonmaleficence. *Autonomy* means that individuals have the right to make decisions for themselves. *Beneficence* means acting to benefit others. *Justice* means fairness. *Nonmaleficence* means doing no harm. Fidelity, truth telling, confidentiality, privacy, and veracity, although important concepts, are not the principles of biomedical ethics. Although doing no harm and doing good are definitions of nonmaleficence and beneficence, respectively, being truthful and respectful are not principles of biomedical ethics.

References: Beauchamp T, Childress J. *Principles of Biomedical Ethics.* 8th ed. New York: Oxford University Press; 2019:99, 155, 217, 267.

American Nurses Association. *Code of Ethics for Nurses with Interpretive Statements.* Silver Spring, MD: American Nurses Association; 2015:23, 45.

Gomella T, Eval F, Bany-Mohammed F. *Gomella's Neonatology: Management, Procedures, On Call Problems, Diseases and Drugs.* 8th ed. New York: McGraw-Hill; 2020:294.

International Council of Nurses. *The ICN Code of Ethics for Nurses.* Geneva: International Council of Nurses; 2021:9. Available at: https://www.icn.ch/system/files/2021-10/ICN_Code-of-Ethics_EN_Web_0.pdf. Accessed January 20, 2023.

5. **(C)** Moral distress is being aware of the right action but feeling powerless and not able to take action. In this scenario the nurse knows that care should be redirected to comfort care, but this is not what the parents want. Ethical dilemma is a situation in which the ethically correct action must be decided. Poor parenting is a judgment. A professional dilemma is an ethical problem that requires an individual to choose a particular course of action (e.g., fraudulent activity at work).

References: American Association of Critical-Care Nurses. *AACN Position Statement: Moral Distress in Times of Crisis.* 2020. Available at: https://www.aacn.org/policy-and-advocacy/aacn-position-statement-moral-distress-in-times-of-crisis. Accessed January 20, 2023.

Mills M, Cortezzo D. Moral distress in the neonatal intensive care unit: what is it, why it happens, and how we can address it. *Front Pediatr.* 2020;10(8):581. doi:10.3389/fped.2020.00581.

American Association of Critical-Care Nurses. *Moral Distress in Nursing: What You Need to Know.* March 2, 2020. Available at: https://www.aacn.org/clinical-resources/moral-distress. Accessed January 20, 2023.

American Association of Critical-Care Nurses. Nurse strong: recognizing and mitigating moral distress. In: *AACN Critical Care Webinar Series.* 2021. Available at: https://www.aacn.org/education/ce-activities/wb0065/nurse-strong-recognizing-and-addressing-moral-distress. Accessed January 20, 2023.

6. **(A)** Breach of confidentiality is the disclosure of information originally disclosed within a confidential relationship. Fidelity is evidenced when promises are kept. Beneficence means acting to benefit others. Information sharing is health care practitioners communicating and sharing complete and unbiased information with patients and families in ways that are affirming and useful. Patients and families receive timely, complete, and accurate information to effectively participate in care and decision-making.

References: Beauchamp T, Childress J. *Principles of Biomedical Ethics.* 8th ed. New York: Oxford University Press; 2019:244.

American Nurses Association. *Code of Ethics for Nurses With Interpretive Statements.* Silver Spring, MD: American Nurses Association; 2015:9-10.

Institute for Patient- and Family-Centered Care. *Patient- and Family- Centered Care Defined.* https://www.ipfcc.org/bestpractices/sustainable-partnerships/background/pfcc-defined.html. Accessed September 25, 2023.

International Council of Nurses. *The ICN Code of Ethics for Nurses.* Geneva: International Council of Nurses; 2021. Available at: https://www.icn.ch/system/files/2021-10/ICN_Code-of-Ethics_EN_Web_0.pdf. Accessed January 20, 2023.

7. **(D)** Ethics committees are multidisciplinary in composition and are designed to ensure emotional stability, objectivity, and consistency. They help facilitate better communication among the medical team and families. The ethics committee is a consultative group only and cannot mandate action or write orders. The ethics committee facilitates the understanding of information about a case. It does not change the plan of care. While discussing the situation with nurse colleagues, informally or formally in a staff meeting, may help the nurse clarify her values and beliefs, resolution to ethical conflicts is best enabled in a forum that includes professionals with expertise in bioethics. Parents have the right to determine what is best for their child. If the nurse shares her personal beliefs with the parents, it can compromise the nurse–patient relationship.

Reference: Sudia T, Catlin A. Ethical issues. In: Verklan T, Walden M, Forest S, eds. *Core Curriculum for Neonatal Intensive Care Nursing.* 6th ed. St. Louis MO: Elsevier; 2021:718.

8. **(C)** Conscientious objection is when a person objects to doing something that goes against their consciousness. Justice means fairness and is not described in the scenario. Respect for autonomy is the right for patients to guide their own fate and does not best describe the nurse's request. Nonmaleficence means do no harm and does not describe the nurse's request.

References: Beauchamp T, Childress J. *Principles of Biomedical Ethics.* 8th ed. New York: Oxford University Press; 2019:42-43.